EVALUATION AND MANAGEMENT OF SPEECH BREATHING DISORDERS

Principles and Methods

EVALUATION AND MANAGEMENT OF SPEECH BREATHING DISORDERS
Principles and Methods

Thomas J. Hixon and Jeannette D. Hoit

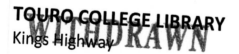
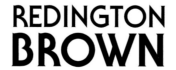
REDINGTON BROWN

Redington Brown LLC
Tucson, Arizona

mw

Evaluation and Management of Speech Breathing Disorders Principles and Methods,
First Edition

Copyright © 2005 Thomas J. Hixon and Jeannette D. Hoit

Redington Brown LLC
5530 Camino Del Celador
Tucson, Arizona 85750

http://www.redingtonbrown.com

Editors: Thomas J. Hixon and Jeannette D. Hoit
Compositor: Todd C. Hixon
Printer: Arizona Lithographers
Binder: Roswell Bookbinding
Illustrations: Michael D. Buffington
Cover Design: Michael D. Buffington

Library of Congress Control Number: 2004099584

ISBN 0-9763513-0-7

Printed and bound in the United States of America

2/8/07

for
Pauline

Contents

Preface

Writing this book was a long labor of love for us. The need for the book is set out in its first chapter and our hope is that the book will go a significant way toward meeting that need. As we worked on the text, we often discussed the debts we owe our mentors. For the first of us, the largest debts are owed to Dr. James Hardy of the University of Iowa and Dr. Jeremiah Mead of Harvard University. For the second of us, the largest debts are owed to the first of us and to Dr. Robert Banzett of Harvard University. We are both grateful to the many clients who have inspired us and taught us along the way. Both their numbers and their contributions to the ideas in this book are large. We are also thankful to the many others whose research and clinical efforts we discuss in the book. We believe there is much between the covers of this book that can be used to help people with speech breathing disorders. We hope that readers will find this to be true.

Thomas J. Hixon and Jeannette D. Hoit
Tucson, Arizona and Pagosa Springs, Colorado

chapter one

Preliminaries

INTRODUCTION

This chapter offers some preliminaries that help to frame the book. These are couched in the form of answers to a series of questions about speech breathing, speech breathing disorders, clinical endeavors, and the focus of the book.

WHAT IS SPEECH BREATHING?

Speech breathing is the process by which driving forces are supplied to the speech production apparatus to generate the sounds of oral communication. This process involves the displacement of structures, the creation of pressures, and the generation of flows within the breathing apparatus. These actions, together with actions of the larynx and/or upper airway, cause the disturbances of air that constitute speech. Speech breathing contributes to the control of such variables as speech intensity (loudness), voice frequency (pitch), linguistic stress (emphasis), and the segmentation (division) of speech into different units (syllables, words, phrases). Speech breathing serves these speech-related functions at the same time it serves ventilatory functions. Thus, although speech breathing is tailored to meet the goals of producing speech, it must also allow for adequate exchange of oxygen and carbon dioxide.

WHAT IS A SPEECH BREATHING DISORDER?

A speech breathing disorder is an abnormality in the process of supplying the energy source for speech production. The term speech breathing disorder is restricted to abnormality of the breathing apparatus proper (i.e., the pulmonary-chest wall unit), and does not include abnormality of the larynx and/or upper airway. A speech breathing disorder may be of functional and/or organic origin. A functional disorder results from inappropriate use of a normal breathing apparatus, whereas an organic disorder results from the sole or combined effects of neural, muscular, or structural abnormalities of the breathing apparatus. Speech breathing disorders may manifest as problems of breathing movement, gas exchange, breathing comfort, or any combination of these.

HOW COMMON ARE SPEECH BREATHING DISORDERS?

Data have not been reported on the prevalence, prevalence rate, or incidence rate of speech breathing disorders. Accordingly, one must rely on personal experience and discussion with other speech-language pathologists to estimate demographic patterns for these disorders. On these bases, it seems reasonable to estimate that, among individuals who present with speech disorders, the prevalence rate of speech breathing disorders is at least 15%. That is, out of each 100 people with clinically significant speech disorders, 15 or more will have problems that are caused, at least in part, by one or more abnormalities of speech breathing. Whatever the precise demographic situation may be, speech breathing disorders are certainly on the increase. This is because increasing numbers of people are attaining ages at which diseases of the nervous system, the major cause of speech breathing disorders, most often occur.

ARE SPEECH-LANGUAGE PATHOLOGISTS PREPARED TO DEAL WITH SPEECH BREATHING DISORDERS?

Many speech-language pathologists have misgivings about their ability to evaluate and manage speech breathing disorders. Some have had no formal preparation. Others say that their preparation was inadequate. Very few take the position that they know as much about evaluating and managing speech breathing as they do about evaluating and managing laryngeal or upper airway functions.

There appear to be several reasons why this area of clinical endeavor has been given inadequate attention in the instruction of speech-language pathologists. Some of these reasons are discussed below.

• The myth persists that resting tidal breathing and speech breathing have similar physical requirements. This myth implies that a client capable of normal resting tidal breathing should be capable of normal speech breathing. Embodied in such a notion is the oft-stated clinical rule "enough to breathe, enough to speak." This rule suggests that if clients are able to breathe on their own they should have an adequate physiological base to produce speech. Those who subscribe to such a rule would have speech-language pathologists believe that only clients who are unable to breathe on their own are likely to have speech breathing disorders.

• There is a common misconception that it is virtually impossible to isolate the function of the breathing apparatus from functions of the larynx and/or upper airway during speech production. This misconception is prominent in textbooks concerned with the evaluation and management of voice disorders and neuromotor speech disorders. Many such textbooks advocate methods of evaluation and management that do not address the function of the breathing apparatus, stating or implying that speech breathing is not amenable to independent analysis or manipulation. This misconception carries with it the notion that, even when speech breathing disorders exist, there is no way to evaluate or manage them in their own right.

• There is a fallacious, but widely accepted, belief that speech breathing exists on a less voluntary or more automatic level than functions of the larynx and upper airway for speech production. This belief extends to the frequently expressed notion that direct attempts should not be made to manage speech breathing disorders, because bringing the client's awareness of breathing to a more conscious level might interfere with the presumed automatic nature of speech breathing. Those who are guided by this belief acknowledge the existence of speech breathing disorders, but view them as something that should be left alone for fear of exacerbating their undesirable influence on speech production.

• The mistaken idea exists that speech breathing is a simple and relatively featureless behavior of the speech production apparatus. A corollary of this idea is that the function of the breathing apparatus is less important than the functions of the larynx and/or upper airway during speech production. Those who embrace these notions tend to relegate speech breathing to a position of lesser importance than the other speech production processes. As a consequence, speech breathing disorders often are given only superficial attention when it comes to evaluation and management and the attitude is imparted that such disorders are not of much importance even when they do exist.

• There is widespread uncertainty about whether or not speech breathing disorders legitimately fall within the domain of speech-language pathology. Underlying this uncertainty is the reasoning that breathing is a life-sustaining function, that speech breathing disorders frequently coexist with breathing disorders, and that concern for these two is more appropriately the province of medicine, physical therapy, respiratory therapy, or other professions. Such uncertainty is seen in the speech-language pathology literature, as reflected by the fact that published reports on clients with speech breathing disorders are concerned almost entirely with the details of medical pulmonary function tests and carry little information about speech breathing per se.

• There are pervasive questions about the propriety of speech-language pathologists working with the breathing apparatus. Torso nudity of clients and physical manipulation of the breathing apparatus by speech-language pathologists are the two concerns raised most often. Guidelines on these issues have not been formalized for speech-language pathologists, nor have the boundaries of usual clinical practice been well-delineated. Without clear standards, many clinical instructors are unsure about such issues and, consequently, often ignore them. Thus, the message conveyed is that the field of speech-language pathology is uncertain about its own role in relation to clients with speech breathing disorders.

• Only recently have extensive data on normal speech breathing become available. Thus, only recently has it become possible to construct a comprehensive account of normal speech breathing that could be used as a standard against which to make clinical decisions about speech breathing disorders. Speech-language pathologists have not, therefore, had access to a comprehensive framework from which to view speech breathing disorders. Consequently, it is no surprise that concerns for the evaluation and management of speech breathing disorders are not yet on equal status with other aspects of the practice of speech-language pathology.

WHAT ARE THE CONSEQUENCES OF BEING UNPREPARED TO DEAL WITH SPEECH BREATHING DISORDERS?

There are significant consequences of being unprepared to deal with speech breathing disorders. These consequences pertain to the field of speech-language pathology, to speech-language pathologists, and to clients who have speech breathing disorders. Some of the more important consequences are discussed here.

• The field of speech-language pathology is being encroached upon by other disciplines when it comes to service delivery for clients with speech breathing disorders. Medicine, physical therapy, respiratory therapy, and other professions often attempt to fill the service-delivery role that speech-language pathology has inadequately embraced. Accordingly, speech-language pathology is often in a less-than-commanding position in a clinical domain that is rightfully its own and for which other professions have no special training. This reflects poorly on the field of speech-language pathology, makes it appear less encompassing than it actually is, and weakens the respect that other professions hold for its contribution to the delivery of healthcare.

• Practicing speech-language pathologists are at risk of appearing incapable of comprehensive service delivery to clients with speech disorders. This has adverse implications for the number of referrals and consultations directed to speech-language pathologists. It also has adverse implications for their professional reputations. To the extent that speech disorders involve multiple parts of the speech production apparatus (breathing apparatus, larynx, and upper airway), those speech-language pathologists who are unprepared to deal with speech breathing disorders are likely to be considered capable of handling only selected aspects of the more complex speech disorders they encounter.

• Time, effort, and other resources can be wasted on clinical endeavors when the speech breathing contribution to speech disorders is not considered in proper perspective. This is especially true when multiple parts of the speech production apparatus are impaired and when the speech-language pathologist concentrates on laryngeal and/or upper airway functions while devoting little or no attention to breathing function. To manage the larynx and/or upper airway without consideration of the breathing apparatus can be unproductive. An analogy is found in trying to teach someone to play a wind-driven pipe organ that has a broken or disconnected bellows pump.

• Inappropriate decisions can result in inappropriate care of clients when speech-language pathologists are not able to evaluate speech breathing disorders. The most disconcerting of these decisions are those involving clients with severe speech disorders who are managed inappropriately through the use of alternative communication when they could profit from management of their speech breathing. Such misdirected management carries with it the negative side effect that too many clients are "biomechanically shelved" for speech production. Unfortunately, an attainable goal of socially useful speech may be forfeited unwittingly.

FOR WHOM IS THIS BOOK INTENDED?

This book is intended for clinicians. It is written mainly for aspiring and practicing speech-language pathologists who are involved in making evaluation and management decisions about clients with speech breathing disorders. It is also written to serve other professionals who participate in such decision-making or who may be involved in the care of clients with speech breathing disorders. These include general practice physicians, nurses, physiatrists, neurologists, laryngologists, occupational therapists, orthotists, physical therapists, pulmonologists, respiratory therapists, and others.

WHAT IS THE PURPOSE OF THIS BOOK?

The purpose of this book is to provide clinicians with a broad-based introduction to principles and methods for the evaluation and management of speech breathing disorders. It is designed to provide a unified account that can be used as a primary source of information for the following: (a) instruction of students of speech-language pathology; (b) continuing education of practicing speech-language pathologists; and (c) further education of other healthcare professionals who provide services to clients with speech breathing disorders. Underlying this stated intent is the desire to move the topic of speech breathing disorders to within the mainstream of clinical thinking and to enhance the quality of services provided to clients with speech breathing disorders.

WHAT TERRITORY IS COVERED BY THIS BOOK?

The bulk of this book is contained in its next six chapters. The territory covered in these chapters is summarized below.

Chapter 2: Foundations of Breathing – This chapter focuses on the foundations of breathing and lays groundwork for understanding other chapters that follow. Discussion is devoted to structural and mechanical bases of breathing. Also considered are adjustment capabilities and control variables of the breathing apparatus. The neural substrates of breathing are given attention and a section is devoted to the nature of breathing for life purposes. Information in this chapter provides the reader with bases for appreciating the complexities of breathing and for extrapolating the principles that underlie breathing in general to various special acts of breathing, including different forms of speech production.

Chapter 3: Normal Speech Breathing – This chapter focuses on information about normal speech breathing and provides a reference against which to compare abnormal function. Breathing for speech purposes is discussed, particularly in relation to extended steady utterances and running speech activities. Attention is given to adaptive control, body position, altered external forces, ventilation and gas exchange, drive-to-breathe, cognitive-linguistic factors, conversational interchange, body type, age, and sex. Normal speech breathing is considered across the human life span, including periods of emergence (infancy), refinement (childhood), and modification (adulthood).

Chapter 4: Evaluation of Speech Breathing – This chapter is concerned with principles and methods for the evaluation of speech breathing. Evaluation is viewed as the foundation on which any sound program of management is built. Consideration is given to the nature of the evaluation task and the types of clients that are most likely to need a systematic speech breathing evaluation. Topics include the case history and the auditory-perceptual examination of speech breathing. The client's perception of his speech breathing is also discussed, as are the physical examination and the instrumental examination of the breathing apparatus. The final section is devoted to an abbreviated bedside screening of speech breathing for use when time is limited or when the client is limited in performance capability or endurance.

Chapter 5: Management of Speech Breathing – This chapter deals with the management of speech breathing and covers topics that draw from behavioral, engineering, and healthcare domains. Discussion is devoted to the nature of the management task and the staging of management. Attention is also devoted to adjusting breathing variables, exteroceptive feedback, and economical valving. Also considered are body positioning, mechanical aids, muscle training, glossopharyngeal breathing, relieving speaking-related dyspnea, monitoring gas exchange, and mouthing and buccal speaking. Other topics include conversational strategies, optimizing the environment, counseling, assistive speech devices, augmentative communication, and alternative communication.

Chapter 6: Ventilator-Supported Speech Breathing – This chapter is concerned with a special type of speech breathing, that found in clients who cannot breathe on their own and who need a ventilator to sustain life. The nature of the task involved in the evaluation and management of such clients is discussed and principles and methods pertinent to such endeavors are considered. Individual sections of the chapter are devoted to different types of ventilators and the evaluation and management of speech breathing in clients who use those types of ventilators. Focus is directed to positive pressure ventilators, negative pressure ventilators, rocking beds, abdominal pneumobelts, and phrenic nerve pacers. The chapter concludes with a comparative summary on the use of these different ventilators.

Chapter 7: Clinical Applications – This chapter presents a series of eight clinical scenarios intended to demonstrate many of the principles and methods discussed in other chapters of the book. These scenarios cover a variety of evaluation and management challenges that illustrate issues pertinent to clients of different ages and with different disorders. Such clinical scenarios provide the reader with an opportunity to fully appreciate the broad domain of speech breathing disorders, their evaluation, and their management. Topics in the chapter focus on speech breathing concerns related to functional misuse of the breathing apparatus, low cervical spinal cord injury, chronic obstructive pulmonary disease, high cervical spinal cord injury, amyotrophic lateral sclerosis, respiratory myoclonus, cerebellar tumor, and muscular dystrophy. The chapter is designed to serve as an experience in practical application for the reader.

REVIEW

Speech breathing is the process by which driving forces are supplied to the speech production apparatus to generate the sounds of oral communication, while simultaneously serving the ventilatory function of adequate oxygen and carbon dioxide exchange.

A speech breathing disorder is an abnormality in the process of supplying the energy source for speech production and may manifest as a problem of breathing movement, gas exchange, breathing comfort, or any combination of these.

Out of each 100 people with clinically significant speech disorders, 15 or more will have problems that are caused, at least in part, by one or more abnormalities of speech breathing.

Many speech-language pathologists have misgivings about their ability to evaluate and manage speech breathing disorders.

There are significant consequences of being unprepared to deal with speech breathing disorders – consequences for the field of speech-language pathology, for speech-language pathologists, and for clients.

This book is intended for clinicians, including aspiring and practicing speech-language pathologists and other professionals involved in the care of clients with speech breathing disorders.

The purpose of this book is to provide clinicians with a broad-based introduction to principles and methods for the evaluation and management of speech breathing.

The remaining chapters in this book consider foundations of breathing, normal speech breathing, evaluation of speech breathing, management of speech breathing, ventilator-supported speech breathing, and clinical applications.

SIDETRACKS

Throughout this book you'll find a series of sidetracks. These are short asides that are related to the issues being discussed. We include these to enhance your reading enjoyment and to make points we just can't seem to resist making. They're intended to be just a dash more lighthearted than the main text. Anyway, they should give you pause for reflection. Or is it paws for reflection?

chapter two

Foundations of Breathing

INTRODUCTION

This chapter focuses on the bases of breathing. The material presented here is foundational to parts of the book concerned with normal and abnormal speech breathing and with the evaluation and management of speech breathing.

STRUCTURE OF THE BREATHING APPARATUS

Figure 2-1 portrays the adult breathing apparatus. This apparatus is located within the torso (body trunk) and consists of two subdivisions, the pulmonary apparatus and the chest wall. These subdivisions are concentrically arranged (one inside the other) and are linked together as a unit.

Pulmonary Apparatus

The pulmonary apparatus is the air-conducting, air-containing, and gas-exchanging part of the breathing apparatus. It provides oxygen to the cells of the body and removes carbon dioxide from them. This apparatus can itself be subdivided into the pulmonary airways and the lungs.

Pulmonary Airways

The pulmonary airways are a complex network of flexible branching tubes through which air can be moved to and from the lungs and between different parts of the lungs. These tubes are patterned like the branches of an inverted deciduous tree.

The trunk of this tree is the trachea (windpipe). The trachea is a tube attached to the bottom of the larynx (voice box) that runs down through the neck into the torso. At its lower end, the trachea divides into two smaller tubes, one running to the left lung and one running to the right lung. These two tubes, called the main stem bronchi, run on and branch into what are termed lobar bronchi. The latter are tubes that extend into the five lobes of the lungs. The branching of the pulmonary airways continues as they divide over and over and extend farther and farther out through the lungs. More than 20 such branchings occur along the pulmonary airways, each leading to smaller and smaller airway structures. These include segmental bronchi, subsegmental bronchi, small bronchi, terminal bronchi, bronchioles, terminal bronchioles, respiratory bronchioles, alveolar ducts, alveolar sacs, and alveoli. The last of these, the alveoli, are extremely small cul-de-sacs of air. They number 300 million or so and are the sites where oxygen and carbon dioxide are exchanged.

Lungs

The lungs are the organs of breathing. They are a pair of cone-shaped structures

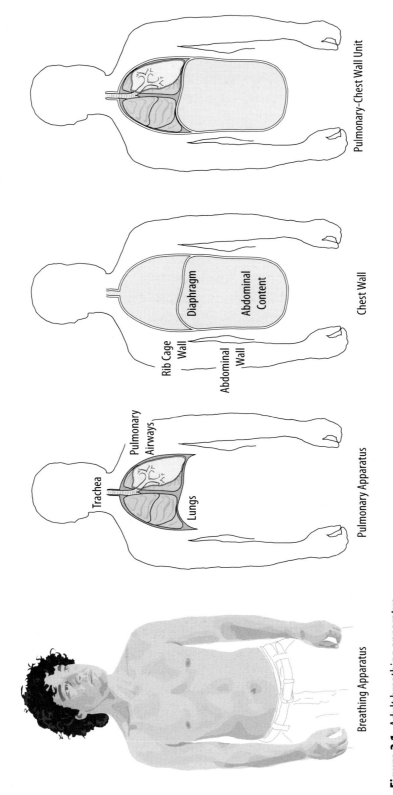

Figure 2-1. Adult breathing apparatus.

Breathing Apparatus

Pulmonary Apparatus

Trachea

Pulmonary Airways

Lungs

Chest Wall

Rib Cage Wall

Abdominal Wall

Diaphragm

Abdominal Content

Pulmonary–Chest Wall Unit

that are porous and spongy. Each lung contains an abundance of resilient elastic fibers and each behaves like a stretchable bag that can change size and shape. The two lungs are not identical. The left lung is smaller than the right. Also, the left lung has two lobes, whereas the right lung has three. Together the two lungs fill much of the upper half of the torso. The outer surface of each lung is covered with a thin airtight membrane called the visceral pleura. A similar membrane covers the inner surface of the chest wall where it contacts the lungs. This membrane is termed the parietal pleura. Together the visceral pleura and the parietal pleura form a double-walled sac that completely encases the lungs. Each pleural membrane is covered with a thin layer of liquid, which lubricates it and enables it to move easily upon its companion membrane. The same layer of liquid links the visceral and parietal membranes together in much the same way that a film of water holds two glass plates together.

Chest Wall

The chest wall encases the pulmonary apparatus by way of a surrounding vertical wall and a floor. This encasement has four parts – the rib cage wall, the diaphragm, the abdominal wall, and the abdominal content. Two of the parts, the rib cage wall and the diaphragm, form an enclosure within the upper torso called the thorax (chest cavity). And two of the parts, the diaphragm and abdominal wall, form an enclosure within the lower torso called the abdomen (belly cavity).

Rib Cage Wall

The rib cage wall encircles the lungs like a cylinder. Its shape is somewhat barrel-like and it consists of a framework of bone and cartilage. This framework is situated within the upper torso and is supported by a back centerpost consisting of 12 vertebrae. These comprise the thoracic segment of the vertebral column (backbone). The ribs extend forward from this back support. They are 24 (12 on each side) flat, arch-shaped bones that slope downward along the sides of the torso, giving roundness to the rib cage. The front ends of the ribs attach to bars of costal (rib) cartilage which, in turn, are connected to a long, flat bone, the sternum (breastbone). The sternum serves as a front centerpost for the rib cage. The typical rib cage includes upper pairs of ribs attached to the sternum by their own costal cartilages, lower pairs sharing cartilages variously, and the lowest two pairs floating without attachments.

The remainder of the rib cage is formed by the pectoral girdle (shoulder girdle). This structure is located near the top of the rib cage. The front of this girdle is formed by the two clavicles (collar bones), each of which is a bony strut extending from the upper sternum over the first rib toward the side and back of the rib cage. At the back, the clavicles attach to two triangularly shaped bony plates, the scapulae (shoulder blades). These complete the pectoral girdle and cover most of the upper back portion of the rib cage. Muscular and nonmuscular tissues fill the spaces between the ribs and cover the inner and outer surfaces of the rib cage wall.

Diaphragm

The diaphragm forms the convex floor of the thorax. This floor is a dome-shaped structure, which looks somewhat like an inverted bowl. Actually, it is somewhat double-domed, the left side being slightly lower than the right. At its center, the diaphragm consists of a tough, thin, flat sheet of nonelastic tissue called the central tendon. The remainder of the diaphragm is made up of a complex sheet of muscle. This muscle forms a broad rim that extends upward to the edges of the central tendon. The bottom of this muscular rim attaches all around the internal circumference of the lower portion of the rib cage wall. The diaphragm separates the thorax and abdomen, and thus, gets its name – diaphragm, meaning "the fence in between."

Abdominal Wall

The abdominal wall forms the casing for the lower half of the torso. Technically, it runs all the way around the torso, although it is often discussed as if it only includes the front and sides of the torso. The casing formed by the abdominal wall is roughly oblong-shaped. Like the rib cage wall, the abdominal wall has a firm back centerpost in the form of the vertebral column. This centerpost consists of 15 vertebrae, 5 each lumbar, sacral, and coccygeal, and extends from near the bottom of the rib cage to the tailbone. The large, irregularly shaped coxal (hip) bones also form part of the abdominal wall near the base of the torso. These two bones, together with the sacral and coccygeal vertebrae, comprise the pelvic girdle (bony pelvis). For the most part, the abdominal wall is constructed of two broad sheets of connective tissue and several very large muscles. The two sheets of connective tissue cover much of the front and back of the abdominal wall and are termed the abdominal aponeurosis and the lumbodorsal fascia, respectively. Muscles are located all around the abdomen – front, back, and flanks – and combine with the abdominal aponeurosis, the lumbodorsal fascia, the vertebral column, and the pelvic girdle to form an encircling cylinder.

Abdominal Content

The abdominal content includes everything inside the abdominal cavity. Although this content consists of a diverse array of structures (e.g., stomach, intestines, and various other organs and glands) it may be thought of as a relatively homogeneous mass. This mass is supported in two ways. It is suspended from above by a suction force beneath the diaphragm and is held in place circumferentially and at its base by the abdominal wall. From a mechanical perspective, the abdominal cavity and the abdominal content are the rough equivalent of an elastic bag filled with water.

Pulmonary-Chest Wall Unit

The pulmonary apparatus and the chest wall are held together as a unit. In this unit, their resting positions are different from their individual resting positions when the two are not linked through their pleural membranes. For example, with the pulmonary apparatus removed from the breathing apparatus, the resting position of the lungs is a collapsed state in which they contain very little air. By contrast, the resting position of the chest wall is a more expanded state.

With the pulmonary apparatus and the chest wall held together by pleural linkage, the breathing apparatus assumes a resting position in which the pulmonary apparatus is somewhat expanded and the chest wall is somewhat compressed. At this resting position, the breathing apparatus is in a mechanically neutral or balanced state. That is, the force of the pulmonary apparatus to collapse is opposed by an equal and opposite force of the chest wall to expand.

> **HANG IN THERE**
>
> We've said that one way the abdominal mass is supported is by being suspended from above by a suction force beneath the diaphragm. The mechanism isn't exactly intuitive, but a simple analogy may help in understanding it. Cut out one end of a can of condensed tomato soup of thick consistency. Quickly turn the can over. Although free to fall, the condensed soup just hangs there and seems to defy gravity. How does it do this? When turning the can over, a suction force is developed between the sealed end of the can and the condensed soup. This force suspends the mass of the soup against gravity. When your breathing apparatus is upright and at rest, your abdominal mass hangs from the undersurface of your diaphragm in much the same manner that condensed soup might hang above a yawning saucepan.

MECHANICAL BASES OF BREATHING

The functional potential of the breathing apparatus lies in its capacity for movement. Such movement can be brought about by forces applied to and by different parts of the apparatus. The forces generated and the movements they create constitute breathing at the mechanical level.

Forces of Breathing

The forces of breathing are of two types – passive and active. Passive force is always present, whereas active force depends on the will and ability of the individual. The passive and active forces of breathing make up the total force of breathing.

Passive Force

The passive force of breathing arises from several sources. These include the

The film that lines the alveoli forms multitudes of liquid-air interfaces. Surface tension at these interfaces causes them to recoil like tiny bubbles. The combined recoil force of all of these interfaces is responsible for as much or more of the total recoil of the lungs as is the actual elastic fabric of the lungs. How do we know that? Because it takes less than half the pressure to fully inflate the lungs when they are liquid-filled than when they are air-filled. The reason for this difference is that in the liquid-filled lungs the normal liquid-air interface of each alveolus is replaced by a liquid-liquid interface whose surface tension is negligible (Comroe, 1965). Submerge the lungs in water (drown them) and all of their recoiling bubbles break. The elastic fabric of the lungs is on its own and the lungs have lost about half of their recoil power. Without bubbles, you'd have troubles.

natural recoil of muscles, cartilages, ligaments, and lung tissue, the surface tension of a special film that lines the alveoli, and the pull of gravity. Such passive force causes the breathing apparatus to behave in a manner analogous to that of a coil spring.

The sign (inspiratory or expiratory) and magnitude of this passive force depend on the amount of air contained within the breathing apparatus. When the amount of air exceeds the amount the apparatus contains at rest, the apparatus recoils toward a smaller size (i.e., it tends to expire). The more air the apparatus contains, the greater the recoil force. By contrast, when the amount of air contained within the breathing apparatus is less than the amount the apparatus contains at rest, the apparatus recoils toward a larger size (i.e., it tends to inspire). The less air the apparatus contains, the greater the recoil force.

The sign and magnitude of the passive force of breathing can be experienced by inspiring fully and relaxing and then expiring fully and relaxing. Following a full inspiration, the breathing apparatus behaves like a stretched spring when released, and following a full expiration, it behaves like a compressed spring when released. Thus, the resting position of the apparatus is analogous to the resting length of a coil spring. And, like such a spring, the more the apparatus is deformed from its resting position, whether stretched or compressed, the greater the passive recoil force it generates in attempting to return to rest.

Active Force

The active force of breathing is vested in the more than 20 muscles that are distributed within the chest wall. The force generated by these muscles arises from the contraction of their fibers.

The sign (inspiratory or expiratory) and magnitude of the active force of breathing are variable and depend on which muscles are in play and in what patterns. The principal limit on the active force that can be generated in either sign is the strength of the breathing muscles involved. The magnitude of the active force that can be generated also depends on the amount of air contained within the breathing apparatus. The more air the apparatus contains, the greater the force that can be produced to decrease the size of the apparatus (i.e., the greater the expiratory force that can be generated). By contrast, the less air the apparatus contains, the greater the force that can be produced to increase the size of the apparatus (i.e., the greater the inspiratory force that can be generated).

The active force of breathing can be experienced at the resting position of the breathing apparatus. The passive force of breathing is zero at this position. Thus, any force generated at the resting position must be the result of muscle activation only. By closing the larynx at the resting position of the breathing apparatus and squeezing as hard as possible (bearing down maximally), one can sense the magnitude of the active force available to decrease the size of the apparatus. And, by closing the larynx and sucking with the apparatus as hard as possible, one can sense the magnitude of the active force available to increase the size of the apparatus.

The contribution of specific breathing muscles to active force generation is not completely understood. Nevertheless, consideration of individual muscle architecture and available evidence about the consequences of muscle activation make it possible to suggest the probable roles of specific muscles in active force generation. This is done below for muscles of the rib cage wall, diaphragm, and abdominal wall, in turn. The function described for individual muscles assumes that only the muscle under consideration is active and that it is shortening during contraction. It should be recognized, however, that the contribution of an individual muscle depends on several factors, including whether or not other muscles are active, the mechanical status of various parts of the chest wall, and the nature of the breathing activity being performed.

Muscles of the Rib Cage Wall

Figure 2-2 depicts the muscles of the rib cage wall in different views. These are defined to include certain muscles of the neck and rib cage proper.

The sternocleidomastoid is a relatively broad, thick muscle located on the front and side of the neck. Its fibers originate in two subdivisions, one at the top surface of the front of the sternum and the other at the top surface of the sternal end of the clavicle. From there, these fibers pass upward and backward and unite to insert into the bony skull behind the ear. When the head is held in a fixed position, contraction of the sternal and clavicular subdivisions of the sternocleidomastoid muscle results in elevation of the sternum and clavicle, respectively. The force generated by contraction of these subdivisions of the muscle, or by the muscle's contraction en masse, is transmitted indirectly to the ribs through their connections to the sternum and clavicle. As a result, the ribs are also elevated.

The scalenus muscle group includes three muscles positioned on the side of the neck. These are the scalenus anterior, scalenus medius, and scalenus posterior. The scalenus anterior originates as four tiny tabs from the third through sixth cervical vertebrae. These tabs converge into a relatively thick bundle that runs downward

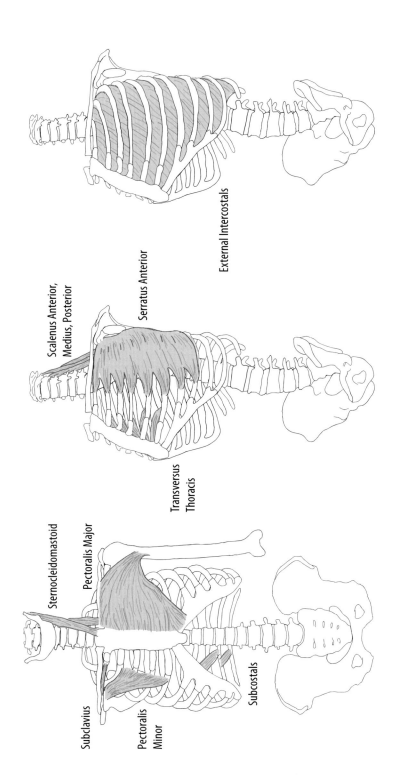

External Intercostals

Scalenus Anterior, Medius, Posterior

Serratus Anterior

Transversus Thoracis

Sternocleidomastoid

Pectoralis Major

Subclavius

Pectoralis Minor

Subcostals

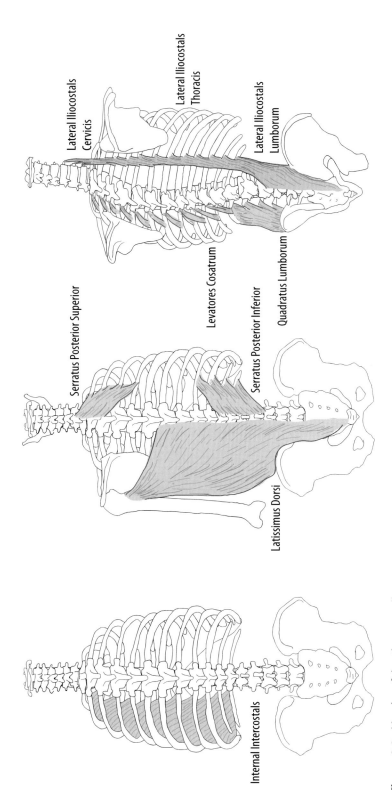

Lateral Iliocostals Cervicis

Lateral Iliocostals Thoracis

Lateral Iliocostals Lumborum

Levatores Cosatrum

Quadratus Lumborum

Serratus Posterior Superior

Serratus Posterior Inferior

Latissimus Dorsi

Internal Intercostals

Figure 2-2. Muscles of the rib cage wall.

and toward the side to insert along the inner border of the top surface of the first rib. The scalenus medius arises as tiny tabs from the lower six cervical vertebrae. Its fibers descend along the side of the vertebral column and, like the scalenus anterior, merge into a single bundle. This bundle inserts along the upper border of the first rib behind the point of insertion of the scalenus anterior. The scalenus posterior arises as tabs from the lower two or three cervical vertebrae. Its fibers converge as they pass downward and toward the side to attach to the outer surface of the second rib. When the head is held in a fixed position, contraction of the scalenus anterior and scalenus medius results in elevation of the first rib. Contraction of the scalenus posterior results in elevation of the second rib.

The pectoralis major is a large, fan-shaped muscle located on the upper front wall of the rib cage. Fibers of the pectoralis major have a complex origin that includes the front surface of the upper costal cartilages, sternum, and inner half of the clavicle. From there, the fibers cross the front of the rib cage wall and converge to insert into the humerus (the major bone of the upper arm). When the humerus is fixed in position, contraction of the pectoralis major draws the sternum and ribs upward.

The pectoralis minor is a relatively large, thin muscle located underneath the pectoralis major. Its origin is from the outer surfaces of the second through fifth ribs near their cartilages. From there, it extends upward and toward the side, where it inserts into the front surface of the scapula. When the scapula is anchored in position, contraction of the pectoralis minor elevates the second through fifth ribs.

The subclavius is a relatively small, narrow muscle that originates on the under-surface of the clavicle. It runs slightly downward and toward the midline, where it attaches to the junction of the first rib and its cartilage. When the clavicle is braced in a fixed position, contraction of the subclavius muscle results in elevation of the first rib.

The serratus anterior is a large, thick muscle situated on the side of the rib cage wall. It originates as several thin, finger-like tabs from the outer surfaces of the upper eight or nine ribs. Fibers pass backward around the side of the rib cage, where they converge to insert into the front surface of the scapula. When the scapula is braced in position, contraction of the serratus anterior muscle raises the upper ribs.

The underline{external intercostals} include 11 muscles that completely fill the outer portions of the rib interspaces. Each is a relatively thin layer of muscle that runs between the lower edge of one rib and the upper edge of the rib immediately below. The individual fibers of each muscle are oriented forward and downward. Collectively, the 11 external intercostals constitute a single, large sheet of muscle that links the ribs to one another and is anchored from above to the first rib, the cervical vertebrae, and the base of the skull. When the muscle in any rib interspace contracts, it elevates the rib immediately below. Other ribs below the elevated rib may also be elevated through the linkage effected by the overall muscular sheet. The external intercostal muscles may activate individually in various rib interspaces or they may activate en masse, depending on the force pattern desired. For activation en masse, the ribs tend to move as a single unit. In addition to effecting elevation of the ribs, contraction of the external intercostal muscles also stiffens the tissue-filled rib interspaces, preventing them from being sucked inward or bulged outward during the lowering or raising of internal pressure, respectively.

The internal intercostals, like the external intercostals, include 11 muscles located within the rib interspaces. These muscles lie underneath the external intercostals and extend from around the sides of the rib cage wall to the sternum. Unlike the external intercostals, the internal intercostals do not fill the interspaces at the back of the rib cage. Fibers of the internal intercostals run downward and backward, from the lower edge of one rib to the upper edge of the rib immediately above. The course of these fibers is at approximately right angles to the course of fibers in the external intercostals. As a group, the internal intercostals constitute a single large sheet of muscle that links the ribs to one another and to the pelvic girdle through several other muscles, mainly those of the abdominal wall. When the muscle in any rib interspace contracts, it pulls downward on the rib immediately above. Other ribs above the depressed rib may also be pulled downward through the linkage effected by the overall muscle sheet. The internal intercostals, like the external intercostals, may activate individually in various rib interspaces or they may activate en masse. For activation en masse, the ribs tend to move in a unitary fashion. Contraction of the internal intercostal muscles also serves to stiffen the tissue-filled rib interspaces. This prevents them from being sucked inward or bulged outward during the lowering or raising of internal pressure, respectively.

The intercartilaginous (between the costal cartilages) segment of the internal intercostals is arranged such that the muscle tissue in that segment exerts an upward pull on the rib cage wall rather than the downward pull exerted by the internal intercostals in their interosseous (between the bony ribs) segment. Thus, the internal intercostals play a functional role in the intercartilagious segment that is similar to that played by their companion external intercostals throughout the rib cage wall. Viewed another way, the two layers of intercostal muscles function similarly toward the front of the rib

---

IN POOR TASTE

The intercostal muscles are the parts of animals you eat when you have ribs. Alfred Packer turned to the human variety in his infamous alleged cannibalism at Lake City, Colorado in 1874. Alfred, also known as Alferd because it was misspelled that way on a tattoo, claimed innocence up to the end. He is immortalized at the University of Colorado. Its Food Service proudly boasts the Alferd Packer Grill. The Grill's menu lists El Canibal, touted as "Boulder's BIGGEST burrito, tacos, nachos, enchiladas, and the best green chile in town." Even alleged crimes may have political overtones. At Packer's sentencing, the judge is reported to have chewed Alferd out (pun intended) because there were only seven Democrats in Hinsdale County, Colorado at the time of the crime, and Alferd was alleged to have eaten five of them. Poor taste, Alferd. Poor taste.

cage, but dissimilarly at other locations.

The <u>transversus thoracis</u> is a thin, fan-shaped muscle located on the inside, front wall of the rib cage. Its origin is at the midline on the inner surface of the lower sternum and the fourth or fifth through seventh costal cartilages. From this origin, it fans out across the rib cage and divides into several muscular tabs that insert into the inner surface of the costal cartilages and bony ends of the second through sixth ribs. The upper fibers of the muscle run almost vertically. The intermediate and lower fibers course at other angles. When the transversus thoracis muscle contracts, it exerts a downward pull on ribs two through six.

The <u>latissimus dorsi</u> is a large muscle located on the back of the body. The fibers of the latissimus dorsi have a complex origin from the lower portion of the vertebral column and the lower ribs. This includes the lower six thoracic, the lumbar, and the sacral vertebrae, as well as the back surfaces of the lower three or four ribs. From this origin, the fibers run upward across the back of the lower torso at various angles to insert into the humerus. When the humerus is held in a fixed position, contraction of the fibers of the latissimus dorsi that insert into the lower ribs will elevate them. Contraction of the latissimus dorsi as a whole, by contrast, compresses the lower portion of the rib cage wall. Therefore, it is not contradictory to view the latissimus dorsi muscle as having the potential to deliver active force of different signs.

The <u>serratus posterior superior</u> muscle is positioned on the upper back portion of the rib cage wall. It is a flat, thin muscle that originates from the back of the vertebral column. Its points of origin include the seventh cervical and the first three or four thoracic vertebrae. Fibers of the serratus posterior superior course downward across the back of the rib cage to insert as muscular tabs into the second through fifth ribs. When the serratus posterior superior muscle contracts, it elevates the second through fifth ribs.

The <u>serratus posterior inferior</u> is a thin, flat muscle located on the lower back portion of the rib cage wall. It originates from the lower two thoracic and upper two or three lumbar vertebrae. Fibers of the muscle slant upward across the back of the rib cage, diverging into four muscular tabs that insert into the lower borders of the lower four ribs. When the serratus posterior inferior muscle contracts, it pulls downward on the lower four ribs.

The <u>lateral iliocostals</u> muscle group includes three muscles located on the back of the body. These are situated to the side of the vertebral column and extend from the cervical region to the lumbar region. The <u>lateral iliocostal cervicis</u> arises from the outer surfaces of the third through sixth ribs. Its fibers course upward and toward the midline to insert into the fourth through sixth cervical vertebrae. The <u>lateral iliocostal thoracis</u> has its origin from the upper edges of the lower six ribs. Its fibers course upward to insert into the lower edges of the upper six ribs. The <u>lateral iliocostal lumborum</u> arises from the lumbodorsal fascia, the lumbar vertebrae, and the back surface of the coxal bone. Its fibers course upward and toward the side to insert into the lower edges of the lower six ribs. Contraction of the lateral iliocostal cervicis muscle results in elevation of the third through sixth ribs, whereas contraction of the lateral iliocostal lumborum muscle results in depression of the lower six ribs. Contraction of the lateral iliocostal thoracis muscle tends to stabilize large segments of the back of the rib cage wall and causes them to move in step with either the rib elevation or the rib depression effected by the cervical or lumbar elements of the overall lateral iliocostals group, respectively.

The levatores costarum are 12 small muscles situated on the back of the rib cage wall. They originate from the seventh cervical and upper eleven thoracic vertebrae. Each muscle extends downward and slightly outward to insert into the back surface of the rib immediately below the vertebra of origin. On the lower rib cage wall, some muscles also extend to the second rib below the vertebra of origin. When an individual muscle of the levatores costarum group contracts, it elevates the ribs into which it inserts. When the levatores costarum contract en masse, their collective action is similar to that effected by en masse contraction of the external intercostal muscles (i.e., the ribs elevate as a single unit).

The quadratus lumborum is a flat, roughly quadrilateral sheet of muscle located on the back of the body. Its fibers arise from the top of the coxal bone and run upward and toward the midline. They diverge into several muscular tabs that insert into the first four lumbar vertebrae and the lower border of the inner half of the lowest rib. When the quadratus lumborum muscle contracts, it pulls downward on the lowest rib.

The subcostals are a group of thin muscles located on the inside back wall of the rib cage. They vary in number from person to person and are most often located and best developed in the lower portion of the rib cage wall. Fibers of these muscles originate near the vertebral column on the inner surfaces of ribs. From there, they course upward and toward the side, inserting into the inner surface of the rib immediately above, or skipping a rib or two and inserting into higher ribs. When the subcostals contract, they pull downward on the ribs into which they insert.

Muscle of the Diaphragm

Figure 2-3 depicts the muscle of the diaphragm. Different views are shown.

The diaphragm is a very large, complex muscle that subdivides the torso into two compartments. It has an extensive origin that includes the internal circumference of the lower rib cage. This origin encompasses the bottom of the sternum, the lower six ribs and their cartilages, and the first three or four lumbar vertebrae. From this internal rim, muscle fibers radiate upward to insert into the circumference of the central tendon. The central tendon is a broad, flat sheet of nonelastic tissue that forms the centermost portion of the structure. When the diaphragm contracts, it pulls downward and forward. This enlarges the thorax vertically. Contraction of the diaphragm also enlarges the thorax circumferentially through elevation of the lower

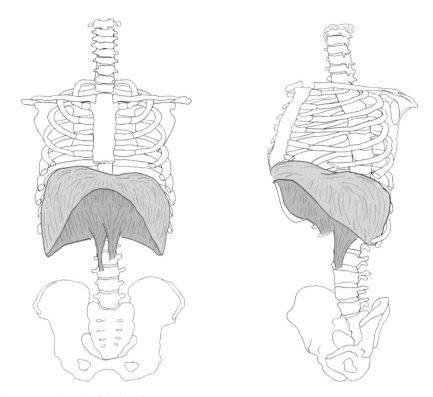

Figure 2-3. Muscle of the diaphragm.

six ribs. The combined action of lowering the base of the thorax and expanding its circumference occurs in patterns that depend, in part, on the relative stiffness of the rib cage wall and abdominal wall, as well as on the pressure developed below the diaphragm.

Muscles of the Abdominal Wall

Figure 2-4 depicts the muscles of the abdominal wall. Different views are shown.

The <u>rectus abdominis</u> muscle is a long, ribbon-like structure located on the front of the lower rib cage wall and the abdominal wall just off the midline. It originates from the upper front edge of the coxal bone and runs vertically upward to insert into the outer surfaces of the fifth, sixth, and seventh costal cartilages and the lower sternum. The muscle is compartmentalized into four or five short segments by tendinous breaks. The mass of the muscle is encased in a fibrous sheath formed by the abdominal aponeurosis. The muscle and its sheath form a centerpost along the front of the abdominal wall. This centerpost is a continuation of the front centerpost formed by the sternum on the rib cage wall. The rectus abdominis muscle has a significant mechanical effect on the lower rib cage wall. When it contracts, it pulls the lower ribs and sternum downward and forces the front of the abdominal wall inward. The compartmentalized segments of the rectus abdominis muscle are also capable of independent contraction.

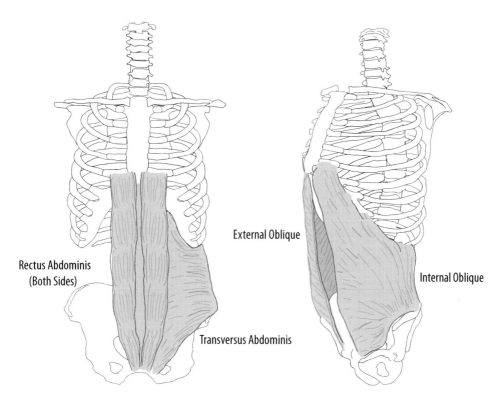

Figure 2-4. Muscles of the abdominal wall.

The <u>external oblique</u> is a broad, flat muscle located on the side and front portions of the lower rib cage wall and the abdominal wall. Fibers of this muscle arise from the upper surface of the coxal bone and from the abdominal aponeurosis near the midline. They course upward across the abdominal wall at various angles. The most prominent course is upward and toward the side, with insertions being in the form of muscular tabs that attach to the outer surfaces and lower borders of the lower eight ribs. As with the rectus abdominis muscle, the external oblique muscle has a significant mechanical effect on the rib cage wall. When it contracts, it pulls the lower ribs downward and forces the front and side of the abdominal wall inward.

The <u>internal oblique</u> is a large, flat muscle situated on the side and front portions of the lower rib cage wall and the abdominal wall. It lies underneath the external oblique. The internal oblique has an extensive origin that includes much of the upper surface of the coxal bone and the lumbodorsal fascia. Its fibers fan out across the abdominal wall to insert into the abdominal aponeurosis and the lower borders of the costal cartilages of the lower three or four ribs. Fibers of the internal oblique muscle run at right angles to those of the external oblique muscle. When the internal oblique contracts, it pulls the lower ribs downward and forces the front and side of the abdominal wall inward. Its functional potential is similar to that of the external oblique.

The <u>transversus abdominis</u> is a flat, broad muscle located on the front and side of the abdominal wall. It lies underneath the internal oblique muscle. The transversus abdominis has a complex origin that includes the upper surface of the coxal bone, the lumbodorsal fascia, and the inner surfaces of the costal cartilages of ribs seven through twelve. Fibers of the muscle run horizontally around the abdominal wall, inserting at the front into the abdominal aponeurosis. The paired left and right transversus abdominis muscles encircle the abdominal wall. When the transversus abdominis contracts, it forces the front and side of the abdominal wall inward.

The four muscles just discussed – rectus abdominis, external oblique, internal oblique, and transversus abdominis – are located on the front and sides of the abdominal wall and are often referred to as "the" abdominal muscles. Recall that the abdominal wall runs all the way around the torso and includes more than just the front and sides. To be complete, therefore, it is important to consider three other muscles that have been discussed above in relation to the rib cage wall – latissimus dorsi, lateral iliocostal lumborum, and quadratus lumborum. These three muscles traverse the abdominal wall at the back and are as much a part of the abdominal wall as they are a part of the rib cage wall. They do not have mechanical advantages on the abdominal wall and cannot effect major displacements of the structure. Nevertheless, they can brace the abdominal wall at the back and vary its stiffness. Accordingly, they are legitimate partners with the other four abdominal muscles in effecting function.

Manifestations of Passive and Active Forces

The passive and active forces of breathing are manifested in two ways. One is through pulls on structures to which they are attached, and the other is through pressures developed at various locations within the breathing apparatus. Pulling forces are distributed within the breathing apparatus in a complicated fashion and their specification is a technical challenge. Fortunately, such forces are uniformly distributed at certain points where they manifest as pressures. The most important of these pressures include the following: (a) alveolar pressure; (b) pleural pressure; (c) abdominal pressure; and (d) transdiaphragmatic pressure. Alveolar pressure is the pressure inside the lungs. Pleural pressure is the pressure inside the thorax but outside the lungs (i.e., between the pleural membranes). Abdominal pressure is the pressure inside the abdominal cavity. Transdiaphragmatic pressure is the difference in pressure across the diaphragm (i.e., the difference between pleural pressure and abdominal pressure).

Movements of Breathing

This section considers the movements of the breathing apparatus, apart from the forces responsible for them. The relation of forces to movements is considered in a separate section on adjustment capabilities. The present section discusses movements as they pertain to the rib cage wall, diaphragm, and abdominal wall.

Movements of the Rib Cage Wall

The rib cage wall is a relatively flexible structure. Much of its flexibility is made possible by its costosternal (between the ribs and sternum) and costovertebral (between the ribs and vertebral column) joints. Movement of its skeletal structure varies somewhat from rib to rib, owing to differences in the lengths and shapes of individual ribs. Nevertheless, two forms of rib movement are typical.

One form of rib movement involves vertical excursion of the front ends of the ribs (and the sternum). Such excursion is either upward-and-forward or downward-and-backward, with a resulting increase or decrease, respectively, in the front-to-back (i.e., anteroposterior) diameter of the rib cage wall. Each rib rotates through the axis of its neck (located at the back near the vertebral column). This pattern of movement is often described as resembling the raising and lowering of the handle on an old-fashioned water pump.

The other form of rib movement involves vertical excursion of the ribs along the sides of the rib cage wall. This action constitutes a rotation of each rib around an axis extending between its two ends. Such excursion is either upward-and-outward or downward-and-inward. The result is an increase or decrease, respectively, in the side-to-side (i.e., transverse) diameter of the rib cage wall. This pattern of movement is often described as resembling the raising and lowering of the handle on a water bucket.

Anteroposterior and transverse movements of the rib cage wall usually occur in phase. Thus, when the anteroposterior diameter of the rib cage wall increases or decreases, the transverse diameter does likewise. The circumference of the rib cage wall also increases or decreases along with increases or decreases in these two diameters.

When the rib cage wall moves, it usually does so with a single degree of freedom. This means that it moves as a single unit, with the movements of different points on its surface being uniquely related. It also means that by monitoring any point on the surface of the rib cage wall, the positions of all other points and the overall configuration of the structure can be specified. There are times, however, when the rib cage wall does not behave with a single degree of freedom. These usually involve instances in which the forces exerted by the rib cage wall muscles are so large that the relations among its anteroposterior, transverse, and circumferential dimensions are altered.

The rib cage wall covers a large portion of the surface of the lungs. Thus, movement of the rib cage wall has a major influence on the movement of air through the pulmonary apparatus. Even a small movement of the rib cage wall can result in the displacement of a large amount of air.

Movements of the Diaphragm

Although hidden from view, movements of the diaphragm can be inferred from the movements of other structures of the chest wall. Both the origin and insertion points of the diaphragm are moveable. That is, the positions of the lower six ribs (origin) and the central tendon (insertion) can be adjusted.

The diaphragm is usually dome-shaped. Two forms of movement can change this shape. One is a decrease in the radius of curvature of the diaphragm. This is manifested as a relative flattening of the structure. This flattening can range from slight to marked. When marked, the configuration of the diaphragm resembles the outline of an inverted pie pan.

The other form of movement is an increase in the radius of curvature of the diaphragm. This is manifested as a more cone-shaped upward projection of the structure. This upward projection can range from slight to marked. When marked, the diaphragm takes on a configuration that resembles the outline of a parabola-shaped bullet nose.

These two forms of diaphragm movement can occur in association with different combinations of relative fixation of the lower ribs and central tendon. For example, the diaphragm can take on a more flattened configuration as a result of elevation of the lower ribs and/or descent of the central tendon. For another example, the diaphragm can take on a more cone-shaped configuration as a result of descent of the lower ribs and/or elevation of the central tendon. When the bottom of the rib cage wall is anchored, the points of origin of the diaphragm are fixed and the movement of the central tendon defines the movement of the diaphragm. By contrast, when the central tendon is firmly anchored, the points of insertion of the diaphragm are fixed and the movement of the rib cage wall defines the movement of the diaphragm.

The diaphragm is in contact with a smaller portion of the lungs than is the rib cage wall. Thus, the diaphragm must go through a greater absolute excursion than the rib cage wall to displace the same amount of air.

Movements of the Abdominal Wall

The usual configuration of the abdominal wall varies from person to person, depending on factors such as body type and abdominal muscle tone. In the upright body position, the abdominal wall is usually distended slightly due to the hydrostatic pressure gradient between the undersurface of the diaphragm and the pelvis. Two general forms of abdominal wall movement can cause departures from this usual configuration. One is an increase in the radius of curvature of the abdominal wall. This is manifested as an increase in the outward protrusion of the wall, in which it becomes increasingly more concave toward the vertebral column. Outward protrusion can range from slight to marked. When such protrusion is marked, the torso (in side view) takes on a shape that resembles one half of a pear that has been sliced vertically.

The other form of abdominal wall movement is a decrease in the radius of curvature of the structure. This is manifested as a flattening of the abdominal wall. Such flattening may range from slight to marked. In some individuals, marked flattening may lead to a configuration in which the front surface of the abdominal wall is actually slightly convex toward the vertebral column (i.e., curved the opposite direction from usual). This extreme positioning is found most often in individuals who are exceptionally lean.

The anteroposterior, transverse, and circumferential movements of the abdominal wall typically occur in phase. As with the rib cage wall, the abdominal wall tends to move as a unit, with the movements of different points on its surface being uniquely related. By monitoring any point on the surface of the abdominal wall, the positions of all other points and the overall configuration of the structure can be specified. Nevertheless, as with the rib cage wall, there are times when the abdominal wall does not behave with a single degree of freedom. These usually involve circumstances in which very large forces are exerted by the abdominal wall muscles and the relations among its anteroposterior, transverse, and circumferential dimensions are altered.

E Pluribus Unum

Although most abdominal walls behave with a single degree of freedom with respect to their movement, not all do. Just as some people are able to wiggle their ears and others can't, some people can make movements with their abdominal walls that others can't. We're reminded of the remarkable belly gymnastics we once saw on television. A woman lying on her back was able to slowly roll a coin (a quarter) up the center of her belly by turning it end over end with her abdominal muscles alone. She apparently did this by using successive activation of the different segments along the vertical axis of her rectus abdominis muscles. We've never been able to find another person who could even remotely accomplish this feat. Maybe that's why it says e pluribus unum on the quarter the woman used. That's Latin for "one of a kind."

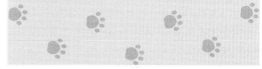

Recall that the abdominal content is essentially incompressible. Thus, the abdominal wall can be viewed as one surface (or side) of a combined structure, the diaphragm-abdominal wall. Functionally, then, the abdominal wall is indirectly in contact with the same surface of the lungs as is the diaphragm. Accordingly, the abdominal wall, like the diaphragm, must go through a greater absolute excursion than the rib cage wall to displace an equivalent amount of air.

The following section extends the present discussion to adjustment capabilities of the breathing apparatus. This shifts the focus from the mechanical bases of breathing to how those bases subserve functional activities.

ADJUSTMENT CAPABILITIES OF THE BREATHING APPARATUS

The breathing apparatus is capable of a wide variety of adjustments. These are made possible by mechanical actions of different parts of the pulmonary apparatus and chest wall. Some of these actions are straightforward and are confined to the parts in which they occur. Others are more complex and may include interplay among the different parts of the breathing apparatus.

Figure 2-5 summarizes both the passive and active forces that may contribute to adjustments of the breathing apparatus. These are shown for the pulmonary apparatus and chest wall, as well as for the three components of the chest wall – rib cage wall, diaphragm, and abdominal wall. The negative signs in the figure represent forces that tend to inspire the breathing apparatus, whereas the positive signs represent forces that tend to expire it. These forces are discussed in sections that follow.

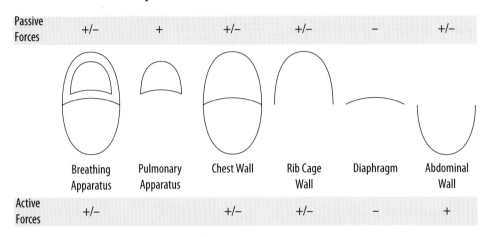

Figure 2-5. Passive and active forces of breathing.

Pulmonary Apparatus

The pulmonary apparatus is a passive participant in all adjustments of the breathing apparatus. It tends to recoil toward a smaller size, like a stretched coil spring. The pulmonary apparatus pulls directly inward on the rib cage wall and directly headward on the diaphragm through its pleural linkage to these two structures. The pulmonary apparatus operates only in the expiratory direction.

Chest Wall

The chest wall can contribute both passively and actively to adjustments of the breathing apparatus. It tends to recoil inward (i.e., in the expiratory direction) at large chest wall sizes, like a stretched coil spring, and to recoil outward (i.e., in the inspiratory direction) at small chest wall sizes, like a compressed coil spring. Thus, it complements the recoil tendency of the pulmonary apparatus at large chest wall sizes and opposes it at small chest wall sizes. Large or small in this context means that the chest wall is at a size that is larger or smaller, respectively, than the size it would assume at rest were it free of its linkage to the pulmonary apparatus.

Muscles of the chest wall can generate active force to cause the breathing apparatus to either inspire or expire at any chest wall size. Muscles of the chest wall that inspire the breathing apparatus are located in the rib cage wall and diaphragm, and muscles that expire the apparatus are located in the rib cage wall and abdominal wall. The ability of the chest wall to generate active force depends on its prevailing size. The force available to inspire the breathing apparatus is greater at small chest wall sizes, whereas the force available to expire the apparatus is greater at large chest wall sizes. Size-dependent force advantages for inspiration and expiration are related to the fact that the muscles generating active force are on more favorable portions of their length-tension characteristics.

Rib Cage Wall

The rib cage wall can contribute both passively and actively to adjustments of the breathing apparatus. The rib cage wall tends to recoil in the expiratory direction at large sizes and in the inspiratory direction at small sizes (except in downright body positions). Thus, it complements the recoil tendency of the pulmonary apparatus at large rib cage sizes and opposes it at small rib cage sizes.

Muscles of the rib cage wall can generate active force in both the inspiratory and expiratory directions. The muscles responsible for delivering inspiratory force are located in superficial layers of the rib cage wall and the muscles responsible for delivering expiratory force are located in deep layers of the wall. The ability of the rib cage wall muscles to generate active force depends on the prevailing rib cage wall size. Larger inspiratory forces are possible at small rib cage wall sizes where inspiratory muscles are on more favorable portions of their length-tension characteristics, and larger expiratory forces are possible at large rib cage wall sizes where expiratory muscles are on more favorable portions of their length-tension characteristics.

The rib cage wall is capable of expansion or compression through its own actions. Such expansion or compression depends, in part, on the movement allowed at the joints between the ribs and the spinal column and on the compliance (stiffness) of the rib cage. The resting position of the rib cage wall is typically near the midpoint of the full range of possible rib cage wall sizes. Therefore, the potential for expansion of the rib cage wall is about the same as the potential for compression (except in downright body positions). The individual adjustment capability of the rib cage wall includes changing its own size in either direction, and doing so in finely graded steps. The smallest muscles of the breathing apparatus are housed within the rib cage wall. This means that the rib cage wall is endowed with tools for precise control and fast action.

Diaphragm

The diaphragm is also capable of contributing both passively and actively to adjustments of the breathing apparatus. When displaced footward, and being less highly domed (i.e., such as at large lung volumes), it develops no recoil. By contrast, when displaced headward and being more highly domed (i.e., such as at small lung volumes), it tends to recoil in the inspiratory direction. This is because the structure undergoes passive stretch from the forces acting across it. Thus, the diaphragm opposes the recoil tendency of the pulmonary apparatus at small volumes.

The diaphragm can generate active force in the inspiratory direction only. Such force generation depends on its configuration. The more highly domed the configuration of the diaphragm, and, thus, the longer its main muscle fibers, the more force the structure is able to exert. This is because its main muscle fibers are on more favorable portions of their length-tension characteristics.

The diaphragm is capable of flattening itself to lessen its dome-like appearance. This flattening is associated with a downward pull on its central tendon. The diaphragm is also capable of pulling headward on its circumferential muscular rim. This is associated with an upward pull on its rib cage wall attachments. The diaphragm is the strongest of all the muscles of the breathing apparatus and its combined pull on the central tendon and rib cage wall can result in major adjustments in its configuration.

Abdominal Wall

The abdominal wall can also make both passive and active contributions to adjustments of the breathing apparatus. The abdominal wall tends to recoil in the expiratory direction at large abdominal wall volumes and in the inspiratory direction at small abdominal wall volumes (except in downright body positions). Thus, it complements the recoil tendency of the pulmonary apparatus at large abdominal wall volumes and opposes it at small abdominal wall volumes.

The abdominal wall is capable of generating active force in the expiratory direction only. This capability depends on the prevailing abdominal wall volume. Greater expiratory forces are possible at large abdominal wall volumes at which the muscles of the abdominal wall are on more favorable portions of their length-tension characteristics.

The abdominal wall is capable of inward movement through its own action. The muscles of the abdominal wall are very strong and can be controlled in various subsets. Adjustment capability of the wall includes not only changing its volume in the expiratory direction, but also doing so in relatively precisely graded steps or holding itself in fixed positions. The abdominal wall is especially well-suited to postural adjustment of the breathing apparatus.

Pulmonary-Chest Wall Unit

Mechanical arrangements between different parts of the pulmonary-chest wall unit play a significant role in how actions of the breathing apparatus are manifested. Several of these arrangements make it possible for one part of the breathing apparatus to bring about adjustments in other parts of the apparatus. Notable among these arrangements are the following: (a) the pulmonary apparatus shares surfaces with the rib cage wall and diaphragm; (b) the rib cage wall, diaphragm, and abdominal wall share points of physical attachment among them; (c) the abdominal content is housed partially within the confines of the domed diaphragm and the lower circumferential encasement of the rib cage wall; (d) the diaphragm resides within the confines of the rib cage wall; and (e) the abdominal content constitutes a hydraulic intermediary between the undersurface of the diaphragm and the inner surface of the abdominal wall.

Action of the rib cage wall can cause adjustments in both the diaphragm and the abdominal wall. For example, when the rib cage wall expands, the circumferential insertions of the diaphragm into the rib cage wall move headward and outward. At the same time, such expansion causes pleural and abdominal pressures to decrease. The decrease in abdominal pressure causes a footward hydraulic pull to be placed on the diaphragm that holds it in position. Simultaneously, the abdominal wall is pulled inward. It is as if the expanding rib cage wall sucks the abdominal wall inward by pulling the abdominal content headward, much in the manner that liquid is pulled upward in a drinking straw. By contrast, when the rib cage wall compresses, the circumferential insertions of the diaphragm into the rib cage wall move footward and inward. Both pleural and abdominal pressures increase during compression of the rib cage wall, causing the diaphragm to flatten and the abdominal wall to be forced outward in the inspiratory direction.

The diaphragm can cause adjustments in the rib cage wall and abdominal wall. To a substantial degree, the magnitudes of such adjustments are related to the prevailing status of the rib cage wall and abdominal wall. When the muscular portion of the diaphragm contracts, its fibers shorten and place pulls on the central tendon and on the lower ribs to which the diaphragm attaches. Whether the central tendon is pulled downward or the ribs are pulled upward depends on the relative fixation of these two attachment points. For example, if the rib cage wall is fixed in position, movement of the diaphragm will be resolved into footward displacement. And, for a contrasting example, if the abdominal wall is fixed in position, movement of the diaphragm will be resolved into headward displacement of the rib cage wall. Usually, neither the rib cage wall nor abdominal wall is rigidly fixed in position. Rather, both will move during contraction of the diaphragm, and the extent of their movement will depend on their relative compliance.

The abdominal wall can effect adjustments in the rib cage wall and diaphragm. More specifically, when the muscles of the abdominal wall contract and displace the abdominal wall inward, the incompressible abdominal content forces the diaphragm headward and increases its radius of curvature. This action also raises abdominal pressure. Headward displacement of the diaphragm causes an upward-lifting force to be applied to the rib cage wall through the muscle fibers of the diaphragm that insert on the lower ribs. At the same time, the associated increase in abdominal pressure causes the lower rib cage wall to move outward in the region known as the area of apposition (i.e., where the muscle fibers of the diaphragm run adjacent to and parallel to the rib cage wall). The combination of upward pull by the diaphragm and outward forcing by abdominal pressure results in passive lifting of the rib cage wall. This adjustment can be appreciated by pulling in the abdominal wall and noting that the rib cage wall expands passively.

Adjustments of the breathing apparatus often seem deceptively simple and there is a tendency to ascribe them solely to the parts of the apparatus in which they occur. As is suggested by the discussion above, the interplay between and among various parts of the breathing apparatus is significant and must be taken into account when trying to specify the actions responsible for any given adjustment.

CONTROL VARIABLES OF THE BREATHING APPARATUS

Acts of breathing involve changes in a number of independent control variables. Three such variables have relevance to the concerns of this book. These are volume, pressure, and shape.

Volume

Volume is defined as the size of a three-dimensional object or region of space. The volume of interest here is that of the air contained within the pulmonary apparatus. This volume is termed the lung volume and its importance lies in the fact that it reflects the prevailing size of the breathing apparatus, the behavior of which is volume-dependent.

Changes in lung volume are manifestations of the summed movements of different parts of the breathing apparatus. These movements cause the air within and around the apparatus to be displaced from the space it occupies (i.e., moved from one place to another). For such movements to be realized as volume displacements, it must be possible for volume to be exchanged back and forth between the lungs and atmosphere through the conducting pulmonary airways. Thus, the laryngeal airway and upper airway must allow air to pass.

Although the volume variable is continuous, it is conventional to delimit certain portions of its range into what are termed lung volumes and lung capacities (Pappenheimer, Comroe, Cournand, Ferguson, Filley, Fowler, Gray, Helmholz, Otis, Rahn, & Riley, 1950). This convention is portrayed in Figure 2-6 through the use of a spirogram, a tracing of lung volume obtained from a device that records volume displacement over time.

There are four lung volumes. Each encompasses a different portion of the volume range without overlap with the other three. The four lung volumes are as follows.

• The tidal volume (TV) is the volume of air inspired or expired during the breathing cycle. Its magnitude is dictated mainly by the oxygen needs of the body and

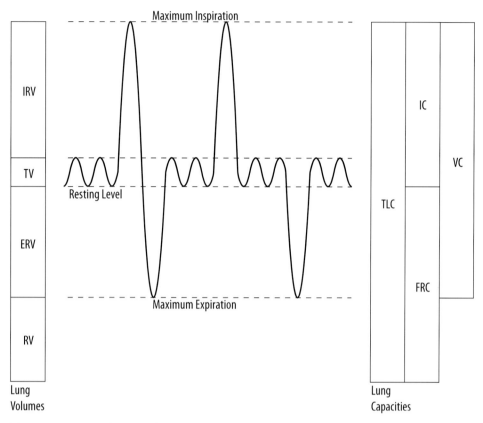

Figure 2-6. Lung volumes and lung capacities.

in the resting individual is termed the resting tidal volume. The term tidal volume is descriptive in that the movement of air in and out of the pulmonary apparatus bears analogy to the flow and ebb of an ocean tide, respectively.

- The inspiratory reserve volume (IRV) is the maximum volume of air that can be inspired from the tidal end-inspiratory level (i.e., the peak of the tidal volume cycle).

- The expiratory reserve volume (ERV) is the maximum volume of air that can be expired from the tidal end-expiratory level (i.e., the trough of the tidal volume cycle).

- The residual volume (RV) is the volume of air contained by the pulmonary apparatus at the end of a maximum expiration. The residual volume is the only one of the four lung volumes that cannot be measured directly, because no matter how forceful the expiration, the pulmonary apparatus cannot be emptied. To estimate the residual volume, indirect measurement methods must be used.

Lung capacities are also four in number. Each capacity includes two or more of the four lung volumes just discussed.

- The inspiratory capacity (IC) is the maximum volume of air that can be inspired from the resting tidal end-expiratory level. This capacity is the sum of the tidal volume and the inspiratory reserve volume.

- The vital capacity (VC) is the maximum volume of air that can be expired following a maximum inspiration. It includes all of the lung volumes except the residual volume.

- The functional residual capacity (FRC) is the volume of air contained by the pulmonary apparatus at the resting tidal end-expiratory level. It includes the expiratory reserve volume and the residual volume.

- The total lung capacity (TLC) is the volume of air contained by the pulmonary apparatus at the end of a maximum inspiration. All four of the lung volumes are encompassed by this capacity.

Pressure

Pressure is defined as a force distributed over a surface (i.e., pressure = force/area). Of present interest is the pressure operating on the air within the lungs – alveolar pressure. This pressure is important because it specifies the magnitude of the mechanical drive provided by the breathing apparatus. Stated otherwise, the alveolar pressure represents the sum of all the passive and active forces operating on the breathing apparatus.

Alveolar pressure is generated by air molecules within the lungs colliding with one another and with the structures of the lungs. Actions of the breathing apparatus that cause these molecules to be less crowded result in fewer collisions and in the pressure in the alveoli being lower. Conversely, actions that cause the same molecules to be more crowded result in more collisions and in the pressure in the alveoli being higher. The actions referred to in these contexts are movements of the breathing apparatus that cause the air contained by the lungs to become either expanded or compressed from the prevailing lung volume (i.e., the space occupied). Lung volume and alveolar pressure are inversely related, provided the pulmonary airways are closed to atmosphere at the larynx or upper airway and provided the temperature of the air contained within the lungs remains constant. Thus, a doubling of the confined lung volume by expansion results in a halving of alveolar pressure, and a halving of the same volume by compression results in a doubling of alveolar pressure.

As with the volume variable, the pressure variable is continuous. It is conventional to display the pressure variable in a volume-pressure diagram. Such a diagram is of analytical value in relating the passive and active forces of breathing to one another, to the summed force expressed in the alveolar pressure variable, and to levels of the lung volume.

Figure 2-7 shows one form of the volume-pressure diagram (Agostoni & Mead, 1964). The amount of air within the lungs (in percent vital capacity, %VC) is displayed on the vertical axis. The alveolar pressure (in centimeters of water, cmH_2O) is shown on the horizontal axis. The solid horizontal line in the diagram represents the resting tidal end-expiratory level of the breathing apparatus. The solid vertical line in the diagram represents atmospheric pressure (i.e., zero, by convention). Points to the left or right of this line represent pressures that are below atmospheric (negative, by convention) or above atmospheric (positive, by convention), respectively. Three curves are shown in the diagram. These represent the volume-pressure relations under the following three conditions: (a) relaxation; (b) maximum inspiration; and (c) maximum expiration.

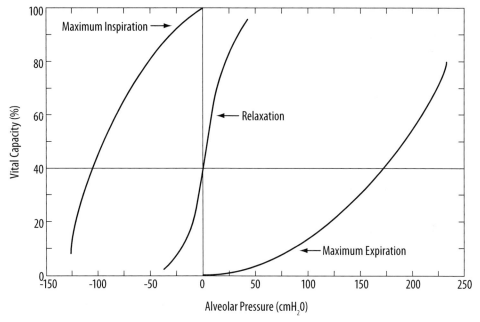

Figure 2-7. Volume-pressure diagram.

The pressure produced entirely by the passive force of the breathing apparatus is designated as the relaxation pressure. The relaxation pressure curve expresses the concepts already considered above, but in a more formal and precise manner. The relaxation pressure is the pressure developed in the pulmonary airways and lungs when the breathing muscles are relaxed. It varies in magnitude depending on how much the lungs are inflated or deflated from the resting tidal end-expiratory level. At lung volumes larger than that at the resting level, relaxation results in a tendency to expire passively through the generation of a positive pressure. This pressure decreases as the lungs are deflated from the total lung capacity to the resting level. Relaxation at lung volumes smaller than that at the resting tidal end-expiratory level results in a tendency to inspire passively through the generation of a negative pressure. The magnitude of this pressure increases (i.e., becomes less subatmospheric) as the lungs are inflated from the residual volume to the resting level. In the mid-range of the vital capacity, the relaxation pressure changes nearly in direct proportion to volume change. At the extremes of the vital capacity, pressure changes more abruptly with volume change. This is because the pulmonary apparatus is stiffer at large lung volumes and the chest wall is stiffer at small lung volumes.

Departures from the relaxation pressure can be accomplished at any lung volume through the use of muscular effort. Pressures lower than the relaxation pressure (i.e., to the left of the relaxation curve) at the prevailing lung volume require that a net inspiratory muscular pressure be added to the relaxation pressure. By contrast, pressures that exceed the relaxation pressure (i.e., to the right of the curve) at the prevailing lung volume require that a net expiratory muscular pressure be added to the relaxation pressure. Net is specified in such descriptions because, although pressures lower or higher than relaxation can be produced solely through inspiratory or expiratory efforts, respectively, it is possible to depart from the relaxation pressure curve with both inspiratory and expiratory forces operating simultaneously, but with one or the other predominating. Also, it is possible to be on the relaxation pressure curve during muscular effort (i.e., to produce a pressure equal to the relaxation pressure at the prevailing lung volume) by exerting inspiratory and expiratory forces that are equal and opposite and cancel. Thus, pressure equal to the relaxation pressure is not proof of breathing muscle relaxation.

The maximum inspiration curve in Figure 2-7 shows the pressure developed in the pulmonary airways and lungs when a maximum inspiratory muscular effort is exerted. This curve represents the greatest negative alveolar pressure that can be developed through the use of muscular effort. The curve also defines the extent to which it is possible to depart from the relaxation pressure in the negative sign at each lung volume. The negative pressure developed during a maximum inspiratory effort depends on lung volume. The maximum inspiratory pressure increases (i.e., becomes less subatmospheric) as the lungs are inflated from the residual volume to the total lung capacity. Greater negative pressure can be produced at smaller lung volumes because the breathing apparatus tends to recoil toward a larger volume with greater force at smaller lung volumes, and because the inspiratory muscles of the breathing apparatus are operating under more favorable length-tension conditions at smaller lung volumes.

The maximum expiration curve in Figure 2-7 shows the pressure developed in the pulmonary airways and lungs when a maximum expiratory muscular effort is generated. The maximum expiration curve reveals the greatest positive alveolar pressure that can be developed through the use of muscular effort. Accordingly, the curve defines the extent to which it is possible to depart from the relaxation pressure in the positive sign at each lung volume. As with the relaxation pressure and the maximum inspiratory pressure, the positive pressure developed during maximum expiratory efforts also depends on lung volume. The maximum expiratory pressure decreases as the lungs are deflated from the total lung capacity to the residual volume. Greater positive pressures can be generated at larger lung volumes because the breathing apparatus tends to recoil toward a smaller volume with greater force at larger lung volumes, and because the expiratory muscles of the breathing apparatus are stretched to more optimum lengths for generating tensions.

Shape

Shape is an outline configuration of an object. It is independent of the size or the volume of an object and for many objects is subject to change. The shape of importance in the present context is that of the chest wall. In this case, shape derives from the combined positioning of the rib cage wall, diaphragm, and abdominal wall. How such positioning influences the surface outline of the rib cage wall and abdominal wall (the two surfaces that can be observed directly) determines the externally expressed geometric shape of the chest wall. Shape is important because it provides information about the prevailing mechanical advantages of different parts of the chest wall.

The shape of the chest wall can be changed substantially and is limited only by the positions that can be assumed by the rib cage wall and abdominal wall. Like the volume and pressure variables, the shape variable is continuous. It is conventional to characterize and delimit the shape variable in terms of relative anteroposterior diameters of the rib cage wall and abdominal wall. Such relative diameters capture the shape of the chest wall, because the rib cage wall and abdominal wall each usually behave with a single degree of freedom with respect to their movement. Thus, the relative diameters of the rib cage wall and abdominal wall are indicative of their prevailing positions and, when combined, are indicative of the prevailing shape of the chest wall.

Figure 2-8 illustrates the conventional way to portray the shape of the chest wall (Konno & Mead, 1967). Shown there is a relative diameter diagram of the rib cage wall and abdominal wall. The diameter of the rib cage wall is displayed on the vertical axis, increasing upward, and the diameter of the abdominal wall is displayed on the horizontal axis, increasing rightward.

The area circumscribed in the diagram depicts the full range of relative diameters, and, therefore, includes all possible shapes that can be assumed by the chest wall. The range of shapes is smaller near the diameter extremes, where the sizes of the rib cage wall and abdominal wall are very large or very small. The range of shapes is larger in the diameter midrange, where the sizes of the rib cage wall and abdominal wall are intermediate. Each point in the diagram represents a unique combination of chest wall shape and size. And any series of points on the diagram (i.e., any pathway) documents the history of chest wall shape and/or size change.

The dashed line in the relative diameter diagram represents the relaxation characteristic of the chest wall. As such, it shows the shape assumed by the chest wall

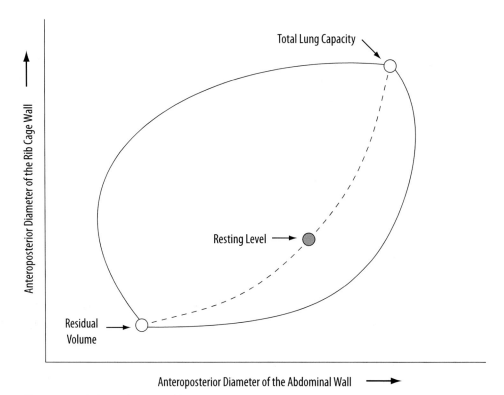

Figure 2-8. Relative diameter diagram.

at different sizes when the breathing muscles are completely relaxed. Circles on the two ends of this relaxation characteristic depict the total lung capacity (TLC) and the residual volume (RV). The filled circle near the middle of the characteristic represents the shape of the relaxed chest wall at the resting tidal end-expiratory level (FRC).

Departures from the relaxation characteristic require that active force be applied to the chest wall. Such active force can be generated in various combinations by the rib cage wall and abdominal wall (Hixon, 1982). Four active force options are possible for achieving chest wall shapes and sizes associated with points lying to the left of the relaxation characteristic on the relative diameter diagram. These include the following: (a) a net inspiratory rib cage wall force; (b) an expiratory abdominal wall force; (c) a net inspiratory rib cage wall force and an expiratory abdominal wall force; and (d) a net expiratory rib cage wall force and a greater expiratory abdominal wall force. Two force options are possible for achieving chest wall shapes and sizes associated with points lying to the right of the relaxation characteristic. They are as follows: (a) a net expiratory rib cage wall force; and (b) a net expiratory rib cage wall force and a lesser expiratory abdominal wall force. And two force options are possible for achieving chest wall shapes and sizes associated with points lying on the relaxation characteristic. These include the following: (a) muscular relaxation (no active force); and (b) a net expiratory rib cage wall force and an equal expiratory abdominal wall force.

NEURAL SUBSTRATES OF BREATHING

Breathing movements are controlled by the nervous system, and the nature of that control differs for different breathing activities. This section describes the neural substrates of breathing with particular focus on those substrates that participate in controlling tidal breathing and special acts of breathing.

Structure of the Nervous System

Figure 2-9 depicts the parts of the adult nervous system that are important to the control of breathing. These reside within two major subdivisions, the central nervous system and the peripheral nervous system.

Central Nervous System

The central nervous system includes the brain, a mass of neural tissue within the skull, and the spinal cord, a long appendage of the brain that extends downward through the vertebral column. Different structures within the central nervous system participate in the control of breathing, depending on whether the breathing activity is automatic, voluntary, or emotionally driven.

The brainstem is responsible for the control of what is often called automatic breathing. Of particular importance to the control of this form of breathing are structures located in the medulla, the region of the brainstem that is contiguous with the spinal cord.

Several structures distributed throughout the brain are crucial to more voluntary forms of breathing. These include the basal nuclei, cerebellum, thalami, and cerebral cortex. Within the cerebral cortex, there are several motor areas believed to participate in the generation of voluntary breathing behaviors, especially the primary motor cortex, premotor cortex, and supplementary motor area, all located in the frontal lobe of the brain. The somatosensory cortex, located in the parietal lobe, is also believed to participate in the control of voluntary breathing behaviors.

Structures within the limbic lobe mediate emotionally driven forms of breathing. These structures are located deep to the cerebral cortex in a phylogenetically old part of the brain.

Peripheral Nervous System

The peripheral nervous system interconnects the central nervous system with other parts of the body. It consists of the cranial nerves and spinal nerves. There are 12 pairs of cranial nerves, 4 of which are important to the control of breathing – IX (glossopharyngeal), X (vagus), XI (accessory), and XII (hypoglossal). These four innervate structures of the larynx, upper airway, and neck.

There are 31 pairs of spinal nerves, 22 of which are involved in the control of breathing. These are listed in Table 2-1 according to the chest wall muscles they

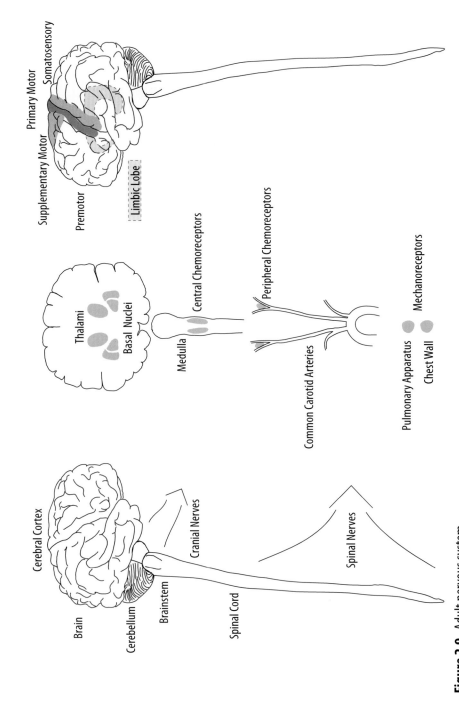

Figure 2-9. Adult nervous system.

innervate. Included are the eight cervical (C) nerves, the twelve thoracic (T) nerves, and the first two lumbar (L) nerves. Each spinal nerve is named for the vertebra above which it exits the spinal cord, except for C1. Successively lower spinal nerves generally innervate muscles from successively lower regions of the chest wall. An exception is the innervation of the diaphragm, which derives collectively from branches of C3-C5 in what is called the phrenic nerve. Table 2-1 lists only the motor innervation to the chest wall (i.e., its efferent innervation, referring to structures that carry neural signals away from the central nervous system). However, the sensory innervation of the chest wall (i.e., its afferent innervation, referring to structures that carry neural signals toward the central nervous system) follows a relatively similar organization. A notable exception is the sensory innervation of the diaphragm. Although primarily vested in the phrenic nerves, sensory innervation of the diaphragm is also supplied by lower thoracic nerves.

Function of the Nervous System

The parts of the nervous system that control the breathing apparatus depend on the nature of the prevailing breathing behavior. Humans exhibit a broad range of breathing behaviors. Such behaviors can be associated with different states – such as being awake, alert, aroused, asleep, conscious, or unconscious – and can be classified in a variety of ways that imply different underlying neural mechanisms. Some of the schemes used to classify breathing behaviors include terms such as automatic, metabolic, reflexive, learned, voluntary, behavioral, purposeful, and emotional, among others. There is no universally accepted way to view or discuss the many manifestations of breathing and their underlying control mechanisms. Thus, for present purposes, the neural control of breathing is examined using a classification scheme that is consistent with the way breathing behaviors are presented in other parts of this book. This scheme uses a simple dichotomy that addresses the control of tidal breathing and the control of special acts of breathing (Comroe, 1965). Also considered is how the control of breathing is managed by the nervous system when several, sometimes competing, neural drives are operating.

Control of Tidal Breathing

Tidal breathing is the most common form of breathing. It is sometimes called automatic breathing, metabolic breathing, or involuntary breathing, and is usually carried out without conscious awareness. Its control is vested in several groups of neurons (nerve cells) located primarily in the medulla of the brainstem (Feldman & McCrimmon, 1999; Lumb, 2000). These groups of neurons are active during either the inspiratory or expiratory phase of the breathing cycle, giving rise to a continuous rhythmic pattern. This network of brainstem neurons is sometimes called the central pattern generator for breathing. The task of this "lower" brain center is to regulate arterial blood gas levels so as to maintain homeostasis. It does this by

Table 2-1. Summary of the segmental origins of the motor nerve supply to the muscles of the chest wall (C = cervical, T = thoracic, L = lumbar). Based on Dickson and Maue-Dickson (1982).

Muscle	Innervation (Spinal Nerve)
Rib Cage Wall	
Sternocleidomastoid	C1-C5
Scalenus Group	C2-C8
Pectoralis Major	C5-C8
Pectoralis Minor	C5-C8
Subclavius	C5-C6
Serratus Anterior	C5-C7, T2-T3
External Intercostals	T1-T11
Internal Intercostals	T1-T11
Transversus Thoracis	T2-T6
Latissimus Dorsi	C6-C8
Serratus Posterior Superior	T2-T3
Serratus Posterior Inferior	T9-T12
Lateral Iliocostals Group	C4-T6, T1-T11, T7-L2
Levatores Costarum	C8-T11
Quadratus Lumborum	T12-L2
Subcostals	T1-T11
Diaphragm	
Diaphragm	C3-C5
Abdominal Wall	
Rectus Abdominis	T7-T12
External Oblique	T8-L1
Internal Oblique	T8-L1
Transversus Abdominis	T7-T12
Latissimus Dorsi	See above
Lateral Iliocostal Lumborum	See above
Quadratus Lumborum	See above

adjusting ventilation (i.e., the amount of air moved in and out of the pulmonary apparatus) so that adequate gas exchange (i.e., oxygen delivery and carbon dioxide elimination) occurs. This lower center can run breathing on its own automatically. It needs no input from "higher" brain centers to maintain homeostasis.

Motor commands from the brainstem travel to breathing muscles via peripheral nerves. When the command signal is strong enough, the muscle fibers innervated by that nerve activate and contract. For example, inspiratory commands from the brainstem activate the diaphragm, the primary muscle of inspiration. Such commands also activate the intercostal muscles, either to stiffen the rib cage wall (during resting tidal breathing) or to serve as supplemental prime movers (during more forceful tidal breathing). Inspiratory motor commands also activate selected muscles of the larynx and upper airway. Activation of these upstream structures serves to lower resistance to inspiratory flow by increasing the size of the airways and stiffening the tissues that line them (to reduce the chances that they will be sucked inward).

Motor commands are not sent blindly through the nervous system. Such commands are strongly influenced by afferent information from a variety of sources. Most afferent information is received and processed unconsciously. Nevertheless, afferent information is sometimes processed to a level of conscious awareness (sensation) or to a level of meaning and association (perception). When the latter occurs, it may be possible to identify breathing-related perceptions, such as the size of the breathing apparatus, movements and forces of breathing, and feelings of breathlessness, to name a few.

The most important afferent information comes from chemoreceptors and mechanoreceptors, structures that are sensitive to chemical changes and mechanical changes, respectively. Chemoreceptors that are relevant to breathing come in two forms – central and peripheral. Central chemoreceptors are located on the anterolateral surfaces of the medulla and respond primarily to changes in the amount of carbon dioxide in cerebral spinal fluid. They provide moment-to-moment updates on the concentration of carbon dioxide. Any change in the level of carbon dioxide stimulates the brainstem breathing center to make appropriate adjustments in ventilation. For example, an increase in the level of carbon dioxide stimulates an increase in brainstem activity and a concomitant increase in ventilation.

The peripheral chemoreceptors important to the control of breathing in humans are located in the carotid bodies at the bifurcation of the common carotid arteries. These are the primary oxygen receptors for the body (conveniently located near the major blood supply to the brain). They also respond to changes in the level of carbon dioxide (although not as strongly as do the central chemoreceptors) and acidity-alkalinity balance in arterial blood. Central and peripheral chemoreceptors generally act synergistically to stimulate adjustments in breathing.

Mechanoreceptors located in the pulmonary apparatus and the chest wall also play an important role in the control of tidal breathing. Those located in the pulmonary apparatus include the following: (a) receptors that respond to the stretching of smooth muscles (such as occurs with an increase in lung volume); (b) receptors that respond to airway irritants (such as smoke, dust, chemicals, or cold air); and (c) receptors that respond to distortions of the alveolar wall (such as might occur when excess fluid surrounds the alveoli). Afferent information from pulmonary mechanoreceptors reaches the central nervous system by way of cranial nerve X.

Mechanoreceptors in the chest wall respond to changes in muscle length (such as occur with changes in rib cage wall or abdominal wall volume) or changes in force (such as occur with changes in inspiratory or expiratory muscular efforts). Afferent signals from chest wall mechanoreceptors reach the central nervous system via spinal nerves. Afferent signals from mechanoreceptors located in the larynx and upper airway can also influence the breathing patterns generated by the brainstem breathing center (Wyke, 1974). For example, irritant stimuli can elicit responses such as coughing and sneezing.

Additional sources of afferent influence on the brainstem-generated breathing pattern come from special senses. Such influence has been found for both visual and auditory stimuli, relayed centrally by cranial nerve II (optic) and cranial nerve VIII (acoustic), respectively. A visual example is that the tidal breathing pattern generated with the eyes open is different from that generated with the eyes closed (Shea, Walter, Pelley, Murphy, & Guz, 1987). An auditory example is that the tidal breathing cycle can differ when generated in silence compared to when generated in the presence of white noise or different types of music (Shea et al., 1987).

Internally generated activity from brain areas outside the brainstem breathing center can have a substantial affect on the tidal breathing pattern (Shea, 1996). Of particular interest here are the effects of cortical activity (critical to the performance of cognitive tasks) and limbic activity (critical to the generation of emotions). Cognitive tasks, such as mental arithmetic, change tidal breathing patterns in ways that usually increase ventilation (Shea, Murphy, Hamilton, Benchetrit, & Guz, 1988; Mador & Tobin, 1991). Also, any con-

ONDINE'S CURSE

The resting tidal breathing that most of us take for granted is a gift that not everyone enjoys all the time. For example, the resting tidal breathing of some people stops when they fall asleep. Those who are born with this condition, called by the imposing name of congenital central hypoventilation syndrome, are at grave risk and usually require ventilatory support during sleep to survive. Their condition is sometimes referred to as Ondine's curse. Mythology has it that Ondine was a beautiful water nymph who married a mortal man. They had what we would today call a pre-nuptial agreement that he would never marry a mortal woman. He didn't keep his word and she became a very vengeful nymph. The terrible price he paid for not keeping his word was that she cursed him to have to think about every breath he took. How she managed to make his central chemoreceptors insensitive to carbon dioxide has been lost in retellings of the tale.

scious (cortical) awareness of breathing alters tidal breathing patterns (Western & Patrick, 1988). This means that just thinking about breathing changes breathing, one reason why truly automatic (unconscious) breathing is so difficult to study. Emotions of all types – excitement, anxiety, anger, fear, joy – also have a profound influence on tidal breathing. In fact, changes in tidal breathing occur so commonly with emotion that they are often considered to be an integral part of the emotional experience (e.g., "It took my breath away!"). Emotions can cause hyperventilation, breath holding, or erratic breathing. Changes in the tidal breathing pattern can be a primary sign (and feelings of breathlessness a primary symptom) of certain psychogenic disorders, such as anxiety disorder or panic disorder. This linkage is so strong that disorders such as these have even been classified as hyperventilation disorders (Gardner, 1996).

Control of Special Acts of Breathing

Special acts of breathing can be thought of as those acts that are not effected for the primary purpose of maintaining homeostasis of arterial blood gases (Shea, 1996). Some special acts of breathing are highly conscious (voluntary), such as breath holding or performing a guided breathing exercise. Other special acts of breathing are learned, well-practiced, and require little conscious awareness of the breathing aspect of the act. Examples of these might be the breathing associated with glass blowing, wind instrument playing, singing, or speaking. Still other special acts of breathing are driven by emotions, such as those seen in crying or laughing. Special acts of breathing are controlled by higher brain centers that either override or bypass activity of the lower (brainstem) breathing center.

A voluntary act of breathing, as with any voluntary motor act, requires the generation of a motor plan. This process is extremely complex and is only partially understood. What is known is that many higher brain centers participate in generating such a plan. These include several subcortical structures, in particular the basal nuclei, cerebellum, and thalami. Another major participant in the development of the motor plan is the cortex, especially the primary motor cortex, premotor cortex, and supplementary motor area. The somatosensory area of the cortex may be important in the interpretation of somatosensory information from the breathing apparatus and related structures. As a behavior becomes learned and less voluntary (less consciously guided), there is believed to be less reliance on cortical participation in the execution of its motor plan.

Many voluntary and learned neural control signals are probably integrated within the brainstem to override the central pattern generator of the lower breathing center. However, there are probably important exceptions to this. Evidence in humans indicates that some cortical neurons make direct connections to spinal neurons so that motor commands from the cortex can reach them directly, bypassing the brainstem altogether (Corfield, Murphy, & Guz, 1998). Even though voluntary or learned control can override (or bypass) activity of the brainstem breathing center, such override has limits. This is clearly demonstrated at the break point of a voluntary breath hold when drive from the brainstem center becomes so strong (in response to danger signals from chemoreceptors) that it is no longer possible to inhibit inspiration.

Special acts of breathing that involve emotional expression are driven by the limbic system. The limbic system has strong connections to the lower (brainstem) breathing center and has a correspondingly strong influence over its output. Limbic influence is evident in its effects on the tidal breathing cycle (as mentioned above), but is perhaps most apparent in its control of special acts of breathing such as crying and laughing. Crying and laughing can override nearly any other voluntary act of breathing, indicating that limbic drive can prevail over cortical drive. It is possible for emotions to continue to influence breathing, even when the voluntary control of breathing is lost (Munschauer, Mador, Ahuja, & Jacobs, 1991). A relevant example is the client who cannot move the abdominal wall voluntarily during speech production or contrived laughter, but whose abdominal wall moves vigorously during spontaneous laughter (Hixon, 1982).

Managing Competing Drives

Perhaps the simplest breathing control problem for the nervous system to solve is one in which tidal breathing occurs at rest. In this case, the goal is to maintain arterial blood gas homeostasis. The control problem presumably becomes more complicated as additional demands are placed on the nervous system. Examples are as follows: (a) needing to blow constantly and forcefully for several seconds (to redirect hot steam while draining freshly cooked pasta); (b) needing to expire through a high resistance at the lips (to whistle to a dog to return home); and (c) needing to use a quick inspiration-slow expiration pattern continually for an hour (to deliver a lecture to a group of university students). These control demands must be met while responding to the ever-present control demands related to maintaining blood gas homeostasis.

Breathing control problems are more difficult to solve when competing drives vie for neural resources. For example, it may be more difficult to maintain the appropriate breathing pattern for delivering a lecture when contending with the emotion of stage fright. In this example, the nervous system is faced with the task of modifying the usual breathing pattern to meet the acoustic goals of speech production, while attempting to minimize the effects of the interfering limbic drive, and, at the same time, maintaining arterial blood gas homeostasis. As another example, it may be more difficult to whistle a tune when hiking at a high elevation than when walking along an ocean beach. In this example, the nervous system is again faced with the task of modifying the usual breathing pattern to achieve an acoustic goal (albeit a less complex one than speech) while maintaining homeostasis in an environment that requires greater-than-usual ventilation to do so.

When managing competing drives, the nervous system must invoke strategies that make it possible to achieve simultaneous breathing-related goals. One strategy for dealing with competing drives is to let one win, at least temporarily. For example, in the case of lecturing with stage fright, the speaker could opt to stop lecturing momentarily to take several deep inspirations. This may help to quell the interfering emotional drive so that speaking can continue more comfortably. Another strategy is to compromise. For example, when whistling a tune at a high elevation, the compromise might be to inspire deeply, whistle during the first part of expiration, finish expiring quickly, and inspire deeply again. In this way, ventilation can increase to meet arterial blood gas needs and whistling can continue with minimal interruption.

BREATHING FOR LIFE PURPOSES

Breathing for life purposes, or tidal breathing, is driven mainly by the need to ventilate (i.e., move air in and out of the pulmonary apparatus). Ventilation serves the life-sustaining process of gas exchange, which consists of the delivery of oxygen to the body and the elimination of carbon dioxide from it. Gas exchange occurs at the alveolar level (so-called external respiration) and at the tissue or cellular level (so-called internal respiration).

Air (consisting of approximately 21% oxygen) is delivered to the alveoli and, from there, oxygen enters the bloodstream and travels to tissues throughout the body. Tissues absorb oxygen from the blood and return carbon dioxide (a byproduct of metabolism) to the blood. The carbon dioxide-rich blood eventually reaches the alveoli where excess carbon dioxide is released and additional oxygen is picked up, and the cycle continues. The rate at which gas exchange occurs depends on the metabolic demand of the body. With higher metabolic demand, more oxygen is required and more carbon dioxide is produced. Metabolic demand increases with exercise, eating, mental activity, and many other variables.

Breathing at rest is associated with a relatively regular inspiration-expiration pattern. Inspiration begins at the resting level of the breathing apparatus. Expansion of the chest wall causes expansion of the lungs and a lowering of alveolar pressure. Air then flows into the breathing apparatus and the lung volume increases. Expiration begins after tidal inspiration ends and results from compression of the lungs and an increase of alveolar pressure. Air then flows out and lung volume decreases to the resting level of the breathing apparatus. These patterns of volume and pressure change are similar across body positions. The only difference is that the resting level of the breathing apparatus changes such that resting tidal breathing encompasses different absolute ranges of lung volumes in different body positions.

Resting tidal breathing is driven by the combination of relaxation pressure and muscular pressure. During inspiration, essentially all of the muscular pressure comes from the diaphragm. This is true for all body positions. Contraction of the diaphragm expands the rib cage wall and displaces the abdominal wall outward. During inspiration in the upright body position, some rib cage wall muscles and abdominal wall muscles are also active (Hixon, Goldman, & Mead, 1973; Loring & Mead, 1982). Rib cage wall muscle activity does not contribute to inspiration as a prime mover, per se, but instead stiffens the rib cage wall (i.e., decreases its compliance) so that it does not get sucked inward when the diaphragm contracts. Thus, the rib cage wall adjusts itself so as to maximize the efficiency of diaphragm function. Likewise, abdominal muscle activity does not contribute to tidal volume change, per se, but serves to maximize the efficiency of diaphragm function. Abdominal muscle activity usually results in inward displacement of the abdominal wall and a concomitant lifting of the rib cage wall. This inward displacement of the abdominal wall moves the diaphragm headward, thereby stretching its fibers so that they are placed on more favorable portions of their length-tension characteristics.

During inspiration in the supine body position, the abdominal wall muscles are relaxed. This is because, in supine, the abdominal wall is already displaced inward and the diaphragm displaced headward by the force of gravity. This gravity-driven inward displacement of the abdominal wall improves the mechanical efficiency of the diaphragm for generating inspiratory pressure, just as abdominal wall muscle activity does for the upright body position.

During resting tidal expiration, the inward movement of the rib cage wall and the abdominal wall is driven by the relaxation pressure of the breathing apparatus. Nevertheless, it is important to recognize that expiration is not entirely passive in the upright body position. This is because the abdominal wall muscles tend to remain active during the entire resting tidal breathing cycle.

Although the general resting tidal breathing pattern is as described above, the details of the pattern can vary from person to person. In fact, the specific resting tidal breathing pattern exhibited by a given person (as characterized by measures such as tidal volume, breathing frequency, inspiratory time, and expiratory time) can be highly individualized. This individualized breathing pattern can be quite stable across days (Shea, Walter, Murphy, & Guz, 1987) and even years (Benchetrit, Shea, Pham Dinh, Bodocco, Baconnier, & Guz, 1989). It can even persist into the deepest stage of sleep (Shea, Horner, Benchetrit, & Guz, 1990). This phenomenon of an individualized and stable breathing pattern is sometimes referred to as the ventilatory personality or respiratory personality (Dejours, 1996; Shea & Guz, 1992). Apparently, each person allows his brainstem to have a say in the expression of his individuality.

REVIEW

The breathing apparatus consists of the pulmonary apparatus and chest wall, the former including the pulmonary airways and lungs and the latter including the rib cage wall, diaphragm, abdominal wall, and abdominal content.

The pulmonary apparatus and chest wall are linked together as a unit through their pleural membranes.

The forces of breathing are passive and active, the former arising from the natural recoil of tissues, surface tension within the lungs, and gravity, and the latter being vested in more than 20 muscles.

The movements of breathing occur throughout the breathing apparatus and result from forces applied to and by different parts of the apparatus.

The adjustment capabilities of the breathing apparatus involve passive and active interplay within and among its different parts and pose a challenge when trying to specify what particular actions are responsible for any given adjustment.

The control variables of the breathing apparatus include lung volume, alveolar pressure, and chest wall shape.

The nervous system controls tidal breathing and special acts of breathing through an array of lower and higher brain centers that mediate movement, perception of movement, and feelings about the need to breathe.

Breathing supports the life-sustaining process of oxygen and carbon dioxide exchange and is characterized by patterns that are relatively individualized and stable at rest, but are influenced in certain ways by body position.

REFERENCES

Agostoni, E., & Mead, J. (1964). Statics of the respiratory system. In W. Fenn & H. Rahn (Eds.), *Handbook of physiology. Respiration 1, Section 3* (pp. 387-409). Washington, DC: American Physiological Society.

Benchetrit, G., Shea, S., Pham Dinh, T., Bodocco, S., Baconnier, P., & Guz, A. (1989). Individuality of breathing patterns in adults assessed over time. *Respiration Physiology, 75*, 199-210.

Comroe, J. (1965). *Physiology of respiration.* Chicago, Ill: Year Book Medical Publishers, Inc.

Corfield, D., Murphy, K., & Guz, A. (1998). Does the motor cortical control of the diaphragm 'bypass' the brain stem respiratory centres in man? *Respiration Physiology, 114*, 109-117.

Dejours, P. (1996). *Respiration.* New York, NY: Oxford University Press.

Dickson, D., & Maue-Dickson, W. (1982). *Anatomical and physiological bases of speech.* Boston, MA: Little, Brown and Company.

Feldman, J., & McCrimmon, D. (1999). Neural control of breathing. In M. Zigmond, F. Bloom, S. Landis, J. Roberts, & L. Squire (Eds.), *Fundamental neuroscience* (pp. 1063-1090). New York, NY: Academic Press.

Gardner, W. (1996). The pathophysiology of hyperventilation disorders. *Chest,*

109, 516-534.

Hixon, T. (1982). Speech breathing kinematics and mechanism inferences therefrom. In S. Grillner, B. Lindblom, & A. Persson (Eds.), *Speech motor control* (pp. 75-93). Oxford, England: Pergamon Press.

Hixon, T., Goldman, M., & Mead, J. (1973). Kinematics of the chest wall during speech production: Volume displacements of the rib cage, abdomen, and lung. *Journal of Speech and Hearing Research, 16*, 78-115.

Konno, K., & Mead, J. (1967). Measurement of the separate volume changes of rib cage and abdomen during breathing. *Journal of Applied Physiology, 22*, 407-422.

Loring, S., & Mead, J. (1982). Abdominal muscle use during quiet breathing and hyperpnea in uninformed subjects. *Journal of Applied Physiology, 52*, 700-704.

Lumb, A. (2000). Control of breathing. In A. Lumb, *Nunn's applied respiratory physiology, 5th Edition* (pp. 82-112). Boston MA: Butterworth Heinemann.

Mador, J., & Tobin, M. (1991). Effect of alterations in mental activity on the breathing pattern in healthy subjects. *American Review of Respiratory Disease, 144*, 481-487.

Munschauer, F., Mador, M., Ahuja, A., & Jacobs, L. (1991). Selective paralysis of voluntary but not limbically influenced automatic respiration. *Archives of Neurology, 48,* 1190-1192.

Pappenheimer, J., Comroe, J., Cournand, A., Ferguson, J., Filley, G., Fowler, W., Gray, J., Helmholz, H., Otis, A., Rahn, H., & Riley, R. (1950). Standardization of definitions and symbols in respiratory physiology. *Federation Proceedings, 9*, 602-615.

Shea, S. (1996). Behavioural and arousal-related influences on breathing in humans. *Experimental Physiology, 81*, 1-26.

Shea, S., & Guz, A. (1992). Personnalite ventiltoire: An overview. *Respiration Physiology, 52*, 275-291.

Shea, S., Horner, R., Benchetrit, G., & Guz, A. (1990). The persistence of a respiratory 'personality' into Stage IV sleep in man. *Respiration Physiology, 80*, 33-44.

Shea, S., Murphy, K., Hamilton, R., Benchetrit, G., & Guz, A. (1988). Do the changes in respiratory pattern and ventilation seen with different behavioural situations reflect metabolic demands? In C. von Euler & M. Katz-Salamon (Eds.), *Respiratory psychophysiology* (pp. 21-28). Basingstoke, United Kingdom: MacMillan Press.

Shea, S., Walter, J., Murphy, K., & Guz, A. (1987). Evidence for individuality of breathing patterns in resting healthy men. *Respiration Physiology, 68*, 331-344.

Shea, S., Walter, J., Pelley, C., Murphy, K., & Guz, A. (1987). The effect of visual and auditory stimuli upon resting ventilation in man. *Respiration Physiology, 68*, 345-357.

Western, P., & Patrick, J. (1988). Effects of focusing attention on breathing with and without apparatus on the face. *Respiration Physiology, 72*, 123-130.

Wyke, B. (1974). Respiratory activity of intrinsic laryngeal muscles: An experimental study. In B. Wyke (Ed.), *Ventilatory and phonatory control systems* (pp. 408-429). New York, NY: Oxford University Press.

chapter three

Normal Speech Breathing

INTRODUCTION

This chapter considers a variety of topics pertinent to normal speech breathing. The topics selected offer a relatively comprehensive coverage of the domain. They also have special bearing on the evaluation and management of speech breathing.

BREATHING FOR SPEECH PURPOSES

Speech breathing is a special act of breathing, one of many that the breathing apparatus performs. There are several forms of speech breathing, two of which are considered here – extended steady utterances and running speech activities. These are chosen because of their importance and because the principles underlying their performance can be extrapolated to other forms of speech breathing. Discussion in this section is limited to the upright body position. Speech breathing in other body positions is considered below in a different section.

Extended Steady Utterances

Extended steady utterances call for slowly changing adjustments of the breathing apparatus. The nature of these adjustments is described here, following the conceptualizations of Hixon (1973).

Volume, Pressure, and Shape Events

Figure 3-1 shows volume, pressure, and shape events for an extended steady utterance produced throughout most of the vital capacity. The utterance is a vowel sustained at normal loudness, pitch, and quality. Data shown are average values. They are also representative of average values for certain other extended utterances, such as repeating a single syllable over and over, counting, and reciting the alphabet.

As shown in the figure, lung volume (in liters, L) decreases at a constant rate during the utterance. Alveolar pressure increases abruptly at the start of the ut-

RAYMOND H. STETSON (1872-1950)

Stetson was a pioneer in the study of speech physiology. One of the tenets of his writing was that speech was a set of movements made audible rather than a set of sounds produced by movements. A great deal of his work was devoted to understanding speech breathing. His investigations were often highly innovative in that he designed much of his own instrumentation and created his own theoretical framework. He posited and tested the notion that each syllable in speech production was accompanied by a so-called "chest pulse" that was controlled principally by muscles of the rib cage wall, with support from muscles of the abdominal wall. Although the details of Stetson's observations were limited by the technology of his era, several of his hypotheses concerning physiological mechanisms have stood the test of time. Stetson once volunteered that he lived for "ideas, to collect ideas." He did that exceptionally well.

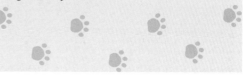

terance, is steady during the utterance, and decreases abruptly at the end of the utterance. Rib cage wall volume and abdominal wall volume decrease at constant and similar rates during the utterance. Together, these latter two reflect the shape of the chest wall.

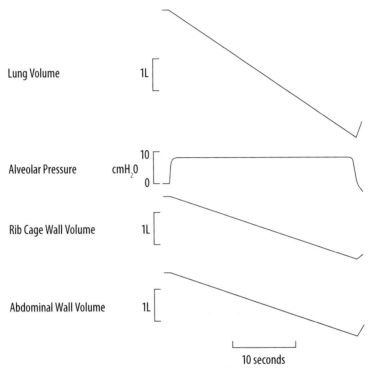

Figure 3-1. Volume, pressure, and shape events for an extended steady utterance produced in the upright body position.

Relaxation Pressure and Muscular Pressure

Both relaxation pressure and muscular pressure contribute to the production of extended steady utterances. Recall that the relaxation pressure represents the passive pressure of breathing, with its magnitude depending on how much air is contained within the pulmonary airways and lungs. This pressure is positive at lung volumes larger than the resting level of the breathing apparatus and negative at lung volumes smaller than that level.

Recall, also, that departures from the relaxation pressure can be achieved at any lung volume through the use of muscular pressure (i.e., muscular effort). Pressure lower than the relaxation pressure results from the exertion of net or solely negative muscular pressure, whereas pressure higher than the relaxation pressure results from the exertion of net or solely positive muscular pressure. Pressure equal to the relaxation pressure results from no muscular pressure (i.e., relaxation) or the exertion of equal negative and positive muscular pressures that cancel one another. Departures from the relaxation pressure reveal the sign and magnitude of the muscular pressure generated by the chest wall.

Figure 3-2 illustrates this for the utterance depicted in Figure 3-1. The alveolar pressure from Figure 3-1 is plotted against lung volume in the upper panel of Figure 3-2 together with the relaxation pressure. The targeted alveolar pressure for the utterance is 8 cmH$_2$O. This pressure is lower than the relaxation pressure throughout the large lung volume range (early in the utterance), equal to the relaxation pressure at one point in the mid volume range (where the two curves intersect), and higher than the relaxation pressure throughout the small lung volume range (late in the utterance). The difference between alveolar pressure and relaxation pressure represents the muscular pressure, the magnitude of which is indicated by the horizontal distance between the utterance tracing and the relaxation pressure curve.

This pressure difference is plotted in the middle panel of Figure 3-2. There, the horizontal axis depicts muscular pressure, with negative values representing inspiratory muscular pressure and positive values representing expiratory muscular pressure. At large lung volumes, negative muscular pressure is added to the relaxation pressure to achieve the targeted alveolar pressure. The magnitude of this negative muscular pressure decreases as utterance proceeds and lung volume decreases. At approximately 60 %VC, the muscular pressure is zero. As lung volume continues to decrease, a positive muscular pressure is required to achieve the targeted alveolar pressure. This positive muscular pressure progressively increases throughout the remainder of the utterance.

For the utterance represented in Figure 3-2, the sign of the muscular pressure generated at large lung volumes is opposite to that of alveolar pressure (i.e., muscular pressure is negative, whereas alveolar pressure is positive). Thus, a negative muscular pressure is being generated during an expiratory activity (extended steady utterance). Such an effort is needed at large lung volumes to counteract the high positive relaxation pressure. The negative muscular pressure generated in opposition to the excessive relaxation pressure represents a braking action.

At intermediate lung volumes (between approximately 60 and 40 %VC), the relaxation pressure is insufficient to meet the requirements of the utterance. Consequently, positive muscular pressure must be used to supplement the relaxation pressure. Within these intermediate lung volumes, the relaxation pressure and muscular pressure are both positive.

For lung volumes smaller than the resting level of the breathing apparatus, positive muscular pressure is required to overcome the negative relaxation pressure and to provide sufficient additional pressure to meet the requirements of the utterance. Positive muscular pressure is high at small lung volumes.

Alveolar pressure demands and muscular pressure demands differ for extended steady utterances of different loudnesses. Utterances that are softer than that illustrated in Figure 3-2 have lower alveolar pressure demands and muscular pressure demands. Thus, more negative muscular pressure is needed to counteract the

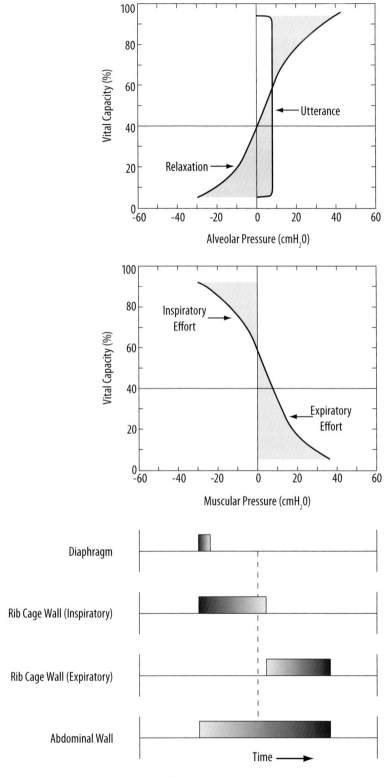

Figure 3-2. Relaxation pressure, targeted alveolar pressure, muscular pressure, and temporal activity of chest wall components for a sustained vowel produced in the upright body position.

relaxation pressure at large lung volumes, and less positive muscular pressure is needed to supplement the relaxation pressure at small lung volumes. By contrast, for louder utterances, less negative muscular pressure is needed to counteract the relaxation pressure at large lung volumes, and more positive muscular pressure is needed to supplement the relaxation pressure at mid and small lung volumes. When the targeted alveolar pressure is sufficiently high, such as for a very loud utterance, positive muscular pressure might be required throughout most or all of the utterance. This is because the relaxation pressure might not exceed the targeted alveolar pressure.

From this discussion, it should be apparent that it is possible to precisely specify the muscular pressure required, given knowledge of the relaxation pressure, the targeted alveolar pressure, and the lung volume at which the utterance is being produced. The important implication is that each alveolar pressure produced during extended steady utterance requires a different muscular pressure at each lung volume.

Actions of the Rib Cage Wall, Diaphragm, and Abdominal Wall

Knowing the sign and magnitude of the muscular pressure used during extended steady utterance, it is relevant to consider how individual parts of the chest wall contribute to the generation of this pressure. Data from a study by Hixon, Mead, and Goldman (1976) have revealed the muscular contributions of these individual parts.

Hixon et al. (1976) studied three male subjects between 36 and 52 years of age. The subjects stood, leaning slightly backward against a tilt table, while changes in rib cage wall volume, abdominal wall volume, and lung volume were estimated using respiratory magnetometers. Pleural, abdominal, and transdiaphragmatic pressures were also estimated from catheter-balloon devices swallowed into the esophagus and stomach and coupled to pressure transducers. Subjects performed maneuvers that allowed determination of the relaxation pressure generated by each part of the chest wall. They then produced sustained vowels and syllable trains at different loudness levels following maximum inspirations. From the data generated, the authors constructed volume-pressure diagrams that allowed them to calculate the contributions of the rib cage wall, diaphragm, and abdominal wall to the generation of alveolar pressure during extended steady utterance production.

For present purposes, data from the volume-pressure diagrams of Hixon et al. (1976) have been distilled into the simple graphic display shown in the lower panel of Figure 3-2. This display represents the temporal activity of four chest wall components that contribute to the generation of the muscular pressure depicted in the middle panel of the figure. These components include the diaphragm (an inspiratory muscle), the inspiratory muscles of the rib cage wall, the expiratory muscles of the rib cage wall, and the abdominal wall (expiratory muscles). The solid bars indicate when each of these four chest wall components is active during the extended steady utterance (the darker the shading within a bar, the greater the magnitude of the muscular pressure). When an inspiratory component is active, the magnitude of its muscular pressure contribution generally decreases with decreases in lung volume (as time progresses). By contrast, when an expiratory component is active, the magnitude of its muscular pressure contribution generally increases with decreases in lung volume (as time progresses).[1] The dashed vertical line in the lower panel of the figure designates the point within the vital capacity at which changeover occurs from the generation of negative muscular pressure to positive muscular pressure by the chest wall.

As shown, the diaphragm, rib cage wall inspiratory component, and abdominal wall are all active at very large lung volumes (i.e., near the start of the utterance). The muscular pressure of the chest wall is negative at very large lung volumes and, as discussed above, represents a braking action that counteracts the excessive positive relaxation pressure. The negative muscular pressure operating at these volumes is a net negative muscular pressure, in which the inspiratory contribution of the diaphragm and rib cage wall exceeds the expiratory contribution of the abdominal wall.

Activity of the diaphragm ceases at a large lung volume (early in the utterance), despite the fact that the relaxation pressure continues to exceed the needed alveolar pressure (i.e., negative muscular pressure continues to prevail). From there, the rib cage wall inspiratory component alone provides the required braking action against the relaxation pressure. The negative muscular pressure operating through the corresponding range of lung volumes remains a net negative muscular pressure, in which the inspiratory contribution of the rib cage wall exceeds the expiratory contribution of the abdominal wall. Activity of the rib cage wall inspiratory component and abdominal wall expiratory component continues throughout the remainder of the range of lung volumes where negative muscular pressure is applied. Inspiratory activity of the rib cage wall continues briefly through a range of lung volumes that involves the application of net positive muscular pressure (corresponding to the portion of the rib cage wall inspiratory activity plot that extends to the right of the dashed vertical line in Figure 3-2).

Note that the zero muscular pressure point in Figure 3-2 (between the negative and positive muscular pressure segments) is a net zero muscular pressure, in which the rib cage wall inspiratory component and abdominal wall expiratory component are equal and opposite and cancel each other. Thus, zero muscular pressure in this

---

[1]The data of Hixon et al. (1976) elucidate how the rib cage wall, diaphragm, and abdominal wall contribute to the generation of muscular pressure during utterance. However, they do not specify how individual muscles contribute to the overall muscular pressure. Such data as are available on individual muscle contributions have come from the use of electromyography, a technique that involves the sensing of electrical activity of muscles through the use of metal electrodes placed over them or inserted directly into them. Unfortunately, the available data are piecemeal and there are many vagaries in trying to form a composite from them. Despite these problems, there is instructive merit in the exercise of trying to construct a composite. The reader interested in such an exercise should find the tutorial provided by Hixon and Weismer (1995) to be a useful starting point.

case does not reflect relaxation of the chest wall muscles.

At the instant the rib cage wall inspiratory component ceases its activity, the rib cage wall expiratory component becomes active. Thereafter, the activities of the rib cage wall expiratory component and abdominal wall expiratory component continue throughout the smaller lung volume range.

Figure 3-2 makes it clear that the breathing apparatus is under continuous active control throughout extended steady utterance. At no time is the apparatus controlled by relaxation pressure alone. Relaxation pressure and muscular pressure are always used in combination.

Each alveolar pressure produced during an extended steady utterance demands a different muscular pressure at each lung volume. Thus, it would be expected that the activity of the four components of the chest wall would also be different for each alveolar pressure produced. This is, indeed, the case. Utterances with higher alveolar pressure demands require less braking by the inspiratory components of the chest wall and earlier and greater activity by the expiratory components of the chest wall than those with lower alveolar pressure demands.

Certain observations made by Hixon et al. (1976) may seem counterintuitive. One such observation is that activity of the diaphragm is dissociated from activity of the rib cage wall inspiratory muscles during utterance production at large lung volumes. Why is the diaphragm not used for inspiratory braking rather than the rib cage wall inspiratory muscles? The answer has to do with the hydraulic properties of the abdominal content in the upright body position.

Inspiratory muscular pressure generation by the rib cage wall causes the rib cage to expand relative to the size it assumes during relaxation at the prevailing lung volume. This expansion causes pleural pressure to decrease. This decrease in pleural pressure acts as an upward-lifting force on the diaphragm and serves to increase support of the abdominal content from above. It also pulls the abdominal wall inward. As pleural pressure decreases, abdominal pressure also decreases. This causes the liquid-filled abdominal content to place a hydraulic pull on the undersurface of the diaphragm. This hydraulic pull by the abdominal content provides a relatively stable mechanism for the inspiratory muscles of the rib cage wall to pull against, and supplants the need for the diaphragm to contract to stay in position. Without this hydraulic mechanism, the inspiratory muscles of the rib cage wall would spend part of their effort pulling the thorax upward along the vertebral column (i.e., moving the breathing apparatus from one place to another, rather than enlarging it).

Another observation of Hixon et al. (1976) that may seem counterintuitive is the simultaneous inspiratory activity of the rib cage wall and expiratory activity of the abdominal wall during negative muscular pressure generation by the chest wall. Why use both inspiratory and expiratory muscles simultaneously during utterance production at large lung volumes when the goal is to provide a braking action? The answer may be that simultaneous inspiratory and expiratory muscle activation enables more economical and precise control of the chest wall than is possible through the use of inspiratory rib cage wall muscles alone.

With the diaphragm inactive, both the rib cage wall and abdominal wall are subjected to identical changes in transmural pressure (i.e., the pressure across each wall). Thus, movement in each part of the chest wall (i.e., rib cage wall and abdominal wall) depends on the prevailing impedance of that part. The inefficiencies that would result from not using simultaneous activity in the two parts can be appreciated by performing some simple maneuvers on a long inflated balloon (representing the breathing apparatus) containing a squeaker in its neck (representing the larynx). If the half of the balloon nearest the squeaker (representing the rib cage wall) is squeezed (to simulate a decreasing rib cage wall volume achieved by a decreasing rib cage wall inspiratory effort), pressure inside the balloon (representing alveolar pressure) will increase and cause the other half of the balloon (representing the abdominal wall) to move outward. However, if both halves of the balloon are squeezed simultaneously (representing decreases in rib cage wall volume and abdominal wall volume), less extensive and slower movement is required of the half representing the rib cage wall to achieve an equivalent pressure adjustment. This also means that an unproductive outward (paradoxical) movement of the half of the balloon representing the abdominal wall is avoided. When both halves of the balloon are moved inward simultaneously, it is possible to have greater precision of control over the pressure inside the balloon.

A final observation of Hixon et al. (1976) that may seem counterintuitive is the occasional reactivation of the diaphragm at very small lung volumes (reported but not shown in Figure 3-2) in the face of very large positive muscular pressures. Why reactivate the diaphragm, an inspiratory muscle, at such moments? It may be that such a strategy reflects an attempt to gain more finely graded control. That is, given that the abdominal drive is substantial at small lung volumes and the muscles of the abdominal wall are significantly shortened, more precise control may be possible by opposing this drive with the diaphragm. The diaphragm, being highly domed at very small lung volumes, is in an excellent mechanical position to "meter out" the abdominal wall drive.

Running Speech Activities

Running speech activities (reading aloud, extemporaneous speaking, and conversational speaking) present a very different set of demands for the breathing apparatus than those just described for extended steady utterances. Discussion in this section considers running speech activities generated in the upright body position.

Volume, Pressure, and Shape Events

The volume, pressure, and shape events associated with running speech activities usually involve more variation than do those associated with the sustained vowel utterance discussed above. The nature of such variation depends on many factors, including the phonetic content of the speech produced (e.g., specific sounds and their serial ordering), prosodic features of the utterances produced (e.g., speaking rate, loudness, intonation, and linguistic stress), and voice quality.

Running speech of normal loudness is most often produced within the midrange of the vital capacity. Such speech generally starts from about twice tidal depth and continues to near the resting tidal end-expiratory level, although some breath groups may encroach upon the expiratory reserve volume. Speaking within this midrange has the advantage of avoiding the lung volume extremes where the breathing apparatus is stiffer and mechanically more costly to control. Also, by speaking at lung volumes that are larger than the resting tidal end-expiratory level, positive relaxation pressure can be used to help drive the larynx and upper airway. When speech is produced at lung volumes that are smaller than the resting level, muscular pressure must be exerted against a negative relaxation pressure.

Alveolar pressure is usually relatively steady during running speech activities, although it may show slight increases during linguistic stress production. At times, alveolar pressure will decrease toward the ends of breath groups. This roll-off of pressure is typically observed at the ends of declarative sentences where loudness and pitch tend to drop.

Rib cage wall volume and abdominal wall volume decrease at relatively constant rates during running speech activities, although the decrease for the rib cage wall is usually faster than that for the abdominal wall. This means that the relative volume contribution of the rib cage wall to lung volume change exceeds that of the abdominal wall.

Running speech activities are usually generated using a chest wall shape that departs from the relaxed shape of the chest wall. Specifically, the rib cage wall is larger and the abdominal wall is smaller than they are when the muscles of the breathing apparatus are relaxed at corresponding lung volumes.

Running speech breathing also may involve a set-up of the chest wall at the beginning of breath groups. This set-up most often occurs during the transition between the end of the inspiratory phase and the beginning of the expiratory phase of speech breathing, and may also carry into the start of speech. The

HEADING OFF SPEECH

The guillotine was once the method of choice for the beheading of condemned prisoners in France. Its sloping blade fell in 1/70th of a second and did its grisly travel through its victim in 1/200th of a second (mercifully brief). Literature from the time of the French Revolution, when the guillotine was used often and publicly, contains mention of prisoner heads talking after being severed from the body. Are these to be believed? Well, it's possible that movements of the speech articulators could have persisted for short durations and that speech could actually have been mouthed. But the usual voice and air sources for speech would not have been available. Once the head and neck were disconnected from the breathing apparatus, any motive force for speech would have been gone (save buccal speech as a remote possibility). All in all, it's a gruesome topic. We address it only because our students sometimes express a morbid curiosity to know.

most common set-up is characterized by inward movement of the abdominal wall and outward movement of the rib cage wall.

Relaxation Pressure and Muscular Pressure

Both relaxation pressure and muscular pressure contribute to the control of running speech breathing. These pressures can be related to one another using the volume-pressure diagram in the same way discussed above for extended steady utterances. When this is done, it is found that the targeted alveolar pressure for running speech activities of normal loudness is higher than the relaxation pressure at all lung volumes through which normal running speech is typically produced. Thus, a positive muscular pressure must be added to the relaxation pressure to achieve the targeted alveolar pressure at each lung volume. The magnitude of this muscular pressure increases as the breath group progresses and lung volume decreases.

Because the sign of muscular pressure for running speech production of normal loudness is continuously positive, no braking is required. The only time braking occurs during running speech production of normal loudness is when the speaker takes a deeper-than-usual breath before initiating speech. Then, a small negative muscular pressure (of decreasing magnitude) may be generated briefly. This changes quickly to a zero muscular pressure and, thereafter, to a positive muscular pressure.

Alveolar pressure demands and muscular pressure demands vary with loudness. For softer speech, lower-than-normal positive muscular pressures are needed to supplement the relaxation pressure within the midrange of the vital capacity (i.e., 60 to 40 %VC). When the alveolar pressure is sufficiently low, such as for very soft speech, a brief period of negative muscular pressure generation might be required. This occurs if the relaxation pressure exceeds the targeted alveolar pressure during the early part of the breath group. By contrast, for louder speech, higher-than-normal positive muscular pressures are needed to supplement the relaxation pressure within the midrange of the vital capacity. This is because the relaxation pressure is less than the targeted alveolar pressure in this lung volume range. Although contrasts made here have used a single range of lung volumes for instructive purposes, loud running speech is often produced at larger lung volumes than is running speech of normal loudness.

Actions of the Rib Cage Wall, Diaphragm, and Abdominal Wall

The muscular pressure generated during running speech production reflects contributions from different parts of the chest wall. These contributions can be determined from the data of Hixon, Mead, and Goldman (1976).

Only the rib cage wall expiratory component and the abdominal wall component are active during most running speech of normal loudness. Both components increase their muscular pressure contribution as speech proceeds, with the positive muscular pressure provided by the abdominal wall substantially exceeding that provided by the rib cage wall at all lung volumes. Only when running speech of normal loudness is initiated from an uncharacteristically large lung volume might inspiratory braking by the rib cage wall occur.

For running speech activities that are softer-than-normal, the magnitude of the muscular pressure provided by the same two components is lower-than-normal. If the utterance is sufficiently soft, some inspiratory braking by the rib cage wall may occur briefly. By contrast, for running speech activities that are louder-than-normal, the rib cage wall expiratory component and the abdominal wall component increase the magnitude of their muscular pressure contributions, the abdominal wall even more than the rib cage wall.

Although the patterns of running speech breathing described thus far are typical, the fact of the matter is that an almost infinite number of muscular strategies can be used to produce running speech. Given the wide range of options available, why choose the option of producing running speech using an expiratory muscular pressure generated by the rib cage wall and an even greater expiratory muscular pressure generated by the abdominal wall? What is to be gained by using a muscular pressure strategy that displaces the abdominal wall inward and elevates the rib cage wall? The answers to these two questions relate to the mechanical efficiencies achieved when using this strategy.

When compared to resting tidal breathing, running speech breathing is characterized by very rapid inspirations and prolonged expirations. This quick inspiration-slow expiration pattern allows the speaker to communicate as much information as possible in as short a time as possible with as little interruption as possible. The preferred muscular strategy observed in normal speech breathing helps to maximize inspiratory speed and enhance expiratory pressure control for this purpose.

Hixon et al. (1976) have shown that inspirations during running speech breathing are driven by activity of the diaphragm alone. Because the diaphragm and abdominal wall cover opposite surfaces of the abdominal content, abdominal muscular pressure has a direct effect on the diaphragm. When the abdominal wall is displaced inward, the diaphragm is displaced headward such that its principal fibers elongate and its radius of curvature increases. The significance of this abdominal-wall-imposed adjustment is that the diaphragm becomes mechanically tuned for producing rapid and forceful inspiratory efforts. Rapid and forceful inspirations are just what are needed to minimize interruptions to the continual flow of running speech production. Thus, what may at first appear to be a costly abdominal wall effort is actually an investment to meet the important inspiratory demands of running speech breathing.

It may seem puzzling that the rib cage wall does not assist the diaphragm during running speech inspirations. Perhaps even more puzzling is the fact that the rib cage wall usually generates a small positive muscular pressure during running speech inspirations. The solution to these apparent puzzles appears to relate to economy of behavior. That is, by maintaining activation of the expiratory muscles (in both the rib cage wall and abdominal wall) during inspiration, they are in a state of readiness for generating expiratory pressure for speech production once the forceful activity of the diaphragm subsides. Because the expiratory muscles are already activated, there is no time lost in activating them after inspiration.

The abdominal wall also tunes the rib cage wall for expiration. When the abdominal wall is displaced inward, the rib cage wall is elevated passively and its expiratory muscle fibers are elongated and placed on more favorable portions of their length-tension characteristics. Furthermore, because abdominal wall muscular pressure exceeds rib cage wall muscular pressure, expiratory activation of the rib cage wall cannot force the abdominal wall outward. If the abdominal wall were to move outward (paradoxically), any gain in rib cage wall efficiency would be lost. Thus, the abdominal wall helps to optimize the function of the rib cage wall for running speech production by elevating it and providing a firm base against which it can operate. It is the abdominal wall that makes it possible for the small and fast-acting muscles of the rib cage wall to effect quick changes in alveolar pressure when needed (such as for stressing). The rib cage wall is especially well-suited to producing quick pressure changes because it contacts a larger portion of the lung than does the abdominal wall.

In summary, the preferred muscular strategy for running speech breathing increases the efficiency of chest wall function. By forcefully and continuously activating the abdominal wall, the shape of the chest wall is mechanically tuned to favor inspiratory function of the diaphragm and expiratory function of the rib cage wall. This strategy maximizes the mechanical advantages of those parts of the chest wall most responsible for forceful and rapid inspirations and for quick expiratory adjustments.

ADAPTIVE CONTROL OF SPEECH BREATHING

Speech breathing is not always carried out in the ways described in the preceding section. Rather, everyday events require that it take place under a variety of circumstances. This means that speech breathing must adapt to changes, some predictable and some not. Wolff (1979) illustrated the concept of adaptive control with the example of a violinist who breaks a string during performance. The violinist can choose to stop playing and replace the broken string. Or he can choose to continue playing with the remaining intact strings of the violin. If he continues to play, he must reprogram his usual fingering and play the notes in a different manner on the instrument. This is adaptation par excellence. Such adaptation capitalizes on the "motor idea" controlling the performance.

Adaptive control can be accomplished without conscious awareness, or it can be willfully achieved. When applied to speech breathing, adaptive control involves a change in one pattern of speech breathing to another pattern that enables the speaker to meet the ventilatory and mechanical goals of the situation. Ventilatory circumstances may change with changes in elevation, when in a smoke-filled room, with extremes in temperature, at different levels of exercise, and with different levels of anxiety. Mechanical circumstances may change when wearing a tight belt or bra, with a significant change in body weight, when in the bear hug of a wrestling opponent, when trying to look slim in a bathing suit, and when riding in an express elevator. Adaptive control capitalizes on the degrees of freedom of performance (different ways to accomplish the same goal) to accommodate to changes in ventilatory and/or mechanical circumstances.

Subsequent sections of this chapter single out special adaptive control issues, including those having to do with changes in body position, gravity, load factor, torso immersion in water, and drive-to-breathe. These are of special relevance to the present book, either for understanding normal function or for dealing with clinical concerns. Considered here is evidence for the general pervasiveness of adaptive control of speech breathing.

Adaptive control of the chest wall during the production of sustained vowels was demonstrated in a study by Bouhuys, Proctor, and Mead (1966). Recall from the previous section that, in the upright body position, the inspiratory muscles of the rib cage wall serve in a braking capacity when the relaxation pressure exceeds the alveolar pressure needed for utterance. Bouhuys et al. reasoned that this particular mechanism might be limited by the strength of the inspiratory muscles of the rib cage wall or by the maximum hydraulic pull of the abdominal content, whichever was less forceful, and that this might have implications for the role of the diaphragm. To test this hypothesis they applied subatmospheric (negative) pressure to the airway opening while a subject sustained a soft vowel through a range of large lung volumes. This application of subatmospheric pressure is the functional equivalent of increasing the prevailing (positive) relaxation pressure. Diaphragm activity was determined from recordings of transdiaphragmatic pressure measured with balloons placed in the esophagus and stomach. Lung volume change was measured using a volume-displacement body plethysmograph.

Bouhuys et al. (1966) found that when the pressure at the airway opening was lowered to -15 cmH_2O (and the prevailing relaxation pressure, thereby, functionally increased by 15 cmH_2O) the diaphragm came into play as a supplemental braking mechanism. And when pressure was lowered to -25 cmH_2O, the diaphragm increased its braking activity in proportion to the change in pressure. Thus, although the diaphragm did not usually contribute much of the braking action, it became a significant control element when the mechanical circumstances changed. Adaptive control was invoked to accomplish the intended goal.

Another experimental example of continuously changing adaptive control of the chest wall during sustained vowel production was offered by Hixon, Goldman, and Mead (1973). They had two subjects (wearing respiratory magnetometers) generate vowels of constant loudness throughout most of the vital capacity while alternately displacing volume back and forth between the rib cage wall and abdominal wall. Hixon et al. found that paradoxical movement of the rib cage wall or abdominal wall occurred nearly continuously. This meant that one part of the chest wall was reducing in size faster than the other part was increasing in size, the implication being that the volume displaced by one of the parts actually exceeded the volume displaced by the lungs. These observations indicated that the interactive performance of the rib cage wall and abdominal wall could be changed dramatically, at will, and with ease, while maintaining a constant alveolar pressure. This work demonstrated not only willful adaptation in control of the chest wall, but also the independence of shape control and pressure control during utterance.

Adaptive control of speech breathing was also demonstrated by Warren, Morr, Rochet, and Dalston (1989). These investigators were interested in determining whether or not the breathing apparatus would attempt to compensate for the loss of air through the nose when the velopharynx was opened. Eight subjects were asked to generate consonant-vowel syllable strings, once as they usually would and once as they "talked through the nose." Warren et al. used a pressure-flow technique to measure oral pressure, calculate velopharyngeal orifice resistance, and estimate velopharyngeal orifice area during the two sets of productions. They also used a respiratory inductance plethysmograph to estimate lung volume change.

Warren et al. (1989) found that when the velopharynx was opened, the volume displaced by the breathing apparatus increased so as to maintain adequate levels of oral pressure to achieve suitable consonant productions. The authors interpreted this as evidence of increased "respiratory effort" (although they did not specifically define this term) and viewed their findings as indicating that the breathing apparatus was under adaptive control and responding to changes in the load being "seen." In this case, the adaptive response was to events occurring downstream of the breathing apparatus. Adaptation, then, is not confined to adjustments among different parts of the chest wall (rib cage wall, diaphragm, and abdominal wall), but can also occur between the breathing apparatus and other downstream components of the speech production apparatus.

DONALD W. WARREN

Warren has been a world leader over the past four decades in the study of speech production aeromechanics. He was cross-trained in dental surgery and physiology and brought a rich interdisciplinary mix to his work. Warren did postdoctoral study with Arthur B. DuBois, one of the world's leading respiratory physiologists. Working with DuBois, Warren pioneered a very clever method for using aeromechanical data to calculate velopharyngeal orifice area in normal speakers. He later expanded the application of this method to a series of studies of individuals with orofacial disorders, particularly cleft palate. Later in his professional career, Warren worked on the development and testing of a novel framework that posited the production of speech as a pressure-regulated performance activity. He is retired and lives in North Carolina where his skill as an expert horseman brings him applause and great joy.

Another example of adaptive control of speech breathing was provided by Hixon and Weismer (1995), who studied the effect of arm folding on speech breathing in three subjects. Each of their subjects read a paragraph, once with his arms at his sides and once with his arms folded across the front of his rib cage wall, while being monitored with respiratory magnetometers. Arm folding caused subjects to use smaller rib cage wall volumes and larger abdominal wall volumes. In most cases, the rib cage wall contribution to expiration increased and the abdominal wall contribution ceased, and, in some cases, the abdominal wall paradoxed (i.e., moved outward during speech production).

Hixon and Weismer (1995) interpreted their findings to indicate a "mechanical surrender" by the abdominal wall to the imposed rib cage wall load. That is, the abdominal wall no longer attempted to lift the rib cage wall as it usually did during running speech production due to the additional weight and restriction imposed by the arms. The authors also suggested that the arms might have been used as surrogate expiratory muscles to squeeze the rib cage wall. That is, the load imposed by the arms may have been neither passive nor constant, but may have been actively adjusted by the subject. The point to be emphasized is that these findings, as with those of Bouhuys et al. (1966), demonstrate adaptive control across different parts of the breathing apparatus when the apparatus is faced with significant changes in mechanical conditions.

BODY POSITION AND SPEECH BREATHING

Speech breathing changes with body position, primarily because of the influence of gravity. Each time the body is reoriented within a gravity field, speech breathing requires an alternate mechanical solution to achieve the desired performance.

In the upright body position, gravity acts in the expiratory direction on the rib cage wall and in the inspiratory direction on the abdominal content and abdominal wall. That is, gravity tends to decrease the size of the rib cage wall and increase the size of the abdominal wall. The gravitational effect is greater on the abdominal wall than on the rib cage wall. Also, the gravitational effect is greater at small lung volumes than at large lung volumes because the height of the abdomen is greater and its wall less stiff. Recall that, in the upright body position, the abdominal content is supported against gravity by the abdominal wall and by the upward-lifting force of negative pleural pressure.

When a shift is made to the supine body position, the gravitational effect becomes expiratory on both the rib cage wall and abdominal wall. This means that the relaxation pressure of the breathing apparatus is greater at any given lung volume in the supine body position than in the upright body position. There is less gravitational effect with changes in lung volume compared to the upright body position because the height of the abdomen is reduced. Importantly, pleural pressure does not have a major role in supporting the abdominal content in the supine body position. Gravity acts on the relaxed abdominal wall and forces the diaphragm headward into the rib cage. The diaphragm moves headward until its own recoil force balances the distending force acting on it. Headward displacement of the diaphragm causes the resting level of the breathing apparatus to shift from its upright value of about 40 %VC to a supine value of about 20 %VC.

Extended Steady Utterances in the Supine Body Position

Figure 3-3 represents a sustained vowel of normal loudness produced throughout most of the vital capacity in the supine body position. The upper panel in the figure depicts the relaxation pressure and the targeted alveolar pressure. Comparison with the analogous panel in Figure 3-2 (for the upright body position) reveals that the relaxation pressure is higher (i.e., the relaxation characteristic in Figure 3-3 is positioned to the right of that in Figure 3-2) and that the resting level of the breathing apparatus (i.e., the lung volume at which the relaxation characteristic intersects zero alveolar pressure) is smaller for the supine body position than for the upright body position. As shown in the middle panel of Figure 3-3, the muscular pressure required to produce the targeted alveolar pressure (8 cmH_2O) changes throughout the utterance. A higher negative muscular pressure (i.e., a more substantial inspiratory muscular effort) is required throughout the large lung volume range for the supine body position than for the upright body position (compare the middle panels in Figures 3-2 and 3-3). Also, this negative muscular pressure must continue to a smaller lung volume in the supine body position than in the upright body position (compare where muscular pressure is zero in the middle panels of Figures 3-2 and 3-3). Further, at small lung volumes, a lower positive muscular pressure is needed in the supine body position than in the upright body position to produce the targeted alveolar pressure (again, compare the middle panels of Figures 3-2 and 3-3).

The muscular pressure needed to produce most targeted alveolar pressures for extended steady utterances undergoes change from negative to zero to positive in both the upright and supine body positions. Thus, at first consideration, it may seem that an identically targeted alveolar pressure could be achieved in the two body positions by using the same muscular strategy, but just adding a different magnitude of muscular pressure at each lung volume in the two positions. However, it is not that simple. The breathing apparatus is operating under very different mechanical conditions in the two body positions. Of principal importance is the fact that gravity's influence on the abdominal content is quite different in the supine body position than in the upright body position and this affects how the components of the chest wall function.

Actions of the Rib Cage Wall, Diaphragm, and Abdominal Wall

The rib cage wall (expiratory component), diaphragm, and abdominal wall

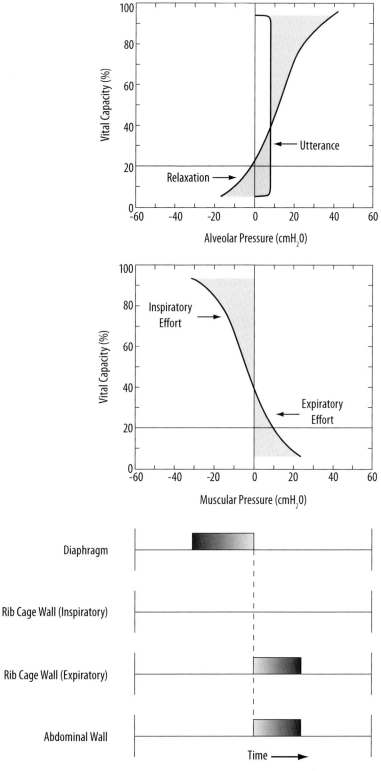

Figure 3-3. Relaxation pressure, targeted alveolar pressure, muscular pressure, and temporal activity of chest wall components for a sustained vowel produced in the supine body position.

contribute to the muscular pressure exerted during extended steady utterance production in the supine body position. The temporal activity of these chest wall components is depicted in the lower panel of Figure 3-3. This depiction is based on the volume-pressure data of Hixon, Mead, and Goldman (1976) and follows the format used in Figure 3-2 for the upright body position.

As shown, only the diaphragm is active at the start of the utterance. It continues to be active throughout the range of lung volumes where muscular pressure is negative. No other component of the chest wall is active within this range of lung volumes. Thus, control of the chest wall is vested entirely in the diaphragm during the initial part of the utterance. This activity of the diaphragm constitutes the braking action needed to counteract the excessive relaxation pressure generated at large lung volumes to meet the alveolar pressure demand of the utterance. The diaphragm provides a graded and progressively decreasing force in this context (the lighter the shading within the bar, the lesser the magnitude of the muscular pressure). At the instant the diaphragm ceases activity, the rib cage wall and abdominal wall initiate expiratory activities. These two components continue their activities throughout the small lung volume range until the utterance terminates.

Each alveolar pressure produced during extended steady utterance demands a different muscular pressure at each lung volume. Also, the activity of different chest wall components differs for different alveolar pressures at different lung volumes. That is, utterances produced with higher alveolar pressures require less braking on the part of the diaphragm than utterances requiring lower alveolar pressures. And utterances produced with higher alveolar pressures exhibit earlier and greater activity of the expiratory components of the chest wall.

In the supine body position, gravity has an expiratory influence on both the rib cage wall and abdominal wall, but the major influence is on the abdominal wall. The abdominal wall is displaced inward and the abdominal content and diaphragm are displaced headward. Abdominal relaxation pressure is high in the supine body position compared to the upright body position due to the effect of gravity on the abdominal content. In the absence of a significant hydraulic pull on the undersurface of the diaphragm, the inspiratory muscles of the rib cage wall cannot contribute much to a lowering of alveolar pressure (without simultaneous activation of the diaphragm). Braking with the diaphragm is the only efficient strategy for counteracting relaxation pressure at large lung volumes in the supine body position because the major component of relaxation pressure in this position comes from the diaphragm-abdomen portion of the chest wall. Thus, an inspiratory control problem is solved by the diaphragm in the supine body position and by the inspiratory rib cage wall muscles in the upright body position. In each case, the inspiratory braking strategy involves the pathway in which the primary gravitational influence on the chest wall is either solely expiratory or more forcefully expiratory than on the remaining pathway.

As with the upright body position, the diaphragm occasionally reactivates at very small lung volumes in the face of very large positive muscular pressures. This reactivation may be a strategy for gaining more finely graded control at a time when the abdominal wall drive is substantial and the muscles of the abdominal wall are significantly shortened.

Running Speech Activities in the Supine Body Position

Recall that running speech activities (reading aloud, extemporaneous speaking, and conversational speaking) in the upright body position present very different demands for the breathing apparatus than those for the production of extended steady utterances. The same is true for the supine body position, as described in this section.

Volume, Pressure, and Shape Events

Running speech of normal loudness in the supine body position, like that for the upright body position, starts from about twice resting tidal depth and continues to near the resting tidal end-expiratory level, with occasional breath groups encroaching upon the expiratory reserve volume. However, volume events in the supine body position occur between about 40 and 20 %VC, rather than between the 60 and 40 %VC associated with the upright body position. This is because the resting level of the breathing apparatus has changed with the shift in body position.

Alveolar pressure events for running speech activities are the same for the supine body position as the upright body position. By contrast, rib cage wall volume and abdominal wall volume events are distinctly different in the two positions. Both of these volumes decrease at relatively constant and similar rates during running speech production, indicating that the two chest wall parts contribute relatively equally to lung volume change. This is unlike the upright body position in which rib cage wall displacement almost always predominates during running speech production.

Running speech activities in the supine body position are generated with a chest wall shape that is quite different from that for the upright body position. Whereas speech in the upright body position is produced with the abdominal wall tucked in and the rib cage wall elevated, the opposite is true for speech produced in the supine body position. That is, the abdominal wall is pushed outward and the rib cage wall is depressed compared to their respective relaxed positions.

Running speech produced in the supine body position may involve a set-up of the chest wall during the transition between the end of the inspiratory phase and the beginning of the expiratory phase of speech breathing, and may also carry into the beginning of utterance. This set-up is most often associated with inward movement of the rib cage wall and outward movement of the abdominal wall. The active posturing element in this case is the rib cage wall, which pushes the abdominal wall outward passively against the force of gravity.

Relaxation Pressure and Muscular Pressure

Both relaxation pressure and muscular pressure contribute to the control of running speech production in the supine body position. Because the targeted alveolar pressure is higher than the relaxation pressure through the range of lung volumes used, a positive muscular pressure must be added to the relaxation pressure to achieve the targeted alveolar pressure at each lung volume. The magnitude of this muscular pressure increases as the breath group proceeds and lung volume decreases.

Running speech produced in the supine body position does not involve braking. Exceptions may occur when the speaker takes a deeper-than-usual breath. When this happens, a small negative muscular pressure (of decreasing magnitude) may need to be generated briefly at the start of the breath group.

Alveolar pressure demands and muscular pressure demands differ for different loudnesses. Softer speech activities require lower alveolar pressures and lower positive muscular pressures at each lung volume, whereas louder speech activities require higher alveolar pressures and higher positive muscular pressures at each lung volume. Also, louder speech activities tend to be generated at somewhat larger lung volumes than activities of normal loudness.

Actions of the Rib Cage Wall, Diaphragm, and Abdominal Wall

Data from the study by Hixon, Mead, and Goldman (1976) indicate that only the rib cage wall expiratory component is active during running speech of normal loudness in the supine body position. This component increases its muscular pressure contribution as speech proceeds.

A different muscular strategy is used for loud running speech. Specifically, loud running speech is produced with activation of both the expiratory rib cage wall component and the abdominal wall component. Recruitment of the abdominal wall in this context prevents paradoxical outward movement of the abdominal wall in the face of a heightened rib cage wall drive. It also preserves the mechanical advantage of the diaphragm for the inspiratory phase of the speech breathing cycle.

Running speech in the supine body position can be produced using a wide variety of muscular pressure combinations and a wide variety of chest wall shapes. Why, then, does the preferred muscular strategy for most running speech in the supine body position include the use of the rib cage wall expiratory component alone? What is special about this muscular pressure strategy and the way it deforms the chest wall?

The answers appear to relate to mechanical efficiencies associated with both the inspiratory and expiratory phases of the speech breathing cycle. Inspirations during running speech breathing in the supine body position, like those in the upright body position, are driven by activity of the diaphragm alone. Recall that, in the upright body position, the abdominal wall is forcefully active and mechanically tunes the diaphragm to maximize its efficiency. By contrast, in the supine body position, gravity drives the abdominal content and diaphragm headward, tuning the diaphragm and supplanting the need for the abdominal wall to be active. Therefore, gravity takes over the role that the abdominal wall muscles perform in the upright body position. While the diaphragm contracts, the rib cage wall maintains a slight expiratory tone. Because the expiratory rib cage wall muscles are already activated, there is no time lost in reactivating them once the expiratory phase begins.

Speech Breathing in Body Positions Other Than Upright and Supine

Focus to this juncture has been on speech breathing in the upright and supine body positions. These are the two most important positions for clinical concerns and the two positions to which most investigative attention has been devoted. Nevertheless, because clients may present in other body positions, it may be necessary to extrapolate mechanism to other body positions. This section suggests some principles to follow when confronted with the need to extrapolate.

One principle to keep in mind is that, as body position changes, the resting level of the breathing apparatus shifts within the vital capacity (recall the 20 %VC shift between the upright and supine body positions discussed above). This principle is illustrated in Figure 3-4 where the resting level of the breathing apparatus is shown for different body positions for a single individual (the first author at 29 years of age). Much of the change in resting level can be attributed to axial displacement of the diaphragm brought about by the influence of gravity on the abdominal content. As the diaphragm is displaced headward, air moves out of the pulmonary apparatus and the resting level of the breathing apparatus shifts to a smaller lung volume. By contrast, as the diaphragm is displaced footward, air is drawn into the pulmonary apparatus and the resting level shifts to a larger volume.

As can be seen in Figure 3-4, movement from an erect standing position to a predominately head-down position causes a significant reduction in the resting level of the breathing apparatus. This is because the diaphragm is displaced progressively more headward. A good rule of thumb is that the resting level will shift in relation to the sine of the angle of tilt of the torso. The prone body position (lying face down) and the side-lying body position (lying face parallel to the wall) do not conform perfectly to this rule because they involve special mechanical circumstances. In the prone body position, the chest wall is mechanically coupled to the surface on which the individual is lying. And, in the side-lying body position, the position of the abdominal content depends on the level of activation of the abdominal wall muscles.

The vertical lines in Figure 3-4 show that the lung volume range through which running speech production occurs is highly dependent on the shift in the resting level of the breathing apparatus. As the resting level changes, so does the range of lung volume events. This is because the lung volume events of running speech production follow the equilibrium level of the breathing apparatus to take advantage of the mechanical efficiencies associated with speaking near that level.

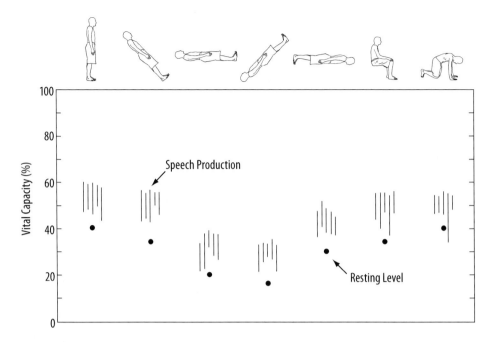

Figure 3-4. Breath groups during running speech production in different body positions. (After Hixon, Goldman, & Mead, 1973)

A second principle to keep in mind when attempting to extrapolate across body positions is that muscular pressure requirements change with changes in relaxation pressure, all else being constant. As the body is tilted from the upright body position toward the supine body position, the relaxation pressure increases at a given lung volume. Thus, the muscular pressure required for utterance production at a given lung volume decreases as the body is tilted toward supine.

A third principle to keep in mind when trying to extrapolate to body positions other than upright and supine is that different chest wall parts assume different roles in supplying muscular pressure as position changes. For example, when inspiratory braking is called for during speech production at large lung volumes, it is likely to be effected by the rib cage wall inspiratory muscles when the body is oriented more toward upright, and by the diaphragm when the body is oriented more toward downright. This shift in responsibility between the rib cage wall and the diaphragm usually occurs at about 45° off-vertical toward supine. For another example, the abdominal wall muscles play an increasingly more prominent role in supporting and posturing the breathing apparatus as body position is shifted toward more upright body positions.

A fourth principle that may aid in extrapolating across different body positions is that the rib cage wall expiratory muscles almost always participate in running speech production, regardless of body position. The rib cage wall has the mechanical advantage of contacting a much larger area of the lungs than does the diaphragm-abdominal wall. This, along with its small and fast-acting muscles, gives the rib cage wall a preeminent role in the generation of muscular pressure for speech production under almost all circumstances.

SPEECH BREATHING UNDER DIFFERENT EXTERNAL FORCES

Speech breathing can occur under special circumstances in which external forces operating on the breathing apparatus are different than those encountered in most everyday events. Three special circumstances relate to gravity, load factor, and torso immersion in water. This section considers the influence of these three on speech breathing as a way of illustrating the importance of different external forces in general.

Gravity

Gravity is the force of natural attraction between bodies. Its magnitude is directly proportional to the product of their masses and inversely proportional to the square of the distance between them. The influence of gravity between Earth and the breathing apparatus can be substantial when body position is changed, and the control of speech breathing can alter dramatically as a result (see previous section). All discussion to this point has assumed that gravitational pull is constant and is between Earth and the breathing apparatus. There are, however, conditions away from Earth in which gravitational pull of a different magnitude prevails. One is space flight. Another is locating to a celestial body that has a mass different from that of Earth.

Space flight involves a change in gravitational pull as the traveler moves toward or away from Earth. Once beyond the influence of Earth's mass, the breathing apparatus is free of the gravitational pull to which it is accustomed and the traveler is weightless. The relaxation pressure of the breathing apparatus for the weightless condition is intermediate to that for the upright and supine body positions on Earth (Agostoni & Mead, 1964). This means that the muscular pressure required to achieve the same alveolar pressure at each lung volume is different under the weightless condition than for either the upright or supine conditions in the gravity field on Earth. Accordingly, the space traveler who is free of the gravitational influence of Earth is faced with a major adaptive challenge. Novel control strategies must be employed in space flight, something that few people have had the opportunity to do. That such strategies can be successful is evident in the many speech transmissions that have been sent back to Earth from space flights.

Up to now, space travelers have stepped on only one celestial body other than Earth. That body is Earth's moon. The moon has a mass that is only about 1/80th that of Earth and a gravitational pull that is only about 1/15th that of Earth. Thus, the relaxation pressure of the breathing apparatus is substantially different in magnitude on the moon than it is on Earth, as are the magnitudes of pulls placed on the individual parts of the chest wall. Those who have spoken on the lunar surface have had to accommodate to these differences and have had to make muscular pressure adjustments accordingly. When people venture to a celestial body other than Earth, it will be necessary to solve novel problems of speech breathing control if the gravitational pull of the visited celestial body is different from that of Earth. Reorganization by the nervous system will undoubtedly be further tested and proven on other extraterrestrial surfaces (probably next on Mars) as it was in the first speech transmission from the moon – "Houston. Tranquility Base. The Eagle has landed."

Load Factor

Most who have flown in an aircraft have an appreciation for the forces operating on them as passengers (as do those who have ridden in fast-moving elevators). A passenger in an aircraft in straight and level flight is subjected to 1 gravity of force, or 1 G. That same passenger may be subjected to a variety of different load factors involving either positive or negative G forces. The precise load borne will depend on the flight trajectory of the aircraft and the abruptness of its aerial maneuvers. Turbulence (atmospheric potholes) may also affect G forces. Positive G forces thrust passengers toward the floor of an aircraft, whereas negative G forces thrust them toward the ceiling. Changes in G forces can be large and rapid and must be accommodated by anyone who wishes to speak while under their influence (e.g., praying out loud while the food tray is crashing off the overhead luggage compartment).

Military fighter pilots have to deal with enormous G forces as a matter of routine. Pulling multiple Gs is a cost for many of their aerial combat maneuvers. Centrifugal force is something they understand intimately. Special flight suits help them cope with some of the cardiovascular consequences of pulling multiple G forces, but they must still make rather remarkable compensations to produce speech that sounds steady and intelligible. When pulling Gs, the external force operating on the breathing apparatus changes markedly. This force also differentially influences individual parts of the chest wall. Muscular pressure solutions by the breathing apparatus must account for these changing external forces at each instant. The nervous system achieves this extraordinary feat of real-time computation and execution. Pilots are not fond of talking during high-G maneuvers and it is no mystery why.

Torso Immersion in Water

Earth is composed mainly of water, and people spend a fair amount of time in it. Being immersed in water has consequences for the breathing apparatus and for speech breathing. Under usual (unimmersed) conditions, a hydrostatic pressure gradient exists within the abdominal cavity. In the upright body position, for example, abdominal pressure progressively increases from the undersurface of the diaphragm to the pelvic girdle (i.e., the deeper down, the higher the pressure). Because of this gradient, the lower abdominal wall tends to distend outward under the influence of the higher abdominal pressure operating on its inner surface (Reid, Loring, Banzett, & Mead, 1986).

This hydrostatic pressure gradient is eradicated when the torso is immersed in water up to the bottom of the sternum. This is because such immersion provides a hydrostatic pressure gradient on the outside of the abdominal wall that is identical to that found within the abdominal content. With the influence of the usual hydrostatic pressure gradient removed, the usual influence of gravity on the abdominal content is altered and the lung volume decreases somewhat (Agostoni, Gurtner, Torri, & Rahn, 1966). The result is a relaxation pressure that closely approximates that associated with weightlessness. That is, there is a higher relaxation pressure at corresponding lung volumes when sitting or standing in water than when sitting or standing out of water (Agostoni & Mead, 1964). In certain portions of the lung volume range, immersion may add as much as 6 to 8 cmH_2O to the relaxation pressure of the breathing apparatus. This means that the muscular pressure demands for speech production are different when the torso is immersed in water than when it is not.

The force exerted on the abdominal wall during immersion to the bottom of the sternum also alters the mechanical circumstances of the muscles of the abdominal wall, diaphragm, and rib cage wall (Reid, Banzett, Feldman, & Mead, 1985; Banzett & Mead, 1995). The operating length of the diaphragm is increased, giving it a contractile advantage, whereas the operating length of the inspiratory muscles of the rib cage wall (particularly the inspiratory intercostals) is decreased, giving them a contractile disadvantage. Also, the operating length of the abdominal wall muscles is decreased, giving them a contractile disadvantage, whereas the operating length of the expiratory muscles of the rib cage wall (particularly the expiratory intercostals) is increased, giving them a contractile advantage. All of this means that the muscular pressures delivered by different parts of the chest wall to control alveolar pressure must be delivered from different-than-usual mechanical advantages for each of the chest wall parts. Immersion in water to above the sternum (e.g., to the neck) has even more complicated mechanical consequences for the breathing apparatus than those already discussed for immersion to the bottom of the sternum (Reid et al., 1986).

Research dealing with immersion has supported the existence of a reflex operational length compensation in breathing muscles that is mechanically based and not locally mediated. Although the mechanism involved remains poorly understood, it is believed to employ afferent information from the breathing apparatus to globally adjust muscle activities (Reid et al., 1985). Whatever the mechanism, each change in the level of immersion brings about a different set of mechanical conditions to which the breathing apparatus must adjust.

VENTILATION, GAS EXCHANGE, AND SPEECH BREATHING

Ventilation is the movement of air into and out of the pulmonary airways and lungs. This movement is continual and is essential to support life. Ventilation goes on during speaking, so that the two go hand-in-hand.

The purpose of ventilation is to allow for gas exchange to occur. Gas exchange takes place within the alveoli and involves the delivery of oxygen to arterial blood (traveling away from the heart) and the collection of carbon dioxide from venous blood (traveling toward the heart). During inspiration, air travels through the pulmonary airways. Some of it reaches the alveoli deep within the lungs to participate in gas exchange. During expiration – which, in the case of speech breathing, involves speaking – air containing excess carbon dioxide is moved out from the alveoli through the pulmonary airways.

Ventilation is usually matched appropriately to the body's metabolic needs. Sometimes, however, there can be too much or too little ventilation. Too much ventilation (hyperventilation) occurs when too much fresh air is moved into and out of the pulmonary apparatus. This, in turn, usually results in too much fresh air being moved into and out of the alveoli (thereby causing alveolar hyperventilation). By contrast, too little ventilation (hypoventilation) occurs when too little fresh air is moved into and out of the pulmonary apparatus. Hypoventilation causes a depletion of oxygen and a build-up of carbon dioxide in the blood and body.

Ventilation and gas exchange can be measured in different ways. For example, ventilation can be measured at the airway opening or at the surface of the chest wall and is usually expressed as lung volume change over time (in liters per minute, LPM). Gas exchange can be measured from arterial blood or estimated from expired air and can be expressed as a partial pressure of oxygen and/or carbon dioxide (in millimeters of mercury, mmHg). Studies of speech breathing have used measures of ventilation and measures of gas exchange, sometimes in combination. The results of these studies, discussed below, indicate that speaking causes hyperventilation. Some of these studies also examined speaking under conditions of high ventilatory drive and are discussed further in the next section.

Bunn and Mead (1971) conducted the seminal study of ventilation and gas exchange during speaking. They studied seven subjects (age and sex unspecified) during resting tidal breathing and speaking. Ventilation was measured as lung volume change using a volume-displacement body plethysmograph. Gas exchange was estimated by sensing the amount of carbon dioxide in air expired from the nose with an infrared sensor coupled to a nasal cannula (actual gas exchange estimates were made during nasal consonant productions). Data were gathered while subjects sat quietly for several minutes and while they read three short paragraphs. The paragraphs included the following: (a) one that contained sounds with large lung volume expenditures (i.e., voiceless fricatives and plosives); (b) one that was loaded with consonants associated with small lung volume expenditures (i.e., nearly all voiced); and (c) one that was phonetically neutral with regard to lung volume expenditures.

Bunn and Mead (1971) reported that their subjects ventilated more while speaking (in air) than during resting tidal breathing for nearly all speaking conditions studied. Ventilation while speaking exceeded ventilation while resting tidal breathing by about 5% for the primarily voiced paragraph, about 15% for the neutral paragraph, and about 30% for the paragraph loaded with voiceless consonants. Estimates of gas exchange showed a reduction in expired carbon dioxide associated with speaking (which was consistent with the speaking-related increase in ventilation observed). They also noted that three of their subjects exhibited periods of apnea (breath holding) immediately after reading. They interpreted these periods of apnea as being a response to the speaking-related hyperventilation.

Meanock and Nicholls (1982) studied ventilation during speaking in eight subjects (including both men and women, ages unspecified). Ventilation was

JEREMIAH MEAD

Mead was the world's foremost leader for many decades in the study of respiratory mechanics. His career was extraordinarily productive and included many fundamental contributions that have influenced our understanding of respiratory biology and the practice of pulmonology. He had a long-standing interest in special acts of breathing, such as singing and speaking, and was instrumental, along with his postdoctoral students, in laying out a framework for understanding such acts. The legacy of his work has had a profound influence on methods currently used in the study of singing and speaking. Those of us fortunate enough to have worked in his laboratory and to have seen his brilliance first hand feel blessed. He played a mean French horn in the Harvard Respiratory Physiology Band and built his own boat that he sails off the coast of Maine where he lives in retirement. Jere Mead is one of our heroes.

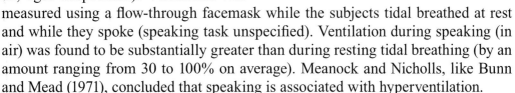

measured using a flow-through facemask while the subjects tidal breathed at rest and while they spoke (speaking task unspecified). Ventilation during speaking (in air) was found to be substantially greater than during resting tidal breathing (by an amount ranging from 30 to 100% on average). Meanock and Nicholls, like Bunn and Mead (1971), concluded that speaking is associated with hyperventilation.

Warner, Waggener, and Kronauer (1983) conducted the only study of ventilation during conversational interchange (rather than during continuous reading). They studied 10 college students (1 man and 9 women, ages unspecified) comprising 5 conversational dyads (pairs). Ventilation was measured using respiratory magnetometers fixed to the rib cage wall and abdominal wall. Members of each dyad were seated together in a room so that they could see each other easily. They sat quietly for 40 minutes and then conversed for 40 minutes.

Rather than reporting measures of total ventilation, Warner et al. (1983) estimated alveolar ventilation by subtracting the estimated dead space (i.e., the volume presumed not to have reached the alveoli, and, therefore, not to have participated in gas exchange) from the inspiratory volume. Their results showed that all 10 subjects ventilated about 40% more during conversation than during resting tidal breathing.

It is important to note that ventilation during conversation included periods of both speaking and listening. Thus, it is unclear exactly how much subjects ventilated during conversational speaking alone (see section on conversational interchange and speech breathing for additional details).

Abel, Mottau, Klubendorf, and Koepchen (1987) studied ventilation in 10 subjects (24 to 29 years, sex unspecified) by recording a signal summed from circumferential changes of the rib cage wall and abdominal wall (presumably closely related to lung volume change). Subjects were studied during periods of resting tidal breathing (lasting from 5 to 15 minutes) and during reading aloud (5 minutes). Results indicated that subjects ventilated more during speaking than during resting tidal breathing, which led Abel et al. to agree with previous investigators that speaking is associated with hyperventilation. The authors also noted that immediately following speaking, inspirations during resting tidal breathing tended to be slower than usual (i.e., longer in duration and lower in flow).

Russell, Cerny, and Stathopoulos (1998) investigated the effects of speech sound pressure level on ventilation in 12 men and 12 women (18 to 30 years of age). Measures of ventilation and gas exchange were obtained using a pulmonary function/cardiopulmonary testing system that was coupled to the subject via a face-mask. Ventilation was measured from flow sensed at the airway opening (mouth and nose). Gas exchange was measured using infrared sensing to determine the amount of oxygen and carbon dioxide in expired gas. Subjects were monitored while resting tidal breathing and while reading continuously, each for 7 minutes. Speech was produced at a comfortable sound pressure level, a low sound pressure level (5 dB below the comfortable level), and a high sound pressure level (10 dB above the comfortable level).

Russell et al. (1998) found that the sound pressure level at which subjects spoke influenced certain ventilation-related variables (with no sex-related differences). They reported that the level of ventilation, the amount of oxygen consumed, and the amount of carbon dioxide produced was greatest during speech produced at the highest sound pressure level. Interestingly, they concluded that their subjects hypoventilated when speaking at a comfortable sound pressure level (a condition that was similar to those used in all other investigations of ventilation and speech breathing). Russell et al. based this conclusion on the observation that the amount of carbon dioxide in expired gas was greater during comfortable speaking than during resting tidal breathing. However, the validity of this conclusion has been challenged by Hoit and Lohmeier (2002) who pointed out that the measurements of Russell et al. were made at the terminations of speech breaths and, therefore, probably provided an artificially high estimate of carbon dioxide in arterial blood. The measures of ventilation (i.e., lung volume change over time) made by Russell et al. for comfortable speech indicated hyperventilation and, thus, were in agreement with those of previous investigations.

Hoit and Lohmeier (2000) studied 20 men (22 to 27 years of age) during resting tidal breathing and speaking. They measured ventilation with respiratory magnetometers fixed to the rib cage wall and the abdominal wall (signals summed to obtain lung volume). They also estimated gas exchange by sensing the amount of carbon dioxide in gas expired from the nose with an infrared sensor coupled to a nasal cannula. Estimates of gas exchange were made by comparing the amount of expired carbon dioxide immediately before and immediately after speaking. This comparison avoided the problems associated with making measurements only during nasal consonant production, as was done by Bunn and Mead (1971), and making measurements at the termination of speech breaths, as was done by Russell et al. (1998). Subjects were asked to sit quietly for 5 to 10 minutes and to read aloud continuously for 10 minutes (at their usual loudness, pitch, and quality). The reading passage was unstructured with respect to volume expenditures (i.e., akin to the neutral paragraph of the Bunn and Mead study). The results of Hoit and Lohmeier indicated that all subjects ventilated more when reading than when resting tidal breathing (an average increase of 100%). A concomitant decrease in the amount of carbon dioxide in expired air was observed following speaking. In general, the greater the increase in ventilation, the greater the decrease in expired carbon dioxide.

When Hoit and Lohmeier (2000) examined individual subject performance, they found that subjects who used large lung volume expenditures per syllable tended to ventilate more than those who did not (accounting for 73% of the variance). Based on this, they speculated that it might be possible to predict ventilation from voice quality. That is, subjects with more breathy voices (and greater gas expenditures per syllable) may ventilate more than those with less breathy voices.

Finally, Hoit and Lohmeier (2000) noted that the usual nature of resting tidal breathing changed after a period of continuous speaking. Specifically, the amount of carbon dioxide in expired air was lower than normal for several minutes, indicating a period of "recovery" following speaking-related hyperventilation. Also, the pattern of breathing (i.e., as reflected in tidal volume and breathing frequency) was decidedly more variable, suggesting that the usual breathing pattern had been perturbed temporarily by the act of speaking. These observations were consistent with those of Bunn and Mead (1971) and Abel et al. (1987) who also reported changes in resting tidal breathing following speaking.

DRIVE-TO-BREATHE AND SPEECH BREATHING

Speech breathing is usually effortless. However, when the demand for ventilation is greater-than-usual, speech breathing can be taxing. Consider, for example, trying to speak during a brisk jog or while climbing a long flight of stairs. Or consider speaking at very high elevations, where the air is thin and little oxygen is available for gas exchange. In such cases, the drive-to-breathe competes with the drive-to-speak. This competition causes a struggle to strike a balance between producing acceptably fluent speech and maintaining adequate ventilation. This struggle is manifested in observable adjustments in speech breathing.

Studies of speech breathing under high drive-to-breathe conditions have used two types of paradigms. One involves speaking during exercise and one involves speaking in gas containing a high concentration of carbon dioxide. Such studies have shown that speech breathing changes under high-drive conditions and that these changes often differ from the changes seen in tidal breathing under high-drive conditions.

In a study of exercise and speech breathing by Otis and Clark (1968), six subjects (age and sex unspecified) were observed while they stood quietly, stood and spoke, walked on a treadmill, and walked on a treadmill and spoke. The speech tasks included counting, reciting the alphabet, reading a list of alphabet letters, and reading or reciting prose or poetry. Ventilation was measured (instrumentation unspecified) throughout the investigation. Otis and Clark found that as exercise demands increased (i.e., as the treadmill increased in speed), ventilation increased and the amount of speech produced per breath decreased. Overall, expiratory flow increased with exercise both because flow during speech production increased and because nonspeech expirations occurred. Speech rate did not change with exercise, but peak speech sound pressure level increased substantially with exercise.

Doust and Patrick (1981) investigated speech breathing during exercise using a paradigm similar to that of Otis and Clark (1968). Six men (average age of 20.8 years) were studied while they walked or ran on a treadmill. Observations were made during tidal breathing and while reading a paragraph under seven treadmill-speed conditions. Ventilation was monitored with a single inductance plethysmograph placed around the rib cage wall and upper abdominal wall. Although this method of monitoring ventilation is problematic on several counts, the overall patterns of exercise-induced change are of interest.

Doust and Patrick (1981) reported the same changes in speech breathing with exercise as did Otis and Clark (1968). In addition, they compared exercise-elevated ventilation during speaking to such ventilation during tidal breathing. They found that when subjects went from exercising to exercising (at the same level) while speaking, ventilation reduced substantially. This was interpreted as evidence that the act of speaking attenuates the usual ventilatory response to the increased metabolic demands associated with exercise. This finding is consistent with those from other studies that have used a carbon dioxide stimulus to increase the drive to breathe, discussed next.

Bunn and Mead (1971) conducted the seminal study of the interaction between the drive-to-breathe and the drive-to-speak. A preliminary description of their work was, in fact, described in the Otis and Clark (1968) publication mentioned above. The general method used by Bunn and Mead is described in the previous section of this chapter as it relates to the study of speech breathing in room air. To examine the influence of an elevated drive-to-breathe on speaking, Bunn and Mead observed their subjects while they breathed a mixture of gas containing 3.0 to 3.5% carbon dioxide (carbon dioxide comprises only 0.03% of room air). Breathing higher-than-usual levels of carbon dioxide increases the drive-to-breathe in a way that resembles exercise or breathing at high elevations.

As expected, Bunn and Mead (1971) found that subjects ventilated more in high carbon dioxide than in air, whether tidal breathing or speaking. Expiratory flow during speaking was found to be greater in high carbon dioxide than in air. And subjects produced nonspeech expirations, usually at the ends of breath groups, when breathing high carbon dioxide. Bunn and Mead found that the carbon dioxide-induced increase in ventilation was much less pronounced for speaking than it was for tidal breathing, suggesting that speaking takes precedence over the drive-to-breathe. This has been interpreted as evidence that the automatic control system (brainstem) can be overridden by the behavioral control system (cortex) to accomplish a behavioral goal such as speech production.

Phillipson, McClean, Sullivan, and Zamel (1978) also used a high carbon dioxide stimulus to increase the drive-to-breathe. Seven subjects (five men and two women, 20 to 40 years of age) were studied while they tidal breathed in a facemask connected to a spirometer. Subjects rebreathed a gas composed of 7% carbon dioxide (93% oxygen) for 4 to 5 minutes (the concentration of carbon dioxide increased as the subject continued to rebreathe the gas mixture). Ventilation was measured from the spirometer and carbon dioxide levels within the mask were measured with an infrared analyzer. During one of the rebreathing trials subjects spoke or read aloud continuously for as long as possible (speaking/reading material unspecified) and on another occasion they read silently.

Phillipson et al. (1978) found their subjects' ventilatory responses (i.e., increases in ventilation) to the carbon dioxide stimulus to be substantially smaller during speaking than during tidal breathing. This is consistent with what Bunn and Mead (1971) had reported earlier. Phillipson et al. also made several new observations. They showed that the ventilatory response to high carbon dioxide during silent reading was similar to that of tidal breathing. Based on this observation, they suggested that it is the motor activity associated with speaking that works to override metabolic demands, not simply the mental processes involved in speaking. In addition, they noted that subjects' end-expiratory lung volumes were unusually large while speaking in high carbon dioxide. Bailey and Hoit (2002) later confirmed this finding. Phillipson et al. also reported that their subjects were considerably "less dyspneic" when speaking than when tidal breathing in high carbon dioxide. Bailey and Hoit later contradicted this finding. Phillipson et al. concluded that their observations supported the idea that the behavioral control system can override the metabolic control system, even when metabolic drive is intense.

Meanock and Nicholls (1982) also studied subjects under different gas conditions. Their general method was described earlier (see section on ventilation, gas exchange, and speech breathing). For this part of their study, subjects tidal breathed and spoke while breathing two levels of carbon dioxide (2% and 4%). Differences in ventilatory response from air to the 2% carbon dioxide condition were similar to those reported previously. That is, although ventilation increased with carbon dioxide for both tidal breathing and speaking, the increase was much smaller for speaking. By contrast, the change in ventilation from the 2% to the 4% carbon dioxide condition was the same for tidal breathing and speaking. Meanock and Nicholls interpreted their findings to mean that the act of speaking does not necessarily change the sensitivity of the breathing control system.

Hale and Patrick (1987) used a rebreathing paradigm similar to that of Phillipson et al. (1978). They studied 12 subjects (sex and age unspecified) as they rebreathed in a facemask attached to a spirometer, beginning with an 8% carbon dioxide (92% oxygen) gas mixture. Subjects tidal breathed, read aloud the low-volume and high-volume expenditure paragraphs of Bunn and Mead (1971), and read silently. The results of the Hale and Patrick study emphasized the effects of increasing levels of carbon dioxide on inspiration as evidenced by increases in inspiratory volume, duration, and flow. The authors concluded that the inspiratory phase of the breathing cycle is highly susceptible to behavioral override during speech production.

Bailey and Hoit (2002) conducted a study to examine how speech breathing is influenced by high ventilatory drive, with special attention to the behavior of the chest wall and to their subjects' perceptions of the experience. Their study included 10 healthy men (18 to 29 years) breathing air and breathing a high carbon dioxide gas (7% carbon dioxide, 93% oxygen). Subjects were seated with a clear plastic dome fitted over the head and into which gas was delivered at a specified flow. Subjects wore respiratory magnetometers on the rib cage wall and abdominal wall so that chest wall behavior could be monitored and volume changes of the rib cage wall, abdominal wall, and lungs could be determined. A transcutaneous blood-gas monitor was used to provide estimates of the amount of carbon dioxide and oxygen in the blood. Subjects tidal breathed and read a paragraph aloud twice under each gas condition.

Their results showed that speech breathing altered substantially to accommodate a high drive-to-breathe. Specifically, speech breathing in high carbon dioxide gas, when compared to speech breathing in air, was associated with the

HOUSE ROCK RAPID

It's a tricky little choke on the Colorado River. Run it right. There's a rock ledge to the left. The water is flowing at 11,000 cubic feet per second. The dory is staunch, but an oar is lost. Wham! We've flipped in an enormous hole. All looks green. We're being recycled like a log against the face of a dam. Breath holding is the best option. We're slamming against the foot well. It's numbing cold. There's no air. Our chests burn. Hours pass in less than a minute. Bang! We're hitting boulders. Remember the safety lecture. "Find the gunwale. Push down and away from the boat." Our lungs are bursting. Suddenly, the green gets lighter. Our life vests move us to the surface like helpless turtles. We're gasping. We're alive. Five heads are bobbing in the water. We get to shore and shake from cold and fear. We paid good money for this experience. Now, more than ever, we appreciate air hunger. Stories. Lunch. Spare sunglasses. 110°F. Life.

following: (a) larger minute volumes; (b) higher inspiratory and expiratory flows; (c) larger lung volume initiations, terminations, and excursions; (d) larger rib cage wall initiations, terminations, and excursions; (e) larger abdominal wall initiations and excursions; (f) shorter expiratory times; (g) shorter speaking times; (h) fewer syllables per breath group; and (i) larger lung volume expenditures per syllable. Also observed were nonspeech expirations, usually at the ends of breath groups, something that never occurred when breathing air. Bailey and Hoit (2002) also found differences in the magnitudes of carbon dioxide-related changes in speech breathing compared to tidal breathing. With carbon dioxide, inspiratory flow increased more, expiratory flow decreased less, and lung volume (and rib cage volume) initiations and terminations increased more during speech breathing than during tidal breathing. Finally, post-experiment queries revealed that the subjects perceived speaking in high carbon dioxide as more difficult (or a related percept) than tidal breathing in high carbon dioxide.

Bailey and Hoit (2002) interpreted their findings as evidence that speech breathing in a high-drive condition is under both metabolic and linguistic control. They went on to speculate that subjects call on both muscular and linguistic strategies when speaking under conditions of higher-than-usual ventilatory drive. Muscular strategies were inferred from their chest wall movement data. Although such inferences are speculative, the evidence suggests that substantially different muscular strategies are used during speaking under a high-drive condition than under a normal-drive condition. This evidence is in the form of larger-than-usual lung volumes, rib cage wall volumes, and abdominal wall volumes, faster-than-usual inspiratory and expiratory movements, and chest wall configurations that are unlike those observed during speech breathing under normal-drive conditions. These behaviors indicate that the rib cage wall muscles may be aiding the diaphragm in generating the large and fast inspirations observed during high drive. The rib cage wall inspiratory muscles may also continue to be active at the beginning of expirations on those occasions when expiration is initiated at extremely large lung volumes (i.e., in excess of 90 %VC). Activation of inspiratory rib cage wall muscles in this case would serve as a brake against the large expiratory relaxation pressures that prevail at such volumes. Although the muscular strategies associated with speech breathing in a high-drive state cannot be specified with certainty, it seems clear that a greater-than-usual motor output is required.

The primary linguistic strategy exhibited by subjects under the high-drive condition was the use of fewer-than-usual syllables per breath group. These syllables were produced with larger-than-usual lung volume expenditures per syllable and with the insertion of nonspeech expirations at the ends of breath groups. Articulation rate was not altered. Such a strategy results in being able to move a large amount of air by reducing the time to the next inspiration. Thus, it is possible to maintain a high level of ventilation while continuing to speak in a relatively uninterrupted manner. Although this is strong evidence that the usual linguistic behavior of speech breathing is altered while under the influence of a high ventilatory drive, it is clear that speech breathing is still under strong linguistic control. Evidence for this can be found in the fact that subjects nearly always paused (for a nonspeech expiration, an inspiration, or both) at sentence, clause, or phrase boundaries. Post-experiment queries indicated that most of the subjects were acutely aware of the competition between ventilatory and linguistic demands and of their attempts to strike a balance between the two. This ventilatory-linguistic competition (demanding mental effort), combined with the presumably greater motor requirements (demanding physical effort) of speech breathing in high carbon dioxide gas, seemed to explain why subjects perceived speaking as more difficult than tidal breathing under the high-drive condition.

COGNITIVE-LINGUISTIC FACTORS AND SPEECH BREATHING

It goes without saying that speech breathing is influenced by what is said, and what is said can range from reciting a poem to reading aloud an unfamiliar passage to explaining an abstract concept. Such speaking activities encompass a wide range of cognitive-linguistic demands. They vary substantially in their mental and memory requirements and differ in the nature and complexity of the language formulation processes involved. When reciting a memorized poem, the linguistic content (including phonological, lexical, and syntactical features) and its parsing are determined ahead of time. When reading aloud, the linguistic content is provided, but the parsing is somewhat free to vary. And when speaking extemporaneously, the content and parsing must be formulated entirely on-line.

It would seem reasonable to predict that such large differences in cognitive-linguistic demands would be accompanied by similarly large differences in speech breathing behavior. Many investigations have considered the potential influence of cognitive-linguistic variables on speech breathing. Some of these have examined the general mechanical behavior of the breathing apparatus during speaking, whereas others have considered more detailed features of the speech breathing cycle.

Surprisingly, cognitive-linguistic demands do not seem to have much affect on the general mechanical behavior of the breathing apparatus. Whether reading aloud or speaking extemporaneously, speech breathing tends to show a similar mechanical patterning. For all of these activities, speech breathing is generated within the midrange of the vital capacity, mostly through lung volumes that are larger than at the resting level of the breathing apparatus, using relatively predictable chest wall shapes, and engaging similar muscular strategies (Hixon, Goldman, & Mead, 1973; Hixon, Mead, & Goldman, 1976; Hoit & Hixon, 1986, 1987; Hodge & Rochet, 1989; Hoit, Hixon, Altman, & Morgan, 1989; Hoit, Hixon, Watson, & Morgan, 1990; Mitchell, Hoit, & Watson, 1996).

Although cognitive-linguistic factors do not influence the general mechanical behavior of speech breathing, they do have a profound influence on certain details of speech breathing performance. This influence spans both the inspiratory and expiratory phases of the speech breathing cycle. Regarding the inspiratory phase, where (within the spoken text) and when (in time) inspirations occur are strongly determined by linguistic structural boundaries. There is substantial evidence that people inspire most often at structural boundaries – especially sentence, clause, and phrase boundaries – when reading aloud (Henderson, Goldman-Eisler, & Skarbek, 1965; Hixon et al., 1973; Grosjean & Collins, 1979; Conrad, Thalacker, & Schonle, 1983; Sugito, Ohyama, & Hirose, 1990; Winkworth, Davis, Ellis, & Adams, 1994; Bailey & Hoit, 2002). People also tend to inspire at structural boundaries when speaking extemporaneously (Henderson et al., 1965; Hixon et al., 1973; Winkworth, Davis, Adams, & Ellis, 1995), although less consistently than when reading aloud. Even when the drive-to-breathe is high enough to cause a conflict between speaking and breathing, inspirations continue to be strongly governed by linguistic structure (Bailey & Hoit, 2002).

Cognitive-linguistic factors also seem to influence depth of inspiration. There is evidence to suggest that deeper inspirations tend to be followed by longer breath groups and that shallower inspirations tend to be followed by shorter breath groups during reading aloud (Horii & Cooke, 1978; McFarland & Smith, 1992; Sperry & Klich, 1992; Winkworth et al., 1994; Whalen & Kinsella-Shaw, 1997; Denny, 2000) and during extemporaneous speaking (Winkworth et al., 1995). This supports the idea that a certain amount of breath-to-breath planning occurs. During reading, planning is in the form of scanning ahead in the written text, and during extemporaneous speaking, planning involves formulating thoughts for their expression.

Cognitive-linguistic factors also influence the expiratory phase of the speech breathing cycle (i.e., the speaking phase), perhaps even more so than the inspiratory phase. To begin, the length of the expiratory phase, whether measured in speech units or temporal units, seems to partially dictate where the speaker terminates the breath group within the vital capacity. That is, longer breath groups tend to terminate at smaller lung volumes and shorter breath groups tend to terminate at larger lung volumes (Wilder, 1983; Hodge & Rochet, 1989; Winkworth et al., 1994, 1995). This, coupled with the fact that inspirations are planned to coincide with linguistic structural boundaries, indicates that a speaker must make an on-line decision during the production of a breath group to continue the utterance to some logical juncture. This can lead to terminating a breath group at a lung volume that is smaller than that associated with the resting level of the breathing apparatus.

Probably the most salient cognitive-linguistic influence on the expiratory phase of the speech breathing cycle is that which relates to processing. Cognitive-linguistic processing has particularly strong effects in the production of speaking activities that require on-line formulation, such as those that involve speaking extemporaneously. Cognitive-linguistic processing can be "heard" in the speech signal as silent pauses and "seen" in speech breathing as breath holds or nonspeech expirations. Silent pauses (usually defined as silences lasting at least 200 to 250 milliseconds) within the expiratory phase of the speech breathing cycle appear to be related to the formulation of upcoming speech (Goldman-Eisler, 1956; Henderson et al., 1965; Reynolds & Paivio, 1968; Lay & Paivio, 1969; Taylor, 1969; Rochester, 1973; Greene, 1984; Greene & Cappella, 1986). Silent pauses accompanied by breath holding have been found to be more prevalent during speaking activities with higher cognitive-linguistic demands than those with lower cognitive-linguistic demands (Webb, Williams, & Minifie, 1967; Mitchell et al., 1996). Nevertheless, the most common type of silent pause is that associated with nonspeech expiration, at least during extemporaneous speaking (Mitchell et al., 1996).

When cognitive-linguistic processing demands are high, less speech is produced per breath group, primarily because of the occurrence of silent pauses accompanied by nonspeech expirations. Yet, lung volume excursions are no different than they are during less demanding speaking activities. This means that the air "wasted" during nonspeech expirations is not compensated for in any way. The result is that the number of syllables produced per breath group is fewer and the overall speech rate is slower (because silent pauses have been added, not because articulation rate has changed) during speaking with higher cognitive-linguistic demands (requiring more formulation) than during speaking with lower demands (Mitchell et al., 1996).

Cognitive-linguistic formulation is not the only explanation for the presence of silent pauses. Such pauses also may be associated with speaker anxiety (Goldman-Eisler, 1955; Siegman & Pope, 1966; Reynolds & Paivio, 1968; Lay & Paivio, 1969; Rochester, 1973). Of course, anxiety might be expected to accompany high-formulation demands, so that both factors could contribute simultaneously to the production of silent pauses in any given situation.

CONVERSATIONAL INTERCHANGE AND SPEECH BREATHING

Most speech breathing occurs within the context of everyday conversations. People engage in conversation much more often than they read aloud, tell a story, give a lecture, or perform other activities that involve continual speaking (without interruption). Even those who have careers with high didactic speaking demands (such as newscasters, teachers, radio disc jockeys, or readers for books-on-tape) probably spend more time conversing with family and friends than they spend in their work-related speaking activities. Thus, conversational speech breathing can be said to be the most common form of speech breathing.

Conversation involves a spoken interchange between two people (or among more than two people). When engaged in conversational interchange, the content and form of one person's speech strongly influence the other person's speech. A person involved in a conversation generally speaks for awhile and then listens for awhile as another person speaks. These periods of speaking and listening usually have an alternating pattern. The specific nature of that pattern is determined by the personalities of the conversational partners, their relationship to one another, the situational context, and many other variables.

The nature of intrinsic rhythms (biological and behavioral) and how they are modified as a consequence of social interaction has generated a great deal of interest. One prominent hypothesis is that during interactions, such as conversational interactions, people seek to entrain their own rhythms with the rhythms of others and that the most enjoyable interactions are those in which individual rhythms are most easily entrained to one another (Chapple, 1970). Given that breathing has a strong intrinsic rhythm and given that breathing is an integral part of conversational speaking, interesting insights can be gained by examining breathing behavior as a window into the nature of the conversational interchange.

A host of studies has examined the nature of conversational interchange, but only two have examined speech breathing directly. One of these was by Warner, Waggener, and Kronauer (1983), who examined long-term oscillations in breathing during conversation, and the other was by McFarland (2001) who focused on cycle-to-cycle changes in breathing.

Warner et al. (1983) made observations of 10 young adults organized into 5 conversational dyads. Each dyad consisted of subjects who considered themselves to be friends. Speech breathing was monitored with respiratory magnetometers while members of the dyad rested and while they carried on a 40-minute conversation. As was reported above (see section on ventilation, gas exchange, and speech breathing), subjects in the Warner et al. study were found to ventilate more when engaged in conversational interchange than when resting tidal breathing. Although it was not clear how much of the overall measured ventilation was associated with speaking and how much was associated with listening, it was clear that either speaking or listening could be accompanied by hyperventilation.

When the Warner et al. (1983) data were examined across time, oscillations in ventilation were found during resting tidal breathing and during conversational speech breathing. That is, ventilation tended to wax and wane with a cycle period that ranged from about 1 to 8 minutes. Oscillations also were noted in the amount of speaking activity for each subject, and such oscillations were closely coordinated with the oscillations of the conversational partner. There was a strong alternating rhythm between partners in the amount of speech produced, such that one member of the dyad tended to be silent while the other member spoke, and vice versa.

The overall finding of the Warner et al. (1983) work was that the rhythmic coupling of speaking activity between conversational partners was much stronger than the coupling between speaking activity and ventilation within individual subjects. This led the authors to conclude that social constraints are more powerful than physiologic constraints (i.e., ventilation) within a conversational context. They also speculated that when an individual's natural oscillations in ventilation are maintained during conversation, that conversation should be perceived as more pleasant than a conversation in which natural oscillations in ventilation are altered. This relates to the idea that the maintenance of one's own intrinsic biological rhythms is an important determinant of the perceived quality of an interaction (Chapple, 1970).

McFarland (2001) studied conversational speech breathing with a focus on turn-taking behavior. His study included 10 dyads consisting of young women. Members of each dyad characterized themselves as friends and equals. Their breathing was recorded with mercury elastic strain gauges placed around the rib cage wall and abdominal wall during the performance of several activities, including a 5-minute scripted dialogue and a 15-minute spontaneous conversation. Data were analyzed to reveal the temporal events of breathing (not the volumetric events) using the rib cage wall data alone. Although occasional paradoxical movement of the rib cage wall may have been misleading, it is reasonable to assume that rib cage wall inspiratory and expiratory movements provided generally good indicators of inspiratory and expiratory movements of the chest wall.

McFarland's (2001) data revealed several patterns. For the scripted dialogue, members of each dyad alternated between reading and listening without overlap of reading events. When subjects listened, as their partners read script, their breathing differed from their resting tidal breathing when not listening. Inspiratory movements of the rib cage wall were shorter during listening than they were during nonlistening resting tidal breathing. That is, inspirations tended to become more "speech like" when listening to a conversational partner speak. Also, there was a tendency for expiratory movements to be longer during breaths that immediately preceded the beginning of a speaking period. That is, expirations during resting tidal breathing tended to become more "speech like" when the listener was preparing to speak.

Speech breathing during spontaneous conversation was found to be much more complex than during scripted dialogue. For example, it was characterized by large variability in the duration of conversational turns, short interjected utterances during listening (apparently confirming the listener's attention to the speaker), and frequent overlaps in utterances. Overlaps in utterances usually consisted of simultaneous speech or laughter and tended to occur at turn-taking junctures in the conversation. During conversational listening, inspiratory patterns resembled those observed during scripted dialogue (i.e., shorter inspiratory movements of the rib cage wall during listening and longer expiratory movements of the rib cage wall during breaths that immediately preceded the onset of speaking). During the actual moments of turn-taking, rib cage wall movements of conversational partners tended to be highly correlated. In some cases, such as when partners laughed simultaneously, rib cage wall movements were positively correlated (i.e., they moved simultaneously in the same direction). In other cases, they were negatively correlated (i.e., they moved simultaneously in opposite directions). Either way, such correlations were indicative of what was referred to as a "coupling" or "synchrony" between the breathing movements of conversational partners.

BODY TYPE AND SPEECH BREATHING

People come in different sizes, shapes, and compositions that give rise to different body types. Some individuals are more endomorphic (fat) than others, some are more mesomorphic (muscular), and some are more ectomorphic (lank). Given such variety, it would seem reasonable to wonder whether or not people with different body types might exhibit different speech breathing behaviors.

Hoit and Hixon (1986) were the first to address this issue empirically.[2] They studied 12 healthy men (18 to 23 years), each of whom fit into one of three different body type groups (4 per group). Each group was characterized by a prominence on one of the three components of body type – high in relative fatness, high in relative musculoskeletal development, or high in relative linearity. Prominence was determined from a combination of physical measurements on a standard anthropometric rating scale (Carter, 1980). Speech breathing was studied using respiratory magnetometers to estimate the volumes displaced by the rib cage wall, abdominal wall, and lungs. Subjects stood upright, leaning slightly backwards against a tilt table, and engaged in conversational speaking and reading aloud of a long passage and a short passage.

Hoit and Hixon (1986) found notable differences across body type groups and interpreted them as support for a linkage between body type and speech breathing performance. The most striking contrasts were between the endomorphic and ectomorphic groups, with the endomorphic subjects exhibiting a high degree of abdominal wall participation and the ectomorphic subjects exhibiting a high degree of rib cage wall participation. Notable patterns were as follows: (a) the endomorphic subjects frequently demonstrated a relative volume predominance of the abdominal wall over the rib cage wall, whereas the ectomorphic subjects usually demonstrated a predominance of the rib cage wall over the abdominal wall; (b) the endomorphic subjects tended to use a wide variety of relative volume contributions of the rib cage wall and abdominal wall within and between breath groups, whereas the ectomorphic subjects did not; (c) the endomorphic subjects used large abdominal wall excursions, whereas the ectomorphic subjects used small abdominal wall excursions; (d) the endomorphic subjects often demonstrated rib cage wall paradoxing (i.e., rib cage wall volume increase) during speech production, whereas the ectomorphic subjects rarely did; and (e) the endomorphic subjects demonstrated large chest wall deformations from relaxation, whereas the ectomorphic subjects showed only small deformations. The speech breathing behavior of the mesomorphic subjects generally fell between the extremes exhibited by the endomorphic and ectomorphic subjects.

Why would subjects of different body types use such different speech breathing

---

[2]Data on body type and speech breathing have also been reported by authors from the University of Queensland. However, these data and other data from the same laboratory on normal and abnormal speech breathing have been shown by Hoit (1994) to be invalid and are not discussed in this book.

behaviors? One possible explanation relates to the inspiratory phase of the speech breathing cycle. Because running speech breathing calls for quick inspirations, it is important to maintain the diaphragm in a highly domed configuration in which its fibers are stretched so it can generate rapid inspiratory pressure changes. Taking as examples the endomorphic and ectomorphic extremes, the diaphragm would be positioned quite differently in individuals whose abdominal walls protrude substantially than in individuals whose abdominal walls protrude only minimally. If an endomorphic individual were to relax the muscles of the abdominal wall, the diaphragm would become flatter and less able to produce quick changes in inspiratory pressure. By contrast, if an ectomorphic individual were to relax the abdominal wall, the configuration of the diaphragm would change relatively little. Therefore, for an endomorphic person, it would seem important to displace the abdominal wall inward to tune the diaphragm mechanically, whereas for an ectomorphic person there would seem to be little need to make such an adjustment. This speculation is supported by the high degree of abdominal wall participation seen in the endomorphic subjects and the insignificant amount of abdominal wall participation seen in the ectomorphic subjects.

Although a body-type effect was borne out by the Hoit and Hixon (1986) data, body type did not account for all of the performance differences observed among the subjects studied. It may be that all of the salient features of body type were not captured by the anthropometric rating method used. It may also be that more between-subject variability could have been accounted for if the components of body type had been combined in some appropriately weighted fashion. Furthermore, it is possible that individuals with identical body types, as measured by standard measurement methods, may demonstrate different torso types that could influence speech breathing. That is, although a body type-speech breathing behavior link is supported by the findings of Hoit and Hixon, the link may not be a direct one. Rather, body type may be related to torso type, which, in turn, may be a major determinant of speech breathing behavior.

AGE AND SPEECH BREATHING

Age changes things, many things. Speech breathing is no exception. Once maturity is reached, speech breathing undergoes a gradual process of modification that continues unnoticed day-to-day. Like other body systems, the breathing apparatus changes in its structure and function throughout adulthood. These changes become pronounced in the senescent years.

The influence of age on speech breathing was first documented in a pair of companion studies of men by Hoit and Hixon (1987) and women by Hoit, Hixon, Altman, and Morgan (1989). These studies examined speech breathing in 60 subjects of average body type, 10 men and 10 women in each of 3 age groups representing the following: (a) young adulthood (25 years, ± 2 years), when general breathing function is at its peak; (b) middle age (50 years, ± 2 years), midway along the age continuum; and (c) senescence (75 years, ± 2 years), when general breathing function has undergone significant change from its peak. The subjects in these studies were required to meet strict health criteria so that if any group differences were found they could be interpreted as being related solely to age differences, not differences in health status. Speech breathing was studied using respiratory magnetometers to estimate the volumes displaced by the rib cage wall, abdominal wall, and lungs. Subjects were seated upright in a chair and were asked to speak extemporaneously and to read a passage aloud.

Results of these investigations revealed several age-related differences in speech breathing, most of which were between the 25-year-old group and the 75-year-old group. The senescent adults, compared to the young adults, generally did the following: (a) initiated breath groups at larger lung volumes and used larger lung volume excursions; (b) initiated breath groups at larger rib cage wall volumes and used larger rib cage wall excursions; and (c) used greater lung volume expenditures per syllable (in both absolute values and when expressed as a percentage of the vital capacity).

These observations did not appear to be linked in any direct way to age-related changes in the structure or function of the breathing apparatus, per se. Rather, they were interpreted to reflect behavioral adjustments made by the senescent subjects. The authors speculated that senescent subjects initiated breath groups at larger lung volumes (and rib cage wall volumes) and used larger lung volume excursions (and rib cage wall excursions) to compensate for anticipated air losses associated with reductions in valving economy at the larynx and/or the upper airway. That is, senescent subjects appeared to use the breathing apparatus to "come to the rescue" of leaky downstream valves.

The idea that age-related reductions in downstream valving economy might help explain the speech breathing behavior of senescent individuals led investigators from the same laboratory to look for direct evidence of such reductions. The laryngeal valve was targeted because it is the first outlet valve "seen" by the breathing apparatus. Specifically, estimates of laryngeal airway resistance during vowel production were determined (using the method of Smitheran & Hixon, 1981) for men (Melcon, Hoit, & Hixon, 1989) and women (Hoit & Hixon, 1992) of various ages. The results for the men showed that laryngeal airway resistance was similar for subjects ranging in age from 25 to 65 years, but that there was a significant reduction in resistance at age 75 years. Thus, for men, the hypothesis was supported that laryngeal valving economy during voicing decreases with age, thereby helping to explain the speech breathing data of Hoit and Hixon (1987). By contrast, the results for the women revealed no significant differences in laryngeal airway resistance during vowel production in subjects ranging from age 25 to 85 years. Thus, in the case of women, a change in laryngeal valving economy for voicing was not a viable explanation for the age-related differences in speech breathing behavior of the Hoit et al. (1989) women. Other explanations were needed.

One possible explanation emerged from a study of age and speech breathing in women conducted by Sperry and Klich (1992). This study included two groups of subjects, one consisting of nine younger women (20 to 28 years) and one consisting of nine older women (62 to 70 years). Respiratory inductance plethysmography was used to estimate lung volume events. Subjects were seated upright and were instructed to read aloud several sentences of various lengths and a passage in which the same sentences were embedded.

Results of the Sperry and Klich (1992) study indicated that the older women, as compared to the younger women, generally did the following: (a) initiated breath groups from larger lung volumes; (b) used larger lung volume excursions; and (c) inspired more often. These characteristics became more pronounced as sentence length increased and as sentences were read in the context of a passage rather than in isolation. The age-related differences in lung volume initiations and excursions were essentially the same as those observed in both men and women by Hoit and Hixon (1987) and Hoit et al. (1989), respectively. To explain the larger lung volume excursions in the older women, Sperry and Klich analyzed speaking behavior within breath groups. They found that the older women tended to exhibit nonspeech expirations at the beginning of breath groups, during pauses within breath groups, and at the end of breath groups.

The observations of Sperry and Klich (1992) and those of Hoit and colleagues (Hoit & Hixon, 1987, 1992; Hoit et al., 1989; Melcon et al., 1989) support the idea that age-related reductions in valving economy influence speech breathing in older adults. These observations offer different specific explanations for men and women. In older men, air wastage occurs during voicing, whereas in older women, air wastage occurs during parts of the breath group that do not involve speaking. There may also be additional sources of reduced downstream valving economy – for examples, air wastage due to slow laryngeal adduction during voiceless-to-voiced articulations, or air wastage due to reduced valving competency of other structures such as the tongue and lips. Such possibilities have yet to be explored.

The existing research indicates that age-related changes in speech breathing generally begin to appear in the seventh or eighth decade of life. Nevertheless, it is important to consider that chronological age is not always a good indicator of biological age and that a more comprehensive understanding of the nature of age-related changes in the physiology of speech breathing might be achieved if it were studied from the standpoint of biological age.

SEX AND SPEECH BREATHING

Until recently, most of what was known about speech breathing had come from the study of men. Although it seemed plausible to assume that this knowledge could be generalized to women, it was as easy to argue that there might be important differences in the speech breathing of women. The fact that the appearance of the breathing apparatus is quite different in men and women and the fact that there are sex-related differences in certain features of speech and language behavior seemed to support this view.

Two studies have been conducted that shed light on whether or not there are sex-related differences in speech breathing. One was the study by Hoit, Hixon, Altman, and Morgan (1989) reviewed in the preceding section. When the data from the 30 women of Hoit et al. were contrasted statistically with the data from the 30 men of Hoit and Hixon (1987), the results showed no sex differences. Specifically, for all age groups studied, there were no significant differences between the sexes for rib cage wall volume events (expressed in percentage of rib cage capacity), abdominal wall volume events (expressed in percentage of abdominal capacity), lung volume events (expressed in percentage of vital capacity), relative volume contribution of the rib cage wall and abdominal wall, syllables per breath group, and lung volume expenditure per syllable (expressed in percentage of vital capacity per syllable).

Only one of the many measures obtained by Hoit et al. (1989) showed a sex-related difference – lung volume expended per syllable [expressed in cubic centimeters (cc) per syllable]. Specifically, the women expended significantly less air per syllable than did the men. Importantly, this was the only volumetric measure included in this study that was expressed in absolute values. All other measures were normalized for each subject. This suggests that the less-air-per-syllable difference, rather than being due to subject sex, per se, was explained by the fact that women are smaller on average than men. Body size (particularly height) is a strong predictor of volumetric measures of breathing because, in general, the larger the body, the larger the pulmonary airways and lungs. Given this, it is likely that if the other volumetric measures (volume initiations, terminations, and excursions of the rib cage wall, abdominal wall, and lungs) had been expressed in absolute values, they would have revealed sex-related differences – that is, size-related differences – as well.

The other study conducted to explore the issue of sex and speech breathing was by Hodge and Rochet (1989). This

His and Her Breathing

We've discussed how speech breathing is pretty much the same in men and women when size differences are taken into account. For the most part, the same is true of most other forms of breathing. So, if men and women don't breathe differently, why then is there a persistent folklore that they do? We can't be sure, but our hunch is that the folklore has been influenced strongly by the physicians who have suggested the difference. Consider that reports on men have often been based on observations made in the upright body position by general practice physicians. By contrast, reports on women have often been based on observations made in the supine body position by obstetricians-gynecologists. The two sexes breathe the same in the same body positions. But, if they have been observed mainly in different body positions, then the differences ascribed to them are not really differences at all. Or maybe you have a better hunch.

study was designed to make comparisons between data collected on women and data available in the literature on men. Hodge and Rochet studied 10 healthy women who were 20 to 32 years of age. Subjects were monitored with respiratory magnetometers while seated upright in a chair and engaged in conversational speaking and the reading aloud of a passage.

Comparisons of their data to existing data on healthy men (Hixon, Goldman, & Mead, 1973; Hoit & Hixon, 1986, 1987) led Hodge and Rochet (1989) to conclude that there were no functional differences in speech breathing between young men and young women. They reached the conclusion that the "use of gender-specific speech breathing normative data appears unwarranted for young adults" (p. 478). Thus, the findings and conclusions of Hodge and Rochet and Hoit et al. (1989) are in agreement.

EMERGENCE OF SPEECH BREATHING

Infancy and early childhood are characterized by rapid growth and development of the breathing apparatus. Speech breathing skill emerges within this context and reflects the natural exploration that occurs before more stable patterns of behavior are laid down.

Most of the information available about the natural course of speech breathing emergence has been provided by a single large-scale investigation. The results of this investigation have been reported in a pair of articles covering the first year of life (Boliek, Hixon, Watson, & Morgan, 1996) and the second and third years of life (Boliek, Hixon, Watson, & Morgan, 1997).

Boliek et al. (1996, 1997) studied 80 healthy infants and young children (40 boys and 40 girls) in a cross-sectional research design that included 5 boys and 5 girls at each of the following ages: 5 weeks (± 3 days); 2.5 months (±3 days); 6.5 months (± 2 weeks); 12 months (± 2 weeks); 18 months (± 2 weeks); 24 months (± 2 weeks); 30 months (± 2 weeks); and 36 months (± 2 weeks). Seventeen infants included in the cross-sectional design were also studied longitudinally as a way to cross check the larger cross-sectional data set. All subjects were within the average to above-average range on developmental milestones related to physical, neuromotor, breathing, speech, language, social-adaptive, and cognitive functions. Breathing was studied using respiratory inductance plethysmography so that estimates could be made of the volumes displaced by the rib cage wall, abdominal wall, and lungs. Subjects were supine or seated, depending on the age of the subject, and vocalizations were generated spontaneously or elicited by an investigator or caregiver using toys or other stimuli.

A total of 3,308 vocalizations was analyzed by Boliek et al. (1996, 1997). For subjects in the first 12 months of life, the preponderance of vocalizations were cries, hiccups, grunts, whimpers, and syllable utterances. By contrast, for subjects from 18 to 36 months of age, vocalizations were primarily syllable, word, or combined (syllable and word) utterances.

Interestingly, breathing behavior did not differ across vocalization types. This was surprising given the wide range of vocalization types studied. Nevertheless, it should be noted that only kinematic features of chest wall behavior were investigated and that vocalization types almost certainly differed with regard to alveolar pressure. For example, cries are usually louder than whimpers, reflecting that alveolar pressure is higher for cries.

No differences were found between the performances of the boys and girls in the Boliek et al. (1996, 1997) study. This finding is consistent with the absence of sex differences found in older children and adolescents (see section in this chapter on refinement of speech breathing) and in adults (see previous section in this chapter).

As expected, Boliek et al. (1996, 1997) found age-related differences in breathing behavior during vocalization. One was that lung volume excursions (expressed in absolute volumes) generally increased with age. This age-related increase could be explained by associated increases in height and concomitant increases in (predicted) vital capacity. When lung volume excursions for vocalizations were normalized (expressed in percentage of predicted vital capacity), age-related differences disappeared.

There was also an effect of body position on breathing behavior. Subjects who were studied in the upright body position (those 6.5 months and older) tended to terminate breath groups at smaller lung volumes, relative to the tidal end-expiratory level, than did subjects who were studied in the supine body position (those 5 weeks and 2.5 months of age). This is best explained by the fact that gravity increases the resting level of the breathing apparatus when shifting from the supine body position to the upright body position, making more expiratory reserve volume available for use in vocalization.

Despite the general effects of age/height and body position observed, the major hallmark of the Boliek et al. (1996, 1997) data was their variability. Breathing adjustments were not stereotypical for any of the vocalization types, either within or between subjects. This variability demonstrated that many degrees

BABIES DON'T GIVE YOU ANY REST

Unlike the resting tidal end-expiratory level of adults, the tidal end-expiratory level of young babies is not determined by passive forces alone. Rather, young babies are known to breathe using a so-called "dynamic" (controlled) tidal end-expiratory level that is larger than their passive level. This changes as they grow, however, and it's believed that sometime during the second half of the first year of life they shift from a dynamic to a passive tidal end-expiratory level. Several factors appear to be implicated in this dynamic control process in babies. These include, among others, laryngeal braking of the expiratory air stream, breath timing reflexes, and active forces provided by the inspiratory muscles of the chest wall. If your experience is that babies don't give you any rest, you're not alone. Babies don't even give themselves any rest.

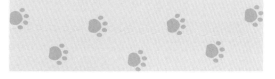

of freedom of performance (possible ways to achieve the desired breathing behavior) were available to the subjects to meet the aeromechanical demands associated with vocalization. Such variability was exemplified by the relative volume contribution data reported by Boliek et al. These data showed that the relative contribution of the rib cage wall to lung volume change during vocalization ranged from rib cage wall paradoxing (i.e., the rib cage wall moving in the inspiratory direction) to abdominal wall paradoxing (i.e., the abdominal wall moving in the inspiratory direction), with nearly all possible rib cage wall and abdominal wall expiratory combinations between these two extremes. The authors interpreted this enormous variability to represent a form of "experimentation" on the part of infants and young children to control a continuously developing breathing apparatus.

The hallmark of variability does not mean that there were not systematic behaviors in subject performance. To the contrary, some strong mechanical effects were demonstrated during the emergence of speech breathing between birth and 3 years of age. For example, the majority of vocalizations were initiated at lung volumes that were larger than the tidal end-expiratory level and within the midrange of the predicted vital capacity. Of these, most were initiated from within one to two predicted tidal depths. Subjects tended to avoid initiating breath groups at the uppermost extreme of the predicted vital capacity.

The research of Boliek et al. (1996, 1997) suggests strongly that the period during which speech breathing emerges is a protracted one. By age 3 years, the assembly of speech gestures by the breathing apparatus has not resolved into consistent patterns. It is known that far more consistent speech breathing behavior is observed in 7-year-old children, but even then it is not fully adult-like (see section in this chapter on refinement of speech breathing). Presumably, sometime between 3 years of age and 7 years of age the variability that is the hallmark of the emergence period begins to decrease.

Another investigation of speech breathing in young children was conducted by Moore, Caulfield, and Green (2001). They studied 11 healthy young children (4 boys and 7 girls) who were 15 months of age. All were developing normally according to parental reports of achievement on gross motor, fine motor, cognitive, speech, and language milestones.

Breathing was monitored with respiratory inductance plethysmography. Signals related to the average cross-sectional areas of the rib cage wall and abdominal wall were recorded (not circumferences, as reported) while subjects were seated in a highchair. Spontaneous and imitative utterances were elicited from the subjects using a variety of toys, books, and games. A total of 297 utterances was analyzed – 125 categorized as babbling, 160 categorized as true words, and 12 categorized as other vocalizations.

Moore et al. (2001) reported a number of consistencies between their findings and those of Boliek et al. (1996, 1997). In particular, they reported that chest wall adjustments were indistinguishable among the different utterance categories. Moore et al. concluded that children of the age they studied (15 months) had not yet developed motor control capabilities beyond those necessary for the most rudimentary of utterances.

Moore et al. (2001) concentrated much of their effort on determining whether or not resting tidal breathing and speech breathing exhibited different coordinative patterns. To do this, they used a time-varying correlational index of coupling between their rib cage wall and abdominal wall measurements that they assumed reflected the synchrony of movement between these two structures. They also used moment-to-moment relations between the two structures to categorize their function (e.g., moving in the same sign or moving in opposite signs). There are significant problems in inferring mechanism on these bases without information about chest wall shape and its history. Nonetheless, the findings of this study remain of interest. Based on the data obtained, Moore et al. concluded that speech breathing is dependent on a different coordinative organization than is resting tidal breathing and that speech breathing emerges as distinct from nonspeech uses of the breathing apparatus (at least resting tidal breathing uses).

Connaghan, Moore, and Higashakawa (2004) reported on an extension of the Moore et al. (2001) study. Connaghan et al. observed four normally developing children (one boy and three girls) longitudinally from age 9 to 48 months at 3-month intervals. Parental reports were taken as evidence of normal development on the same milestones used in the Moore et al. study. Breathing was studied using respiratory inductance plethysmography, while subjects were seated upright in a highchair or at a play table. Spontaneous and imitative utterances were elicited in the manner described by Moore et al. A total of 1,456 utterances was analyzed – 85 categorized as babbling and 1,371 categorized as true words. Data analysis procedures were the same as those used by Moore et al.

The findings of Connaghan et al. (2004) generally agreed with those of Moore et al. (2001). Of particular interest were developmental changes noted in the longitudinal data. Connaghan et al. reported that resting tidal breathing showed little change in coupling between the rib cage wall and the abdominal wall across the developmental period studied. However, speech breathing exhibited a substantial decrease in coupling during the same period. Specifically, an increase in the frequency of rib cage wall paradoxing and decrease in rib cage wall and abdominal wall coupling during expiration were observed as the children grew older. The changes noted were gradual and were interpreted by Connaghan et al. to be related, in part, to anatomical and biomechanical changes attendant to development.

REFINEMENT OF SPEECH BREATHING

Once the rudiments of speech breathing skill are laid down in infancy and early childhood, a good deal of refinement occurs before the adult skill level is reached.

The process is relatively slow and extends from the emergence period through adolescence.

A study by Hoit, Hixon, Watson, and Morgan (1990) has provided most of the data on this refinement process. This study included 80 normal, healthy children and adolescents, 40 boys and 40 girls, 10 each of each sex, representing 4 age groups – 7, 10, 13, and 16 years (± 3 months). Age 7 was chosen as the lower end of the range because children of that age are essentially adult-like in phonological skill, but are still developing motor skill. Age 16 was selected as the upper end of the range because adolescents of that age have completed all stages of puberty and presumably are adult-like in their motor skill. To take into account possible influences of puberty, all of the 7- and 10-year-old subjects were without signs of having entered puberty, whereas all of the 13- and 16-year-old subjects had a history of signs of having entered puberty. Speech breathing was studied with respiratory magnetometers to estimate the volumes displaced by the rib cage wall, abdominal wall, and lungs. Subjects were seated upright and engaged in extemporaneous speaking and oral reading activities appropriate to their reading-proficiency level.

Hoit et al. (1990) found speech breathing to be similar for the two sexes. The few significant differences between boys and girls did not relate directly to sex, but rather could be accounted for on the basis of size of the speech production apparatus and speech fluency. Therefore, sex was not an important variable during the refinement period. This conclusion, combined with those discussed for infants, young children, and adults, suggests that speech breathing performance is the same for both sexes across the entire life span.

Age-related differences were found for many of the speech breathing measures. General patterns of differences were similar for extemporaneous speaking and reading and the great majority of differences were between the 7-year-old group and the older groups (10, 13, and 16 years). Specifically, the 7-year-old subjects, when compared to the older subjects, tended to do the following: (a) initiate and terminate breath groups at larger lung volumes, rib cage wall volumes, and abdominal wall volumes; (b) use larger lung volume excursions and rib cage wall volume excursions during breath groups; (c) use larger lung volume expenditures per syllable (in both absolute and normalized forms); and (d) produce fewer syllables per breath group.

Hoit et al. (1990) speculated that their 7-year-old subjects used larger lung volumes (and rib cage wall volumes) because young children are known to speak at higher sound pressure levels (Stathopoulos, 1986) and use higher driving pressures during speech production than older children and adolescents (Bernthal & Beukelman, 1978; Stathopoulos & Weismer, 1985; Stathopoulos & Sapienza, 1993). By using larger lung volumes, the 7-year-old children would be able to take advantage of the higher relaxation pressures available at those volumes. Such a strategy would augment the positive muscular pressure used in producing alveolar pressure for speech production. The use of larger lung volumes for speaking probably ends soon after 7 years of age, given that there is no evidence of this behavior in the 10-year-old children studied by Hoit et al., nor was it observed in the 8 to 10-year-old children studied by Russell and Stathopoulos (1988).

Perhaps even more intriguing was the observation that the 7-year-old subjects of Hoit et al. (1990) initiated and terminated spoken breath groups at larger abdominal wall volumes than their older counterparts. In fact, there were occasions when some of the 7-year-old subjects spoke using abdominal wall volumes that were larger than abdominal wall volumes associated with relaxation. Comparisons across the four age groups showed that abdominal wall volume initiations and terminations became progressively smaller with increasing age. The authors interpreted this trend to indicate that as children grow older they assume a chest wall shape for speech production that is increasingly deformed from the relaxation configuration. This shape is such that abdominal wall vol-

JAMES F. CURTIS

Curtis had an eminent and distinguished career as a speech scientist. He did not publish extensively on speech breathing, but he had an enormous influence on its study through his students at the University of Iowa. Curtis was intimately involved in a large group of dissertations about speech breathing and strongly guided them to their final forms. Among these were the works of Arkebauer, Cooker, Eblen, Hardy, Hixon, Kneil, Kunze, McGlone, Netsell, and Shrum. He was a superb and detailed editor. Much of his style he attributed to his mentor, Grant A. Fairbanks. Curtis created anxiety at national conferences because he could cut to the heart of any weakness in a research design and verbalize it faster than a speeding bullet. He retired to Montana where he built a log home and where he loves to hunt and fish. He is a very kind person and is currently a national leader on environmental issues in the Sierra Club.

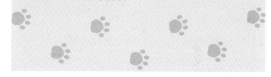

umes are increasingly smaller and rib cage wall volumes are increasingly larger at prevailing lung volumes. As discussed in relation to the adult breathing apparatus (see section in this chapter on breathing for speech purposes), this shape serves to position the different parts of the breathing apparatus so that they are at favorable mechanical advantages for producing inspiratory and expiratory muscular pressures.

The remaining speech breathing differences found between the 7-year-old group and the older age groups, as well as among the older age groups, were not interpreted to be directly related to subject age. Rather, these differences were believed to be linked to the size of the speech production apparatus, speech fluency, and cognitive-linguistic skill (including oral-reading skill). Puberty did not prove to have a significant influence on speech breathing, given that the major changes in speech breathing took place prior to the onset of puberty, sometime between the ages of 7 and 10 years.

Hoit et al. (1990) had the opportunity to compare performance of the children and adolescents in their study with those from the 25-year-old men (Hoit & Hixon, 1987) and 25-year-old women (Hoit, Hixon, Altman, & Morgan, 1989) previously studied using similar procedures. Results indicated that speech breathing is adult-like (in pattern, but not in absolute volumes) with respect to rib cage wall volume, abdominal wall volume, and lung volume events by age 10, and with respect to events related to syllable production by age 16. It would appear, then, that there are two types of refinement in speech breathing, one having to do with control of the breathing apparatus and one having to do with control of cognitive-linguistic function. Hoit et al. (1990) concluded that general background control of the breathing apparatus for speech production is mature long before the breathing apparatus and its downstream valves and airways have reached their adult size and prior to the attainment of adult-level linguistic abilities. Apparently, control of the breathing apparatus, once established, is maintained and is relatively unperturbed by the ongoing changes in structure and the continuing elaboration of spoken communication skill that accompany late childhood and adolescence.

REVIEW

Speaking is a special act of breathing, one of many that the breathing apparatus performs.

Both relaxation pressure and muscular pressure are involved in the control of speech breathing.

The muscular pressure required at any moment during speech production depends on the relaxation pressure available at the prevailing lung volume and the targeted alveolar pressure.

Each alveolar pressure produced during speech production requires a different muscular pressure at each lung volume.

The activity of individual parts of the chest wall (rib cage wall, diaphragm, and abdominal wall) may change for the generation of different alveolar pressures at different lung volumes during speech production.

The control strategy for running speech breathing is distinct from that for other forms of breathing and is designed to enhance function during both the inspiratory and expiratory phases of the breathing cycle to facilitate oral communication.

Speech breathing is highly adaptive and accommodates to changing ventilatory and mechanical demands, sometimes with and sometimes without conscious awareness on the part of the speaker.

Speech breathing is influenced by body position, primarily because gravity affects the relaxation pressure of the breathing apparatus, the resting level of the apparatus, and the mechanical advantages of different parts of the chest wall.

Changes in gravity, load factor, and hydrostatic pressure differential within the abdomen (as in water immersion) can significantly influence the adjustments required to meet speech breathing demands.

People hyperventilate when they speak, as evidenced from measures of ventilation (more air moved into and out of the breathing apparatus during speaking than during resting tidal breathing) and from measures reflecting gas exchange (less carbon dioxide in expired air associated with speaking than associated with resting tidal breathing).

When the drive-to-breathe becomes strong enough to compete with the drive-to-speak, such as during exercise or when inspiring high levels of carbon dioxide, speech breathing is a difficult task to perform and is characterized by large volumes, high flows, and a limited quantity of speech per breath group.

Cognitive-linguistic factors influence speech breathing in a variety of ways that include when an inspiration will occur, what depth the inspiration will be, how long the following expiration (speaking) will be, how often silent pauses (both breath holding and expiratory pauses) will occur, and how much speech will be produced per breath group.

Conversational speech breathing is strongly influenced by the conversational partner and the nature of the interaction between partners, with both long-term and short-term synchronies being established.

Body type has a significant influence on speech breathing, with individuals high in relative fatness (endomorphic) showing a high degree of abdominal wall participation, individuals high in relative linearity (ectomorphic) showing a high degree of rib cage wall participation, and individuals high in relative musculoskel-etal development (mesomorphic) showing a mixture of these behaviors.

Age-related changes in speech breathing begin to appear in the seventh or eighth decade of life (as a compensation for the reduced valving economy of downstream structures) and take the form of larger lung volume and rib cage wall volume initiations, larger lung volume and rib cage wall volume excursions, and greater average volume expenditures of air per syllable.

Sex does not significantly affect speech breathing in that women and men show similar speech breathing patterns at similar ages when measures are normalized to take size into account.

Speech breathing emerges over a protracted period, is characterized by a high degree of variability in performance, involves a control mechanism that is distinct from those for nonspeech breathing activities, is the same for boys and girls, and has not yet resolved into consistent patterns as late as 3 years of age.

Speech breathing undergoes refinement throughout childhood and adolescence, with its adult-like motor skill component being nearly fully achieved by 10 years of age and before the onset of puberty, and its cognitive-linguistic skill component being nearly fully achieved by 16 years of age.

REFERENCES

Abel, H., Mottau, B., Klubendorf, D., & Koepchen, H. (1987). Pattern of different components of the respiratory cycle and autonomic parameters during speech. In G. Sieck, S. Gandevia, & W. Cameron (Eds.), *Respiratory muscles and their neuromotor control* (pp. 109-113). New York, NY: Alan R. Liss.

Agostoni, E., Gurtner, G., Torri, G., & Rahn, H. (1966). Respiratory mechanics during submersion and negative pressure breathing. *Journal of Applied Physiology, 21,* 251-258.

Agostoni, E., & Mead, J. (1964). Statics of the respiratory system. In W. Fenn & H. Rahn (Eds.), *Handbook of physiology. Respiration 1, Section 3* (pp. 387-409). Washington, DC: American Physiological Society.

Bailey, E., & Hoit, J. (2002). Speaking and breathing in high respiratory drive. *Journal of Speech, Language, and Hearing Research, 45,* 89-99.

Banzett, R., & Mead, J. (1995). Reflex compensation for changes in operational length in inspiratory muscles. In C. Roussos (Ed.), *The thorax* (2nd ed.), Vol. 85, Part A (pp. 987-1006), in the series C. Lenfant (Ed.), *Lung biology in health and disease.* New York, NY: Marcel Dekker.

Bernthal, J., & Beukelman, D. (1978). Intraoral air pressure during the production of /p/ and /b/ by children, youths, and adults. *Journal of Speech and Hearing Research, 21,* 361-371.

Boliek, C., Hixon, T., Watson, P., & Morgan, W. (1996). Vocalization and breathing during the first year of life. *Journal of Voice, 10,* 1-22.

Boliek, C., Hixon, T., Watson, P., & Morgan, W. (1997). Vocalization and breathing during the second and third years of life. *Journal of Voice, 11,* 373-390.

Bouhuys, A., Proctor, D., & Mead, J. (1966) Kinetic aspects of singing. *Journal of Applied Physiology, 21,* 483-496.

Bunn, J., & Mead, J. (1971). Control of ventilation during speech. *Journal of Applied Physiology, 31,* 870-872.

Carter, J. (1980). *The Heath-Carter somatotype method* (3rd ed.). San Diego, CA: San Diego State University Press.

Chapple, E. (1970). *Culture and biological man.* New York, NY: Holt, Rinehart, and Winston.

Connaghan, K., Moore, C., & Higashakawa, M. (2004). Respiratory kinematics during vocalization and nonspeech respiration in children from 9 to 48 months. *Journal of Speech, Language, and Hearing Research, 47,* 70-84.

Conrad, B., Thalacker, S., & Schonle, P. (1983). Speech respiration as an indicator of integrative contextual processing. *Folia Phoniatrica, 35,* 220-225.

Denny, M. (2000). Periodic variation in inspiratory volume characterizes speech as well as breathing. *Journal of Voice, 10,* 23-38.

Doust, J., & Patrick, J. (1981). The limitation of exercise ventilation during speech. *Respiration Physiology, 46,* 137-147.

Goldman-Eisler, F. (1955). Speech-breathing activity – A measure of tension and affect during interviews. *British Journal of Psychology, 29,* 53-63.

Goldman-Eisler, F. (1956). The determinants of the rate of speech output and their mutual relations. *Journal of Psychosomatic Research, 1,* 137-143.

Greene, J. (1984). Speech preparation processes and verbal fluency. *Human Communication Research, 11*, 61-84.

Greene, J., & Cappella, J. (1986). Cognition and talk: The relationship of semantic units to temporal patterns of fluency in spontaneous speech. *Language and Speech, 29*, 141-157.

Grosjean, F., & Collins, M. (1979). Breathing, pausing, and reading. *Phonetica, 36*, 98-114.

Hale, M., & Patrick, J. (1987). Ventilatory patterns during human speech in progressive hypercapnia. *Journal of Physiology, 394*, 60P.

Henderson, A., Goldman-Eisler, F., & Skarbek, A. (1965). Temporal patterns of cognitive activity and breath control in speech. *Language and Speech, 8*, 236-242.

Hixon, T. (1973). Respiratory function in speech. In F. Minifie, T. Hixon, & F. Williams (Eds.), *Normal aspects of speech, hearing, and language* (pp. 75-125). Englewood-Cliffs, NJ: Prentice-Hall Publishers, Inc.

Hixon, T., Goldman, M., & Mead, J. (1973). Kinematics of the chest wall during speech production: Volume displacements of the rib cage, abdomen, and lung. *Journal of Speech and Hearing Research, 16*, 78-115.

Hixon, T., Mead, J., & Goldman, M. (1976). Dynamics of the chest wall during speech production: Function of the thorax, rib cage, diaphragm, and abdomen. *Journal of Speech and Hearing Research, 19*, 297-356.

Hixon, T., & Weismer, G. (1995). Perspectives on the Edinburgh study of speech breathing. *Journal of Speech and Hearing Research, 38,* 42-60.

Hodge, M., & Rochet, A. (1989). Characteristics of speech breathing in young women. *Journal of Speech and Hearing Research, 32*, 466-480.

Hoit, J. (1994). A critical analysis of speech breathing data from the University of Queensland. *Journal of Speech and Hearing Research, 37*, 572-582.

Hoit, J., & Hixon, T. (1986). Body type and speech breathing. *Journal of Speech and Hearing Research, 29*, 313-324.

Hoit, J., & Hixon, T. (1987). Age and speech breathing. *Journal of Speech and Hearing Research, 30*, 351-366.

Hoit. J., & Hixon, T. (1992). Age and laryngeal airway resistance during vowel production in women. *Journal of Speech and Hearing Research, 35*, 309-313.

Hoit. J., Hixon, T., Altman, M., & Morgan, W. (1989). Speech breathing in women. *Journal of Speech and Hearing Research, 32*, 353-365.

Hoit, J., Hixon, T., Watson, P., & Morgan, W. (1990). Speech breathing in children and adolescents. *Journal of Speech and Hearing Research, 33*, 51-69.

Hoit, J., & Lohmeier, H. (2000). Influence of continuous speaking on ventilation. *Journal of Speech, Language, and Hearing Research, 43*, 1240-1251.

Hoit, J., & Lohmeier, H. (2002). No postscript needed: A post postscript on Russell, Cerny, and Stathopoulos (2002). *Journal of Speech, Language, and Hearing Research, 45*, 1138-1140.

Horii, Y., & Cooke, P. (1978). Some airflow, volume, and duration characteristics of oral reading. *Journal of Speech and Hearing Research, 21*, 470-481.

Lay, C., & Paivio, A. (1969). The effects of task difficulty and anxiety on hesitations in speech. *Canadian Journal of Behavioral Sciences, 1*, 25-37.

McFarland, D. (2001). Respiratory markers of conversational interaction. *Journal of Speech, Language, and Hearing Research, 44*, 128-143.

McFarland, D., & Smith, A. (1992). Effect of vocal task and respiratory phase on prephonatory chest wall movements. *Journal of Speech and Hearing Research, 35*, 971-982.

Meanock, C., & Nicholls, A. (1982). The effect of speech on the ventilatory response to carbon dioxide or to exercise. *Journal of Physiology, 325*, 16P-17P.

Melcon, M., Hoit, J., & Hixon, T. (1989). Age and laryngeal airway resistance during vowel production. *Journal of Speech and Hearing Disorders, 54*, 282-286.

Mitchell, H., Hoit, J., & Watson, P. (1996). Cognitive-linguistic demands and speech breathing. *Journal of Speech and Hearing Research, 39*, 93-104.

Moore, C., Caulfield, T., & Green, J. (2001). Relative kinematics of the rib cage and abdomen during speech and nonspeech behaviors of 15-month-old children. *Journal of Speech, Language, and Hearing Research, 44*, 80-94.

Otis, A., & Clark, R. (1968). Ventilatory implications of phonation and phonatory implications of ventilation. In A. Bouhuys (Ed.), *Sound production in man* (pp. 122-128). New York, NY: Annals of the New York Academy of Sciences.

Phillipson, E., McClean, P., Sullivan, C., & Zamel, N. (1978). Interaction of metabolic and behavioral respiratory control during hypercapnia and speech. *American Review of Respiratory Disease, 117*, 903-909.

Reid, M., Banzett, R., Feldman, H., & Mead, J. (1985). Reflex compensation of spontaneous breathing when immersion changes diaphragm length. *Journal of Applied Physiology, 58*, 1136-1142.

Reid, M., Loring, S., Banzett, R., & Mead J. (1986). Passive mechanics of upright human chest wall during immersion from hips to neck. *Journal of Applied Physiology, 60*, 1561-1570.

Reynolds, A., & Paivio, A. (1968). Cognitive and emotional determinants of speech. *Canadian Journal of Psychology, 22*, 164-175.

Rochester, S. (1973). The significance of pauses in spontaneous speech. *Journal of Psycholinguistic Research, 2*, 51-81.

Russell, B., Cerny, F., & Stathopoulos, E. (1998). Effects of varied vocal intensity on ventilation and energy expenditure in women and men. *Journal of Speech, Language, and Hearing Research, 41*, 239-248.

Russell, N., & Stathopoulos, E. (1988). Lung volume changes in children and adults during speech production. *Journal of Speech and Hearing Research, 31*, 146-155.

Siegman, A., & Pope, B. (1966). Ambiguity and verbal fluency in the TAT. *Jour-

nal of Consulting Psychology, 30, 239-245.

Smitheran, J., & Hixon, T. (1981). A clinical method for estimating laryngeal airway resistance during vowel production. *Journal of Speech and Hearing Disorders, 46,* 138-146.

Sperry, E., & Klich, R. (1992). Speech breathing in senescent and younger women during oral reading. *Journal of Speech and Hearing Research, 35,* 1246-1255.

Stathopoulos, E. (1986). Relationship between intraoral air pressure and vocal intensity in children and adults. *Journal of Speech and Hearing Research, 29,* 71-74.

Stathopoulos, E., & Sapienza, C. (1993). Respiratory and laryngeal measures of children during vocal intensity variation. *Journal of the Acoustical Society of America, 94,* 2531-2543.

Stathopoulos, E., & Weismer, G. (1985). Oral airflow and intraoral air pressure: A comparative study of children, youths, and adults. *Folia Phoniatrica, 37,* 152-159.

Sugito, M., Ohyama, G., & Hirose, H. (1990). A preliminary study on pauses and breaths in reading speech materials. *Annual Bulletin of the Research Institute of Logopedics and Phoniatrics, 24,* 121-130.

Taylor, I. (1969). Content and structure in sentence production. *Journal of Verbal Learning and Verbal Behavior, 8,* 170-175.

Warner, R., Waggener, T., & Kronauer, R. (1983). Synchronized cycles in ventilation and vocal activity during spontaneous conversational speech. *Journal of Applied Physiology, 54,* 309-317.

Warren, D., Morr, K., Rochet, A., & Dalston, R. (1989). Respiratory response to a decrease in velopharyngeal resistance. *Journal of the Acoustical Society of America, 86,* 917-924.

Webb, R., Williams, F., & Minifie, F. (1967). Effects of verbal decision behavior upon respiration during speech production. *Journal of Speech and Hearing Research, 10,* 49-56.

Whalen, D., & Kinsella-Shaw, J. (1997). Exploring the relationship of inspiration duration to utterance duration. *Phonetica, 54,* 138-152.

Wilder, C. (1983). Chest wall preparation for phonation in female speakers. In D. Bless & J. Abbs (Eds.), *Vocal fold physiology: Contemporary research and clinical issues* (pp. 109-123). San Diego, CA: College-Hill Press.

Winkworth, A., Davis, P., Adams, R., & Ellis, E. (1995). Breathing patterns during spontaneous speech. *Journal of Speech and Hearing Research, 38,* 124-144.

Winkworth, A., Davis, P., Ellis, E., & Adams, R. (1994). Variability and consistency in speech breathing during reading: Lung volumes, speech intensity, and linguistic factors. *Journal of Speech and Hearing Research, 37,* 535-556.

Wolff, P. (1979). Theoretical issues in the development of motor skills. *Symposium on developmental disabilities in the pre-school child.* Chicago, Ill: Johnson and Johnson Baby Products.

chapter four

Evaluation of Speech Breathing

INTRODUCTION

This chapter focuses on the evaluation of speech breathing. Although issues pertinent to overall evaluation are discussed, only those that are directly related to breathing are covered in depth. Those who are new to the field of speech-language pathology, or who are otherwise unfamiliar with the components of a speech evaluation, should supplement their reading through other sources.

This chapter proceeds with a brief description of the nature of the task involved in the evaluation of speech breathing, followed by a description of the types of clients that present with speech breathing disorders. Next, discussion centers on breathing-related aspects of the case history. Then, consideration is given to the auditory-perceptual examination of speech breathing and the evaluation of speaking-related dyspnea. Thereafter, physical examination of the breathing apparatus is described, followed by discussion of instrumental examination of speech breathing. The chapter concludes with suggestions for a bedside screening of speech breathing.

NATURE OF THE TASK

A speech breathing evaluation should accomplish several goals. It should first help the clinician determine if a speech breathing disorder exists. If it turns out that it does not, this portion of the evaluation would be complete and the speech-language pathologist would move on to examine other speech production subsystems and seek other potential sources for the client's speech-related problems. If, however, a speech breathing disorder is identified, the evaluation should provide qualitative and quantitative information that enables the clinician to draw meaningful conclusions about its nature and severity.

A thorough and carefully performed speech breathing evaluation should reveal the status and functional capabilities of a client's breathing apparatus. At the completion of a speech breathing evaluation, the clinician should be equipped to do the following: (a) offer a reasonable diagnosis when appropriate; (b) develop a rational, effective, and efficient management plan; (c) monitor the client's progress over the course of management; and (d) provide a reasonable prognosis as to the extent and speed of improvement to be expected. A competently performed and documented evaluation will serve the client well by providing information important to his care. Such an evaluation may also be important if legal testimony is required to address personal injury or malpractice claims.

Speech breathing evaluation is often not an easy task. One reason is that speech breathing disorders do not always exist in isolation, but are often accompanied by disorders in other parts of the speech production apparatus. In such cases, the speech-language pathologist must sort out the contribution of the breathing apparatus from the contributions of the larynx and/or upper airway. One focus of this chapter is to suggest strategies for doing this.

Another reason that a speech breathing evaluation may be challenging is that a client's behavior is often not a manifestation of disease alone, but also reflects his adaptation to disease. Part of the evaluation task, therefore, is to sort out the direct influence of the disease from what the client may be doing to cope with the disease. It is especially important to determine if the client's coping behaviors are maladaptive. If they are, such behaviors may need to be managed.

Finally, clients with speech breathing disorders may pose special challenges for still other reasons. For example, clients with cognitive impairments may not be able to follow instructions or accurately report their symptoms or perceptions. This complicates the evaluation, as well as the client's management.

CLIENTS

Clients with speech breathing disorders come in many forms. They encompass the human life span and include both sexes. Their speech breathing disorders can have a wide range of causes, as discussed below.

Some speech breathing disorders have functional bases. That is, there may not be an identifiable organic sign that explains a client's speech breathing behavior. Functional misuse of the breathing apparatus may be observed in clients who use speech extensively in their work activities, such as salespersons, teachers, preachers, sportscasters, newscasters, actors, and singers. Functional misuse disorders may manifest as undesirable speech breathing habits. Such habits are often straightforward to evaluate and manage. Clients who exhibit them are usually motivated to change them because their livelihoods may be at stake. Of course, not everyone with a functional misuse disorder relies extensively on speech for work activities. Some clients show up without employment-threatening complaints, but with complaints nonetheless.

Some speech breathing disorders have functional bases, but are not necessarily related to misuse of the breathing apparatus. Most of these have a psychogenic disorder at their root. Examples include malingering (pretending to be ill or injured) and conversion reaction (loss of voluntary control over sensory or motor functions as a result of emotional conflict). Malingering may be used for personal gain, whereas conversion reaction may somatize (convert to physical dysfunction) some psychic pain. Malingering may present a significant forensic challenge for the speech-language pathologist. Conversion reaction may be even more challenging, because it can masquerade in a variety of signs and symptoms.

Other speech breathing disorders have structural bases. Many of these are congenital and relate to maldevelopment of the skeletal framework of the breathing apparatus. Examples include pectus excavatum (funnel chest), pectus carinatum (pigeon chest), and bifid sternum (split breastbone), all of which can influence speech breathing performance when severe. Others include scoliosis (abnormal lateral curvature of the spine), kyphosis (abnormal posterior concavity of the spine), and spina bifida (defective closure of the bony encasement of the spinal cord). Skeletal fractures, displacements, and acquired deformities (through injury or disease) may also contribute to speech breathing disorders, as may the sequelae of certain surgical procedures (e.g., breast amputation). Structural problems such as these are often accompanied by compensatory behaviors. Such behaviors are often beneficial. However, sometimes compensatory behaviors limit the client's performance and may need to be addressed in management.

A structural problem not included in the present discussion is the surgical removal of the larynx (i.e., laryngectomy). Although a client with a laryngectomy could be classified as having a speech breathing disorder because he has a tracheostomy (opening in the anterior neck), the source of the disorder is not the breathing apparatus proper. Therefore, speech breathing associated with laryngectomy is not discussed in this book.

Speech breathing disorders may also be associated with chronic diseases of the pulmonary airways and lungs. Those that accompany asthma, emphysema, or sarcoidosis are examples. The first two obstruct the flow of air and impair gas exchange, especially emphysema, whereas the last one stiffens the lungs and increases the work of breathing. Clients with diseases such as these often complain of breathing discomfort (dyspnea) and may alter their breathing behavior in attempts to relieve their discomfort. Speech breathing problems can be so severe that they limit vocational options. For example, teachers with pulmonary disease have been known to retire early because of speaking-related breathing discomfort (Lee, Loudon, Jacobson, & Stuebing, 1993).

The most common types of speech breathing disorders are those with neuromotor bases. Neuromotor disorders come in many forms and result from maldevelopment, injury, or disease (often progressive) that affects the nervous system and/or the muscle system. Nervous system and/or muscle system problems may impair function of the breathing apparatus alone, but often they also impair function of other subsystems of the speech production apparatus. Nervous system disorders can also cause sensory dysfunction. For example, impairment of the ability to sense position and movement of the breathing apparatus may affect the control of speech breathing. Impairment of hearing sensitivity is another example of sensory dysfunction that can influence the control of speech breathing.

There are many neuromotor disorders that can impair speech breathing. Cerebral palsy, in its different forms, is an example of a neuromotor disorder caused by maldevelopment. Cerebral palsy is associated with high-risk births and can affect speech breathing from infancy to senescence. Spinal cord injury, most prevalent in young men, can have a profound influence on speech breathing behavior. Numerous nonprogressive and progressive diseases and conditions can cause neuromotor-based speech breathing disorders. Examples of these include muscular dystrophy, peripheral neuropathy, stroke, Parkinson disease, multiple sclerosis, amyotrophic lateral sclerosis, tumors, and many others. The array of breathing signs attendant to such disorders is diverse. Commonly encountered ones include weakness, inaccurate movement, dyscoordinated movement, and involuntary movement.

Finally, there are conditions that cause impairments of the breathing apparatus that are so severe that the client must rely on a ventilator to sustain life. Clients with high cervical spinal cord injury, certain progressive neuromotor diseases, or severe chronic obstructive pulmonary disease are examples of those who may require a ventilator. Clients who use ventilators present a special challenge because evaluation and management considerations require that the client and the ventilator be viewed as a single system (see Chapter 6).

SPEECH BREATHING CASE HISTORY

The case history is a critical part of any speech-language evaluation and much has been written about how to obtain a case history. It is not the intent here to duplicate what others have already covered in depth. Rather, the present focus is on portions of the case history that pertain specifically to breathing and speech breathing. The material presented in this section can be used to supplement existing case history procedures and forms.

The way in which a case history is obtained is influenced by how much information is already available. There are times when the speech-language pathologist knows almost nothing about a client, as with the client who arrives without a diagnosis, without medical records, or without any other information that would offer a point of departure in taking the case history. Alternatively, a client may have a confirmed diagnosis and medical records that document a condition that appears to be causally related to his speech breathing disorder. In a sense, a confirmed diagnosis makes the taking of the case history easier. However, it also increases the possibility that the clinician may jump to the conclusion that the given diagnosis is the only cause of the client's speech breathing disorder and, thereby, fail to explore other important avenues.

Whenever possible, the client's history should be obtained using an interview format. An interview format offers the clinician access to information communicated verbally and nonverbally. The client's choice of words, tone of voice, hesitations, facial expressions, and body language all convey information that might otherwise be missed. Furthermore, it is during the case history interview that the clinician often has her first chance to listen to the client's speech and begin the auditory-perceptual examination.

Whenever possible, the case history should be obtained directly from the client. Nevertheless, there are situations in which case histories must be obtained from someone else. Usually this someone else is a parent, in the case of a child, or a spouse, in the case of an adult. Exactly how the questions and probes are formed depends on who is being interviewed. For purposes of the discussion to follow, it is assumed that the speech-language pathologist has no prior information about the client, that the case history is obtained using an interview format, and that the client is an adult who is able to provide the information requested.

Items in the speech breathing case history are given in Form 4-1 at the end of the chapter. They are divided into the following sections: (a) alerting signs and symptoms; (b) airway risk factors; (c) medical evaluations, diagnoses, and treatments; (d) breathing and speaking experiences; and (e) client perceptions of speech breathing. Each section includes space to write explanatory comments.

The speech breathing case history interview begins with the clinician stating that she will be asking the client about his breathing and that breathing

> **YOU CAN OBSERVE A LOT JUST BY WATCHIN'**
>
> This is our favorite of all the quotes attributed to former New York Yankees baseball player Yogi Berra. We often repeat it to students who encounter types of clinical cases that seem not to have been dealt with in the literature. Where do I go to read about this? How should I structure my evaluation? Where will I find the best management ideas? Can you tell me what to do? Well, these are the times that speech-language pathology is really fun. Novelty challenges you. So, you shouldn't always expect cases to fit nicely into the conceptual bins you've made for yourself. These are times when you let your experiences, your occult faculties, and your good judgment step back together and "observe a lot just by watchin'." Apply the principles you're learning one at a time. Slow down and attend to the person in front of you. Nobody else will encounter a case exactly like this one. Yogi knew what he was talking about.

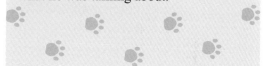

may or may not be related to his speech problems (see language near the top of Form 4-1). Such a statement is intended to give the client an unbiased context in which to respond to queries. Without such a statement, the client may feel compelled to report breathing problems merely to please the clinician.

Alerting Signs and Symptoms

The first section of the speech breathing case history is designed to identify signs and symptoms that could alert the clinician to potential respiratory, laryngeal, cardiac, and neural problems. Specifically, the clinician asks the client if he has recently experienced any of the following: (a) frequent coughing; (b) persistent hoarse voice; (c) coughing up mucus; (d) coughing up blood; (e) wheezing in the chest; (f) difficulty breathing; (g) chest pain or chest ache; and (h) numbness, weakness, coordination problems, or involuntary movements. These items cover a broad range of problems that require medical referral. If the client answers affirmatively to any of the items listed, referral should be made to the appropriate specialty physician. If a client reports chest pain or chest ache, referral should be made to a cardiologist. If there is a report of coughing up mucus, referral should be made to a pulmonologist. If there is a report of a persistent hoarse voice, referral should be made to a laryngologist. And, if there is a report of numbness, weakness, or other potential neural signs or symptoms, referral should be made to a neurologist. A client may answer affirmatively to more than one of these items. For example, he might report wheezing in the chest and chest ache, paired sign and symptom that might be indicative of congestive heart failure. Or he might report wheezing and coughing up mucus, paired signs that might be indicative of chronic bronchitis. The first report might suggest referral to a cardiologist, whereas the second might suggest referral to a pulmonologist. Coughing up blood (i.e., hemoptysis) can be especially serious and demands immediate medical attention from an emergency room physician.

Airway Risk Factors

The next section is designed to ascertain the client's airway risk factors. Included in this section are questions regarding smoking history and exposure to environmental irritants, significant contributing factors in obstructive pulmonary disease. The questions on smoking ("Have you ever smoked?" "If so, when did you start smoking?" etc.) are designed so that the clinician can calculate the client's smoking history in pack years (the number of packs per day times the number of years). For example, 2 packs a day for 10 years is 20 pack years. The questions on airway irritants are included because the client's responses may influence the management plan. When pursuing this line of questioning, the clinician should appear as nonjudgmental as possible. If the client senses that the clinician disapproves of smoking, for example, he may not be forthright in his answers.

Medical Evaluations, Diagnoses, and Treatments

Medical evaluations, diagnoses, and treatments are the topics covered in the third section of the speech breathing case history. This section begins with asking the client if he has seen any of several healthcare professionals, including a pulmonologist, laryngologist, cardiologist, neurologist, respiratory therapist, physical therapist, and speech-language pathologist. If the client responds affirmatively, additional information should be sought about the outcome of any evaluation and the nature of any management. It may also be necessary for the clinician to obtain relevant names and contact information so that she can request records.

The next item in this section includes the lead-in question "Has a doctor ever diagnosed you with any of the following?" The wording of this question is such that it is meant to discourage the client from merely rendering his own opinion regarding the nature of his condition. The list of possible diagnoses is designed to reveal the client's medical history with emphasis on breathing, cardiac, and neural conditions. This list of diagnoses is long, but not exhaustive. Brief descriptions of each are given below. Some are adapted from Kersten (1989).

- Hay fever (or pollen allergy) is an allergic reaction affecting the upper airway. It can result in nasal airway obstruction and hyponasal and/or denasal voice quality.

- Asthma is constriction of the pulmonary airways (both large and small) usually caused by allergic reaction and often resulting in coughing, wheezing, and shortness of breath.

- Chronic bronchitis is characterized by excess mucus production and structural alterations of the bronchi and is caused by smoking, air pollution, environmental irritants, infection, and genetic factors.

- Emphysema is characterized by destruction of the alveolar walls and enlargement of air spaces and is caused by the same factors as chronic bronchitis.

- Chronic obstructive pulmonary disease (COPD) is a nonspecific term that includes chronic bronchitis and emphysema.

- Cystic fibrosis is a genetic disease that affects many body organs, including the lungs, and causes excess secretion of abnormal mucus and airway obstruction.

- Pneumothorax is the presence of gas in the space between the visceral and parietal pleura and is often caused by trauma.

- Arthritis (in shoulders, spine, or hips) is inflammation of joints. When it occurs in joints of the torso, it can restrict movements of the breathing apparatus.

- Scoliosis or kyphosis (or kyphoscoliosis) is a progressive musculoskeletal deformity which results in angulation of the spine and can limit and alter movements of the breathing apparatus.

- Pneumonia is an inflammation of lung tissue and is usually accompanied by fluid-filled alveoli. There are infectious and noninfectious causes of pneumonia.

WHEEZE

Asthma is a complex disorder. How you get it is an intriguing mystery. Children who grow up on farms have significant protection against asthma compared to their counterparts who grow up in cities. Believe it or not, livestock, poultry, dogs, and cats are believed to confer some of this protection. Most people confronted with this possibility find it to be counterintuitive. You might think it would be just the opposite, with children from farms having less protection against asthma than children from cities. Current medical thought has it that the development of the immune system is important in the prevention of asthma (Martinez, 2001). Just as your eyes need light and your ears need sound to develop normally, so it seems that your immune system must have endotoxins to develop normally. More insults lead to more rapid development. That is, you get more experience in fending things off. All of this is great news for animals lovers like us.

• Diffuse interstitial fibrosis is a general term encompassing a variety of conditions associated with thickening or fibrosis (scarring) of the alveolar interstitium (connective tissue located between the alveoli and capillaries).

• Coccidioidomycosis (or valley fever) is primarily a disease of the lungs that is common in the southwestern United States and is caused by a fungus. Fatigue, cough, chest pain, and generalized muscle and joint aches are signs and symptoms.

• Tuberculosis (often called TB) is an infectious disease that usually attacks the lungs. Signs and symptoms can include cough, chest pain, fatigue, weight loss, and fever.

• Tumor in the lung or chest cavity can be benign or malignant. The degree to which it restricts lung volume depends on its size and location.

• Pulmonary edema is extra fluid in the lungs, a common complication of cardio-pulmonary disease. It is life-threatening in its acute form.

• Congestive heart failure is a condition in which the pumping action of the heart weakens and causes a reduction in blood circulation and a build-up of fluid in the lungs and other body tissues.

• Adult respiratory distress syndrome (ARDS) is a nonspecific term for conditions causing injury to the alveolar capillary units with consequences similar to pulmonary edema.

• Pulmonary embolism is an embolic occlusion (e.g., blood clot, air bubble) of pulmonary blood vessels. It can cause hypotension and rapid, shallow breathing.

• Muscular dystrophy is a genetic disease of the muscles that causes weakness or paralysis.

• Myasthenia gravis is an autoimmune disease that destroys receptors for acetylcholine (a neurotransmitter that stimulates skeletal muscle contraction) and causes weakness or paralysis.

• Amyotrophic lateral sclerosis (ALS, or Lou Gehrig's disease) is characterized by death of motor neurons throughout the nervous system and causes weakness or paralysis.

• Post-polio syndrome is characterized by progressive weakness that begins decades after apparent recovery from poliomyelitis.

• Multiple sclerosis causes destruction of myelin in the central nervous system which can result in weakness, dyscoordination, and sensory changes.

• Parkinson disease is caused by death of selected neurons in the basal nuclei and can be associated with muscle rigidity, paucity of movement, tremor, and impaired scaling of motor commands.

• Dystonia is caused by abnormalities in the basal nuclei and is characterized by sustained contraction of muscles. Dystonia can cause breathing difficulty if contractions occur in the muscles of the breathing apparatus or larynx.

• Tremor is caused by central nervous system dysfunction and is characterized by rhythmic oscillations of muscle activity. Tremor can affect breathing if it is manifested in the muscles of the breathing apparatus.

• Stroke is a vascular event that can cause hemiplegia or quadriplegia and concomitant weakness or paralysis of the muscles of the breathing apparatus.

• Spinal cord injury can cause weakness or paralysis of the muscles of the breathing apparatus, the extent of which depends on the location of the injury.

• Other breathing disease, other heart disease, and other nervous system disease are general terms that are designed to elicit other diagnoses not included in the present list of terms.

If the client answers "yes" to any of these diagnoses, the clinician should request additional information. "When were you given this diagnosis?" "Who gave you this diagnosis?" "Were you treated for it?" If yes, "What was the treatment?" and "Was it successful?" The latter two should elicit responses regarding medications, surgeries, and, perhaps, alternative treatments such as vitamin therapy, massage, and acupuncture, among others. In certain cases (e.g., asthma), follow-up questions might include, "Are there certain times of day that it is better or worse?" "Are there certain situations that make it better or worse?" "Is it generally getting better, getting worse, or staying the same?" It also may be informative to ask if any of these conditions show up in the family history. If so, inquire as to which family members have or had the condition. It is sometimes revealing to ask the client, "Do you have any other medical problems that might affect the way you breathe?" in case a contributing condition has been overlooked. The client is also asked "Do you have any psychological conditions that might affect the way you breathe?" For example, the client might have panic attacks that affect breathing. Even if the client denies psychological problems, it is prudent to probe for any psychogenic issues that might be causal or associated with a speech breathing disorder.

The next few questions concern relevant medications, surgeries, and other treatments that might relate to speech breathing. Responses to these questions can have important implications for management. For example, if a client's breathing comfort fluctuates with medication dosage, it may be necessary to teach the client one speaking strategy for periods of comfortable breathing and another speaking strategy for periods of uncomfortable breathing. As another example, if a client has had surgical implantation of a feeding tube, he would not be a candidate for management with certain forms of abdominal support. The presence of a tracheostomy may influence certain aspects of speech breathing evaluation and management, as may the use of oxygen, an abdominal wall binder, or a back support. It is relevant to note that abdominal wall binders are used to help control hypotension in certain clients, such as those with cervical spinal cord injury. The presence of such a binder also alters the mechanical behavior of the breathing apparatus and may provide a fruitful option for management in some clients (see section on mechanical aids in Chapter 5).

Breathing and Speaking Experiences

The next section focuses on the client's breathing and speaking experiences. The first question, "Do you ever have problems with your breathing?" is a critical one. This question is designed to allow the client to describe, in his own words, any breathing problems he has experienced or is currently experiencing. In clients who are knowledgeable about their problems and are gregarious, this question can elicit a great deal of information. The clinician should make note of any words and phrases used by the client to describe his breathing problems. In other clients, it will be necessary to probe further with additional questions. A series of follow-up questions is provided for this purpose to help the clinician understand the nature of the client's breathing problems. If the client denies having problems with his breathing, the clinician may skip the follow-up questions. However, if she suspects that the client is being less than forthcoming, she may want to ask a few of the follow-up questions as a way to probe further.

The second major question of this section is "Do you ever have problems with your breathing while speaking?" It is possible for the client to deny problems with breathing in general (first question), but report problems with breathing while speaking. Or he may report problems with neither or both. If the client answers affirmatively to this latter question, the clinician should continue queries along this line by asking the list of follow-up questions provided in the form.

The last few questions in this section are designed to glean additional information about the client's breathing and speaking experiences. They include questions about special training that might involve attention to breathing and about the client's speech intelligibility in various contexts. The question of "How well do people understand you when you speak?" requires that the client evaluate his speech from the listeners' perspective. Responses to this question can range from "They understand everything I say" to "I always have to repeat myself." Of course, such statements vary widely in their accuracy and should be verified by interviewing those with whom the client interacts. The client may report that communication with specific individuals is more difficult than with others, alerting the clinician to examine potentially important variables that could account for such differences (e.g., hearing loss in the listener, noise in the environment). For clients who report using a speech recognition system, the clinician should measure and document the accuracy with which the system recognizes the client's speech so that the effects of speech breathing management on its accuracy can be determined later.

The final two questions of this section are intentionally general and open-ended. The question "Is there anything else you would like to tell me about your breathing or your speech?" is included to give the client the opportunity to offer additional information that was not elicited by previous questions. This question can evoke an unexpected response (e.g., "I don't really care about my speech. I don't like to talk to people anyway."), or it can lead to additional discussion of a previously raised topic. In most cases, it will merely elicit a "No." The last question – "What do you hope I can do for you?"– introduces the topic of management and allows the client to express his desires and expectations regarding potential management goals. For example, the client might tell the clinician that he would like to be able to speak in longer sentences, speak well enough to go back to work, or be able to talk on the telephone with his grandson. Responses such as these should help in the development of the management plan.

> **A ROUND OF A-PAWS**
>
> Some clients who have physical impairments have canine companions that are trained to help them with routine daily activities. Such animals are usually under voice command. One of the questions of our evaluation protocol asks "How well do people understand you when you speak?" Those clients who have canine companions should also be asked "How well does your dog understand you when you speak?" Service dogs are an important part of the lives of people who have them and their motivational potential to improve a client's speech and/or language can be significant. Those with speech or language problems have been known to work on their problems more intently to better communicate their wishes to an animal helper. As a clinician, you should always be on the lookout for ways that a service dog might be able to help you achieve your clinical goals. Service dogs can be great speech-language pathology aids.

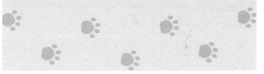

Client Perceptions of Speech Breathing

This final section should be administered to any client who reports that he experiences problems with his breathing. It should also be administered to a client who denies breathing discomfort, but who the clinician suspects may be withholding information or who may be unaware of his problems.

This part of the speech breathing evaluation allows the clinician to gain insight into the symptoms (client perceptions) associated with speech breathing disorders.

The remainder of the evaluation (auditory-perceptual examination, physical examination, and instrumental examination) is directed primarily toward revealing the signs (observable indicators) of speech breathing disorders. Sometimes symptoms and signs relate to each other in predictable ways, but sometimes they do not. A client may report only minor symptoms, but exhibit very deviant speech breathing signs. Or a client may report extreme speech breathing symptoms, but exhibit only mildly abnormal signs, or even no signs. A client may be so effective at compensating for the underlying disorder that his speech and associated speech breathing appear to be normal. If a client perceives problems with his speech breathing, it must be assumed that a speech breathing disorder exists, whether or not signs of a disorder are apparent to the clinician.

Dyspnea is the term often used in medical and scientific contexts to mean breathing discomfort. Dyspnea is an umbrella term that encompasses a wide variety of symptoms. Research on dyspnea has revealed that certain words and phrases tend to be associated with certain physiological and psychological states. The last section of Form 4-1 includes a list of dyspnea-related words and phrases designed to determine the nature of the client's dyspnea. For each percept listed, the client is asked, "Do you ever experience (*percept*) while speaking?" If the client responds that he does not experience a given percept, the item is left blank, and the clinician proceeds to the next item. If his response is affirmative, the item is checked (to the left of the word or phrase), and the client is asked, ". . . in what situation(s)?" Examples of client responses might be, "When I'm trying to walk and talk at the same time" or "When I have to speak for a long time" or "When I have to speak in front of people and I feel nervous." After noting the client's response on the form, the clinician then asks the client "How strong is the (*percept*)?" while offering him the choices of mild, moderate, severe, and intolerable (noted on the form as m, M, S, and I, respectively). The potential significance of affirmative responses to each percept is discussed below.

A "frequent awareness of breathing" can serve as a general alert that a client may be experiencing dyspnea. Healthy individuals are seldom conscious of their breathing, except during activities that require physical exertion (e.g., walking up stairs) or guided breathing (e.g., yoga exercises). Thus, an affirmative response to this item indicates that a problem may exist, but does not necessarily offer clues as to its nature. The client may mention that he thinks about his breathing more when he is not speaking. This may be because speaking acts as a cognitive distracter. Alternatively, awareness of breathing may be more pronounced during speaking because the performance demands are greater than for many other breathing activities.

The percepts "hunger for air," "uncomfortable urge to breathe," "breathlessness," and "shortness of breath" are usually judged to reflect similar phenomena. The advantage of including all of these terms is that a given client may find one to be more meaningful than the others. These percepts are most closely associated with changes in blood gas composition, such as elevation in the amount of carbon dioxide in the blood. Two potential sources for these percepts have been suggested (Banzett, Lansing, Reid, Adams, & Brown, 1989; Banzett, Lansing, Brown, Topulos, Yager, Steele, Londono, Loring, Reid, Adams, & Nations, 1990; Lansing, Im, Thwing, Legedza, & Banzett, 2000; Moosavi, Topulos, Hafer, Lansing, Adams, Brown, & Banzett, 2000). One suggestion is that they arise from chemoreceptor activity. Recall that chemoreceptors activate in response to changes in the amount of carbon dixoide and oxygen in the blood and elsewhere. Another suggestion is that they arise from motor commands originating in brainstem centers. It is believed that these commands are sent in parallel to breathing muscles (to increase ventilation) and to cortical sensory areas (where conscious perception occurs). This latter mechanism is called corollary discharge. Air hunger can be relieved by stimulation of mechanoreceptors in the pulmonary airways and lungs, such as occurs with the larger and faster breathing movements that accompany increased ventilation (Manning, Shea, Schwartzstein, Lansing, Brown, & Banzett, 1992). Percepts such as hunger for air, uncomfortable urge to breathe, breathlessness, and shortness of breath are commonly associated with cardiopulmonary disease, but can also be associated with many other conditions. Hunger for air and its related percepts are apt to place ventilation in competition with speaking (see section on drive-to-breathe and speech breathing in Chapter 3). If the percept becomes overwhelmingly strong, the client may cease to speak altogether so as to dedicate all resources to ventilation.

Dyspnea can also take on a character of increased work and effort. Two exemplars of work/effort percepts in the checklist are "hard work to breathe" and "high effort to breathe." The mechanisms underlying these work/effort percepts differ from those of hunger for air. These percepts appear to have two potential sources (Lansing et al., 2000). They may arise from chest wall muscle mechanoreceptor activity (activity that signals change in muscle length and tension), such as occurs with large and fast breathing movements. Work/effort percepts may also arise from corollary discharge from cortical motor centers (i.e., copies of cortical motor commands are sent to cortical sensory areas and are perceived). The corollary discharge hypothesis has received the most empirical support (Campbell, Gandevia, Killian, Mahutte, & Rigg, 1980; Gandevia, Killian, & Campbell, 1981; Moosavi et al., 2000). Work/effort-related percepts may signal pulmonary disease such as emphysema or asthma. Or they may signal neuromotor disease or injury that impairs the force production capabilities of chest wall muscles (e.g., muscular dystrophy or spinal cord injury) or the generation of appropriately scaled motor commands (e.g., Parkinson disease). The magnitude of work/effort may be especially great during speaking because greater muscular pressure is required for speaking than certain other breathing activities.

Closely related to work/effort percepts are those reflecting weakness and fatigue. The checklist items corresponding to this percept category are "weak breathing muscles" and "tired breathing muscles." Clients who respond affirmatively to the work/effort percepts will most likely respond affirmatively to weakness/fatigue percepts as well. Weakness and fatigue are often seen in association with neuro-motor disease, for example, myasthenia gravis.

A report of "difficulty breathing in" can be associated with a variety of breathing disorders. This percept could signal weakness of inspiratory muscles caused by neuromotor disease or injury. Or it could signal high airway resistance, such as that found in emphysema or asthma. In the case of emphysema, difficulty breathing in can be further exacerbated by the fact that clients with this disease tend to be chronically hyperinflated. Hyperinflation places inspiratory muscles at a mechanical disadvantage and also requires that inspiratory efforts be great enough to overcome high (expiratory) relaxation pressures. In all of these examples, difficulty breathing in is usually greater when inspiring rapidly than when inspiring slowly. This is because muscles must generate rapid pressure change and because airway resistance is greater (worse) at higher flows than at lower flows. Difficulty breathing in is also a cardinal symptom in clients with paradoxical vocal fold dysfunction. Paradoxical vocal fold dysfunction is characterized by adductory vocal fold movements during inspiration (paradoxical to the normal abductory vocal fold movements during inspiration) that result in constriction or occlusion of the airway with concomitant reduction or cessation of flow. This disorder is often misdiagnosed as asthma (Newman, Mason, & Schmaling, 1995). However, it differs from asthma in the following three ways: (a) asthma is associated with wheezing in the pulmonary airways, whereas paradoxical vocal fold dysfunction is associated with inspiratory stridor generated at the larynx; (b) asthma is characterized by difficulty breathing out, whereas paradoxical vocal fold dysfunction generally is not; and (c) asthma is sometimes associated with a hoarse voice (due to the asthma itself and/or to topical corticosteroids used in its treatment), whereas paradoxical vocal fold dysfunction generally is not. Nevertheless, it is important to note that individuals with paradoxical vocal fold dysfunction often have concomitant asthma (Newman et al., 1995). Paradoxical vocal fold dysfunction does not appear to have a single cause, but instead may be associated with a variety of neurogenic and psychogenic etiologies (Maschka, Bauman, McCray, Hoffman, Karnell, & Smith, 1997).

"Difficulty breathing out" could signal that a client has a condition that causes airway constriction during expiration, such as might occur with obstructive airway disease. Airway resistance associated with constriction is greater (worse) at higher flows. Difficulty breathing out could also signal expiratory muscle weakness, especially if such difficulty is experienced during high pressure/low flow expiratory events (e.g., singing, playing an oboe) or during expiration of the expiratory reserve volume.

If a client reports experiencing "tightness in chest," there is a strong possibility that the underlying cause is asthma (Simon, Schwartzstein, Weiss, Fencl, Teghtsoonian, & Weinberger, 1990). This percept probably arises from stimulation of pulmonary receptors secondary to active constriction of the airways. Asthma can also be associated with air hunger and work/effort percepts, especially as its severity increases (Schwartzstein & Cristiano, 1996).

"Difficulty coordinating breathing movements" usually has a neurogenic origin. Such coordination difficulties are sometimes associated with dyspnea. For example, dyspnea has been reported to accompany dystonia (a neurogenic disorder characterized by action-triggered sustained muscle contractions) when the contractions occur in muscles of the breathing apparatus and larynx (Braun, Abd, Baer, Blitzer, Stewart, & Brin, 1995). Dyscoordinated breathing movements can result from events such as inappropriate timing of diaphragm contraction (e.g., during expiration) or inappropriate adduction of the vocal folds (e.g., during inspiration). In a client with dystonia, the perception of difficulty coordinating breathing movements is commonly accompanied by a perception of increased breathing effort. Dyspnea is often greater during speech breathing than during other forms of breathing because speaking usually exacerbates the involuntary movements of dystonia. Examples of other disorders that might be accompanied by difficulty coordinating breathing movements include the following: (a) respiratory dyskinesia (seen in association with basal nuclei impairment); (b) respiratory dyspraxia (seen in association with cortical and subcortical damage to areas involved in motor planning); (c) respiratory ataxia (seen in association with cerebellar damage); (d) paradoxical vocal fold dysfunction (of unknown cause); and (e) certain psychogenic phenomena.

"Need to think about breathing" is a distinguishable percept, although it may be closely related to work/effort percepts (e.g., "hard work to breathe" and "high effort to breathe") (Lansing et al., 2000). The need to think about breathing has a concentration component that may become noticeable during the performance of certain types of shared breathing tasks. For example, speaking while experiencing air hunger may require noticeable "mental effort" and "concentration" to maintain expected speech patterns while also satisfying ventilatory demands (Bailey & Hoit, 2002).

"Feelings of distress with breathing" are common in clients who are experiencing any form of dyspnea, and "feelings of panic with breathing" are also experienced by some. These percepts tap directly into the emotional or affective component of dyspnea (although other percepts presented here also embody some degree of affect in their meanings). There are cases in which a breathing disorder appears to have a psychological/emotional cause, as in anxiety disorder, panic disorder, or psychogenic hyperventilation syndrome (Bass, Kartsounis, & Lelliott, 1987; Gardner, 1996). More often, the relationship between the psychological/emotional aspects and the organic aspects of a breathing disorder are exceedingly complex. Dyspnea can elicit feelings of anxiety and panic, which, in turn, can cause the dyspnea to worsen. Blood gas imbalances associated with certain diseases can impair cognitive function and alter mood state, which may further exacerbate dyspnea. The primary value of determining a client's perceptions of his feelings of distress and panic with breathing may be to help guide the clinician in making appropriate referrals (e.g., to a psychiatrist, psychologist, or counselor) and in designing speech breathing management.

Although a wide selection of percepts is offered in the list provided, there may be other terms that better describe the perceptual experiences of a client. If a client volunteers additional terms, they should be noted on the form along with information regarding situations and strength.

At the end of this section, the client is asked, "Which of the words or phrases just discussed (*list percepts selected*) best describes your breathing problems while you are speaking?" The clinician should remind the client of his choices and encourage him to select the single best percept. There may be cases in which it is appropriate for the client to select two, especially if they are equally important to him and if they reflect different underlying mechanisms. For example, the client might select "shortness of breath" and "feelings of distress with breathing" because they reflect different perceptual phenomena. By contrast, the client should be encouraged to select only one percept if his two favorites are within the same general category, such as "hunger for air" and "shortness of breath." Upon completion of this part of the case history interview, the speech-language pathologist should have a single percept (or, at most, two percepts) that can be used during later parts of the speech breathing evaluation (see section on evaluation of speaking-related dyspnea in this chapter) and during management (see Chapter 5).

AUDITORY-PERCEPTUAL EXAMINATION OF SPEECH BREATHING

The ear is an essential clinical tool. In fact, it is the final arbiter for determining the influence of a speech breathing disorder on speech. Auditory-perceptual examination can offer the speech-language pathologist important clues for understanding the nature of a client's speech breathing disorder.

The premise underlying the auditory-perceptual examination of speech breathing is that speech carries information about the breathing behavior that contributed to its generation. That is, certain transformations between breathing behavior and speech are straightforward enough that the clinician should be able to "hear" what the breathing apparatus is doing. A speech-language pathologist listening to a client speak is like an automobile mechanic listening to an engine run as the first step in diagnosing an engine problem.

A skillful auditory-perceptual examination can lay the groundwork for the remainder of the speech breathing evaluation by suggesting areas of focus for the physical examination and instrumental examination. Of course, even if the auditory-perceptual examination turns out to be unremarkable, it is still possible that the physical and instrumental examinations may uncover abnormalities that are being masked by the client's behavioral compensations.

Even the most skilled clinician will encounter ambiguity when attempting to infer what speech breathing (physiological) events could be responsible for generating speech (acoustic) events. One reason is that certain acoustic events can arise from more than a single physiological source. For example, there may be laryngeal and/or upper airway contributions to the disorder that mask or confound the breathing contributions. Another reason for ambiguity may be that the speech sample is not adequate for making physiological inferences. This may occur with clients who present with cognitive, language, or speech impairments that limit their output, or who are unwilling or unable to cooperate with the examination.

Despite these potential limitations, the auditory-perceptual examination is a powerful clinical tool. It can be used to glean the following information: (a) a global impression of the degree of speech breathing abnormality; (b) insight into how individual breathing control variables – volume, pressure, and shape – may contribute to the speech breathing abnormality; and (c) information about a client's adjustment capabilities through the use of prescribed speech tasks.

Global Ratings

The auditory-perceptual examination should begin by forming a global impression of the client's speech breathing disorder. This is when the speech-language pathologist determines if an abnormality exists at the auditory-perceptual level of observation, and if so, how severe it is. When making a global judgment, it is important to focus the severity rating on the speech breathing abnormality alone. The clinician should ignore, as much as possible, any laryngeal and/or upper airway components that might contribute to the speech abnormality.

Global ratings should be assigned while the client is performing the following three running speech activities: (a) reading aloud; (b) extemporaneous speaking; and (c) conversational speaking. For the reading activity, a declarative passage should be used that is within the reading capability of the client and elicits a large number of breath groups that vary in syllable number. One such reading passage for adults is shown below. This passage consists of 12 sentences ranging in length from 7 to 53 syllables and typically elicits between 15 to 25 breath groups when read by normal speakers.

The California Passage

California is a unique state. It is one of the few states that has all the geographical features found in the rest of the country including deserts, forests, mountain ranges, and beaches. Its beaches draw thousands and thousands of people each year particularly during the summer months when the sun is shining, the skies are blue, and the ocean is warm enough to swim in. Surfers are often in the water by daybreak. Of course there are many other things to do besides surfing such as sailing, swimming, water skiing, kite flying, and sun bathing. In the winter the mountains of California are favorite vacation spots. Here, snow skiing is the sport. There are many places in California to snow ski but the largest and most popular is Mammoth Mountain. Because of its popularity the property surrounding the Mammoth ski resort is extremely expensive. Unfortunately, the threat of earthquakes in this area is very high. In fact, earthquakes are common occurrences in many parts of California. Because of this, there are people who are afraid that someday a large piece of the state will fall into the Pacific Ocean. The possibility of a serious earthquake such as the one that demolished San Francisco in 1906 frightens some people enough that they choose not to visit California just for that reason.

(Hoit & Hixon, 1987)

When reading, the client is provided with all the required linguistic material so that he is relieved of the need to formulate while he is speaking. In this sense, reading is less demanding than are those activities that require linguistic formulation. However, for certain clients, reading may present other challenges, especially for those with reading impairments or visual impairments. If a client exhibits significant reading difficulty, inferences about his speech breathing may be difficult to interpret. In such cases, it is advisable to omit reading from the examination.

For the extemporaneous speaking activity, the client is asked to speak on a given topic for approximately 2 to 3 minutes. This activity is not linguistically constrained like reading. Thus, the client has more flexibility in how breath groups are chunked, when to pause, and when to inspire. There is less expectation that the client will speak continually, without pauses, than during the reading activity. Extemporaneous speaking is usually best elicited by suggesting topics to the client of the "tell me about" variety, such as "Tell me about your family," "Tell me about your job," or "Tell me about your favorite vacation." The topic(s) selected should not be emotionally loaded or cognitively taxing. If they are, the client's speech breathing may reflect emotional responses or cognitive struggle which could mask his more typical speech breathing behavior. The goal of this activity is to elicit relatively continual speaking from the client with minimal interruption from the clinician. To keep the client's speech flowing, the clinician may need to use probes such as "Go on" or "Tell me more about that." With certain clients, the request for an adequate speech sample can be made directly. For example, the clinician might say, "Now I need to listen to you speak on your own for a while, so I'd like you to tell me something that you can talk to me about for several minutes." When making judgments about extemporaneous speaking, it is important to keep in mind that extemporaneous speaking requires on-line linguistic formulation that could interact with speech breathing performance. For example, if the client pauses frequently, it may be because he needs to inspire frequently. However, it may also be because he requires processing time to formulate his spoken message. Thus, the speech-language pathologist needs to attempt to discern the underlying reasons for the client's breathing behavior.

Conversational speaking, the third activity, consists of generally alternating patterns of speaking and listening between the client and a conversational partner. Conversational speaking is the most common of all speaking activities, requires linguistic formulation, is less self-directed than extemporaneous speaking, and entails that the client follow the rules of conversational interchange (e.g., pragmatic and temporal). Often, in the context of a speech breathing evaluation, the client's conversational partner is the clinician. This has the advantage that the clinician is able to control the nature of the conversation, but it has the disadvantage that she must attempt to make simultaneous auditory-perceptual judgments of the client's speech. One solution is to record the conversation on audiotape or videotape and make judgments later. Another solution is to ask a client's family member or another clinical staff member to engage in conversation with the client while the clinician makes auditory-perceptual observations. As with extemporaneous speaking, the topics under discussion should be relatively neutral in emotionality and should not impose heavy cognitive demands. A conversation of 2 to 3 minutes should suffice, assuming that the client shares at least half of the speaking load.

Form 4-2 can be used to record auditory-perceptual judgments. The first three sections are devoted to judgments associated with running speech activities: reading aloud, extemporaneous speaking, and conversational speaking. The first item in each of these sections is designated for the recording of global judgments. A 5-point rating scale is provided which spans from normal (0) to profoundly abnormal (-4). Space is available for comments if the clinician wishes to elaborate on the reasons for her rating.

Variable-Based Ratings

Variable-based ratings are made on the same speech performances as are global ratings. Variable-based ratings reflect a more analytical level of auditory-perceptual observation and are focused on the three control variables introduced in Chapter 2 – volume, pressure, and shape. These are, of course, physical variables that can be measured with instrumentation. Nevertheless, they also have auditory-perceptual correlates that can be useful in helping to define the nature of a speech breathing disorder.

Auditory-Perceptual Correlates of Volume

The volume of interest is the lung volume displaced (i.e., expended) during the expiratory phase of the speech breathing cycle. It can be thought of as the volume stroke, much like the stroke of a violin bow (in one direction). The strongest auditory-perceptual correlate of volume displacement during speech performance is breath group length. In this context, breath group length can be defined as either the amount of time (e.g., seconds) it takes to produce a breath group or the quantity of speech (e.g., number of syllables) produced in a breath group. As a general rule, the greater the perceived length of a breath group, the greater the lung volume expended.

When rating breath group length, the speech-language pathologist must first decide if the client's breath group lengths are generally normal or abnormal. If they are abnormal, then she needs to judge if they are abnormally short or abnormally long and to what degree of severity. The auditory-perceptual rating form contains scales for recording ratings of breath group length for each of the three running speech activities (reading aloud, extemporaneous speaking, and conversational speaking). The center point of each rating scale ("0") indicates normal breath group length. Ratings to the left of center indicate abnormally short breath groups (of increasing severity) and ratings to the right of center indicate abnormally long breath groups (of increasing severity). Space is available to add written comments.

Although breath group length is strongly correlated with lung volume displacement, it is important to recognize that the behaviors of the larynx and upper airway also influence breath group length. If the larynx and/or upper airway offer an abnormally high or abnormally low resistance, lung volume may be expended at a lower-than-normal or higher-than-normal rate, respectively. Judgments of voice quality can provide clues regarding downstream resistance, with a breathy quality indicating an abnormally low resistance and a pressed quality indicating an abnormally high resistance. Also, if articulation rate is abnormally fast or abnormally slow, breath group length may be perceived as longer or shorter than it actually is. In cases where articulation rate is abnormal, the better indicator of breath group length is the perception of duration rather than the number of syllables per breath group. Finally, it is important to realize that breath group length (as measured in syllables) generally decreases with age in adults (see section on age and speech breathing in Chapter 3). Thus, the clinician should not expect senescent clients to produce as many syllables per breath group as young clients.

Judgments of breath group length can also be confounded by the fact that speech production does not always occur throughout the entire breath group. This calls for differentiating between the breath group (i.e., the entire expiratory phase of the speech breathing cycle) and the speech portion of the breath group. Usually the breath group and its speech portion are the same because speech is produced during the entire expiration. However, sometimes the speech portion of the breath group is shorter than the entire breath group. For example, some clients expire during the initial part of the breath group and then start to speak. Other clients speak during the initial part of the breath group and then expire. And still other clients may not be able to generate enough pressure to speak at all. In cases such as these, breath group length cannot be estimated from the number of syllables or the speech duration. Instead, length judgments must be made from other available cues, such as the duration of nonspeech expirations or movements of the chest wall.

A client may exhibit abnormal breath group lengths for many reasons. Short breath groups can result from neuromotor impairment of inspiratory muscles (e.g., from spinal cord injury or muscular dystrophy) or reduced compliance of the breathing apparatus (e.g., from scoliosis or severe scarring). Such reduced inspiratory strength or increased stiffness of the breathing apparatus during inspiration can restrict the amount of air available for speech production during expiration. Or the speech portions of breath groups may be short and followed by nonspeech expirations. This behavior often occurs in association with disorders that cause dyspnea (e.g., chronic obstructive pulmonary disease), because it allows the client to maintain a high level of ventilation while speaking. When clients are restricted in their breath group lengths or speech lengths, whatever the cause, they do not have the capability to alternate between short and long utterances and, therefore, lack the variability that is characteristic of normal speech. Whereas short breath groups generally have physical causes, long breath groups usually have functional or psychogenic causes. These causes may range from a maladaptive habit (e.g., a newscaster operating under strict time limitations) to a sign associated with psychogenic disorder (e.g., someone with anxiety disorder that avoids reciprocity in a conversation by "talking nonstop").

Auditory-Perceptual Correlates of Pressure

Control of average alveolar pressure and variation in that pressure are important aspects of normal speech breathing. The strongest auditory-perceptual correlate of average pressure is average loudness and the strongest auditory-perceptual correlate of variation in pressure is loudness variability. In general, the higher the average pressure, the louder the speech, and the larger the pressure swing, the greater the loudness variability. Loudness variability is included in the auditory-perceptual examination because it has important implications for speech steadiness, linguistic stress, and expressiveness.

The auditory-perceptual examination form contains separate items for recording judgments of average loudness and loudness variability. If both perceptual features are normal, the clinician records a rating of "0" for each. If the client's average loudness is abnormal, the clinician indicates on the rating form if it is abnormally soft (by rating to the left of "0") or abnormally loud (by rating to the right of "0"). If the client's loudness variability is abnormal, the clinician rates it as abnormally even (by rating to the left of "0") or abnormally variable (by rating to the right of "0").

Although loudness is strongly related to pressure, it is important to bear in mind that adjustments of the larynx and upper airway also contribute to loudness. Increases and decreases in laryngeal opposing pressure (i.e., squeezing force) often accompany increases and decreases in alveolar pressure to effect loudness change. Increases and decreases in the openness of the upper airway (mouth opening in particular) also change loudness.

There are many abnormal loudness signs that reflect abnormal alveolar pressure control. Softer-than-normal speech suggests that alveolar pressure is abnormally low. Taken to the extreme, the absence of speech can indicate that pressure is so low that vocal fold oscillation is impossible. The inability to produce adequately high pressure is usually caused by muscular weakness associated with neuromotor impairment (e.g., amyotrophic lateral sclerosis, Guillain-Barre syndrome). Of course, softer-than-normal speech can also be a behavioral sign of an emotional disorder or a personality trait. Louder-than-normal speech is a manifestation of higher-than-normal pressure and can be associated with a neuromotor disorder (e.g., spastic cerebral palsy), a hearing impairment, or a certain personality type (e.g., aggressive). Loudness variability can also be abnormal in several ways. It can be abnormally even, indicating smaller-than-normal variation in alveolar pressure. Abnormally even pressure variability is associated with some central nervous system disorders (e.g., parkinsonism). When loudness variability is excessive, such as when bursts of loudness occur, it is most likely to be caused by a hyperkinetic disorder (e.g., Huntington's chorea, dyskinetic forms of cerebral palsy). Loudness can also fluctuate rhythmically, reflecting corresponding changes in alveolar pressure (e.g., tremor, myoclonus). Or loudness can fade across the breath group, suggesting a gradual decrease in pressure. This often occurs when alveolar pressure is generated solely by the prevailing relaxation pressure, such as with muscle paralysis (e.g., cervical spinal cord injury).

Auditory-Perceptual Correlates of Shape

The shape of the breathing apparatus is important to both the inspiratory and expiratory phases of the speech breathing cycle. The auditory-perceptual correlates for shape are inspiratory duration and the loudness component of linguistic stress. Form 4-2 provides places for the clinician to rate inspiratory duration as normal ("0"), abnormally short (to the left of "0"), or abnormally long (to the right of "0"). The loudness component of linguistic stress is best reflected in ratings of loudness variability (discussed above under auditory-perceptual correlates of pressure).

Recall that the normal shape of the breathing apparatus in the upright body position is characterized by a smaller abdominal wall volume and a larger rib cage wall volume than those associated with relaxation at the prevailing lung volume. Inward displacement of the abdominal wall causes the diaphragm to be stretched and displaced headward, thereby improving its capacity to produce quick and forceful inspiratory adjustments. However, if the abdominal wall is distended (such as with abdominal muscle weakness), the diaphragm is correspondingly flattened and loses its usual mechanical advantage for producing quick and forceful inspirations. Because the diaphragm cannot produce as rapid an inspiration as usual (given the same neural input), the time to produce the inspiration is longer. Also, in cases where the rib cage wall is weak and highly compliant, action of the diaphragm may cause the rib cage wall to be sucked inward. This, in turn, causes a substantial increase in the work of breathing and, unless there is a compensatory augmentation of neural drive, the inspiration may be abnormally slow.

Inspirations during running speech breathing are typically about half a second in duration. If the clinician perceives inspirations to be routinely much longer than this, she should consider the possibility that the shape variable may be compromising the function of the diaphragm. It is important to realize, however, that there are other factors that could contribute to abnormally long inspirations. One is abnormally large inspiratory volume displacement. If the client inspires a very large volume of air, the time it takes to inspire probably will be longer than usual. It should be possible to detect large inspiratory volume displacements by watching the movements of the chest wall. Another potential contributor to abnormally long inspirations can be higher-than-normal airway resistance. High resistance can be imposed by the larynx (as in paradoxical vocal fold dysfunction) or pulmonary airways (as in obstructive pulmonary disease). High resistance should be relatively easy to recognize by the noise generated during inspiration. Another possible source of high resistance is the nasal pathway. However, it would be unusual for this to influence inspiratory duration because once nasal pathway resistance is high enough, the natural response is to switch from nose breathing to mouth breathing. It is also possible for inspiration to be abnormally short in duration. Short inspirations are almost always associated with small inspiratory volumes. Small inspiratory volumes can be normal (such as catch breaths) or they can be indicative of inspiratory muscle weakness.

The shape of the breathing apparatus also has consequences for the ability to generate quick loudness increases for linguistic stress production. The normal chest wall shape for upright speech breathing facilitates linguistic stress production in two ways. One is that the expiratory muscles of the rib cage wall are stretched and placed at mechanical advantages for generating rapid increases in muscular pressure. When chest wall shape is abnormal, the abdominal wall usually protrudes outward and the rib cage wall volume is smaller than usual. At this smaller volume, the expiratory muscles of the rib cage wall are short and mechanically disadvantaged for generating force. The second reason that the normal chest wall shape facilitates linguistic stress production relates to the supportive role played by the abdominal wall. Under normal circumstances, abdominal wall muscles are activated and the abdominal wall is less compliant (stiffer) than it would be without such activation. Because the abdominal wall is stiff, the rib cage wall is able to push against it to generate quick muscular pressure change. When the abdominal wall is abnormally compliant (floppy), the rib cage wall does not have a firm base to operate against. Instead, when the expiratory rib cage wall muscles contract, that contraction causes the abdominal wall to move outward rather than to raise alveolar pressure.

When a shape abnormality contributes to longer-than-normal inspirations and impaired linguistic stress, this is usually attributable to paresis or paralysis of the abdominal wall muscles. Abdominal muscle paresis or paralysis is caused by neural impairment (e.g., spinal cord injury, degenerative neuromotor diseases).

Prescribed Variable-Based Adjustments

If problems are noted in the control of breath group length, loudness (average or variability), or inspiratory duration during running speech activities, the auditory-perceptual examination should go on to include prescribed speech activities. The prescribed speech activities described below are designed to help determine the capabilities of the breathing apparatus and clarify the nature of the underlying problem(s) by using a variable-based approach. Such activities are intended to reveal the client's adjustment capabilities by manipulating the speech end-product in ways that are known to depend on certain adjustments of the breathing apparatus. Not all of the activities described in this section should be used with every client. It is up to the clinician to determine which of these activities, if any, are appropriate for any given client.

Ratings of the client's performance on the prescribed speech activities can be recorded on Form 4-2. A 5-point rating scale is used, ranging from normal (0) to profoundly abnormal (-4).

Volume (Breath Group Length)

Prescribed activities for volume focus on manipulations of breath group length. They are intended for clients who exhibit abnormalities in breath group length or in the length of the speech portion of their breath groups.

For clients who exhibit shorter-than-normal breath group lengths or speech lengths, the following activities are suggested. Ask the client to "Take in a deep breath and go as long as you can before taking in another breath" as the prelude to the following activities: (a) breathing out through pursed lips; (b) sustaining a vowel; and (c) counting aloud. The purpose of these activities is to determine the maximum breath group length that the client is able to generate. Breathing out through pursed lips allows the clinician to assess breath group length in the absence of speech production demands. Breath group length (volume displacement) is judged by listening to the noise generated at the lips and watching the movements of the chest wall. Sustaining a vowel allows the clinician to observe the interaction between the breathing apparatus and the larynx for voice production in the absence of upper airway influences. Counting aloud engages all speech production subsystems in an activity that has minimal cognitive-linguistic demands. If the client does not appear to be putting forth his best effort, the speech-language pathologist may encourage him with prompts such as "Be sure to take in the biggest breath you can" or "Be sure to keep going until you are completely out of air." These activities will offer the clinician insights into the breath group length capabilities of the client under various conditions. This does not mean that the client will be able to (or should) use his maximum breath group lengths during everyday speaking activities.

For clients who exhibit longer-than-normal breath group lengths, it is instructive to determine if the client is able to reduce the length of his breath groups under controlled conditions. Before performing the prescribed activities, the client is asked to breathe quietly and notice the size of his breaths. Assuming he is using his usual resting tidal volume, he is then asked to make his breaths a little bigger. The clinician coaches him until his tidal volume appears to encompass the normal speech breathing range. The client is then asked to perform the three activities described above – breathing out through pursed lips, sustaining a vowel, and counting aloud – while using this lung volume range. Thus, to perform this activity appropriately, the client will need to reduce the lung volume range through which he usually operates. If the client is able to perform these prescribed activities, similar activities may be incorporated into management.

Pressure (Loudness)

Prescribed activities for pressure involve loudness manipulation as an indicator of the ability to control pressure. These activities are designed for clients who exhibit lower-than-normal loudness, higher-than-normal loudness, abnormally even loudness, and/or abnormally variable loudness.

The first two prescribed activities for pressure involve manipulations of the average pressure. First, the client is asked to "Use your loudest possible comfortable voice" and to "Use your softest possible voice" while performing the following activities: (a) sustaining a vowel; and (b) counting aloud. After observing the client's initial performance, the clinician may decide to coach the client in ways designed to improve his performance. For example, she might encourage him to "Take a deeper breath before beginning to speak" as a way of determining if an increase in lung volume might help him to generate higher pressure.

The next four prescribed activities are designed to test how well the client can change pressure within a breath group. For these activities, the client is asked to sustain a vowel and alter his loudness according to the following instructions: (a) "Begin with your usual loudness, then gradually make your voice louder and louder;" (b) "Begin with your usual loudness, then gradually make your voice softer and softer;" (c) "Begin with your usual loudness, then abruptly make your voice louder;" and (d) "Begin with your usual loudness, then abruptly make your voice softer." It will probably be necessary for the clinician to demonstrate these activities.

The last activity is designed to determine if the client can maintain a targeted pressure. For this activity, the client is asked to sustain a vowel at "your usual loudness and hold it as steady as you can." This activity should reveal any rhythmic or arrhythmic fluctuations in pressure if they exist. It is important that the client not attempt this using a loud voice, because increased loudness may mask the presence of pressure-driven unsteadiness. A certain degree of unsteadiness is normal, so the clinician must judge whether any unsteadiness detected is greater than would be expected in a normal voice. Also, the clinician needs to be careful to sort out fluctuations in loudness (which are primarily related to pressure fluctuations) and pitch (which are primarily related to changes in laryngeal muscular tension).

Shape (Inspiratory Duration)

Prescribed activities for shape focus primarily on inspiratory duration. These are intended for clients who exhibit abnormally long inspirations.

The prescribed activity for shape is designed to elicit rapid inspirations. Specifically, the client is instructed to "Count as quickly as you can until I tell you to stop. You may take as many breaths as you need." During the client's performance of this activity, the clinician should judge inspiratory duration, as well as note the loudness component of the client's linguistic stress capability. Next, the clinician alters the client's shape by placing her hands over the client's anterior abdominal wall and exerting a firm inward force. She then asks him to perform the activity again, while she judges whether or not inspiratory duration has changed. She should also note if the imposed shape adjustment increases linguistic stress generation capability and average loudness.

EVALUATION OF SPEAKING-RELATED DYSPNEA

Recall that the final part of the case history is devoted to eliciting information about the client's perceptions of speech breathing (see section on client perceptions of speech breathing in Form 4-1). Some clients will deny breathing-related discomfort (dyspnea) and will exhibit no signs of such discomfort during the case history interview. When this occurs, the clinician may decide to skip the present part of the evaluation. Other clients will report experiencing dyspnea. For those who do, completion of the client perceptions part of the case history should yield a single term (or two, at the most) that best represents the quality of that dyspnea as experienced during speaking. That term, whatever it may be for a particular client (e.g., "breathlessness," "hard work to breathe"), should be the term used for obtaining client perception ratings during the present part of the evaluation.

Client-generated dyspnea ratings should be obtained during the running speech activities portion of the auditory-perceptual examination. Specifically, dyspnea ratings should be obtained immediately following reading aloud, extemporaneous speaking, and conversational speaking. Although all of these activities involve running speech breathing, they differ in the nature of their speech breathing demands. Reading aloud calls for continual speaking with no natural breaks of substantial duration. Also, reading aloud dictates the linguistic content and punctuation, which, in turn, strongly influence the length of breath groups and the timing of inspirations. Extemporaneous speaking allows the client much greater flexibility than reading aloud. When the client is free to formulate the linguistic content, as he is during extemporaneous speaking, he is also free to insert a greater number of natural pauses during which he can catch his breath. Conversational speaking involves alternating speaking and listening. Thus, conversational speaking may be less taxing to the client because listening periods can be used to concentrate on ventilation alone. If a client is experiencing speaking-related dyspnea, it is likely that the dyspnea will be more pronounced during continual, linguistically constrained speaking (reading aloud), less pronounced during relatively continual but not linguistically constrained speaking (extemporaneous speaking), and least pronounced during intermittent speaking (conversational speaking). However, it is also possible that a client could feel stressed by the demands of a conversation and, therefore, experience his worst dyspnea during conversational speaking.

Dyspnea ratings are obtained immediately after the client completes a speaking activity and are recorded on Form 4-2. Specifically, the clinician asks the client to "Rate your _____ while you were speaking" and inserts the dyspnea-related term selected previously by the client (for example, "Rate your urge to breathe while you were speaking."). The client selects from one of the rating descriptors (none, mild, moderate, severe, intolerable) and the clinician records the client's rating in the appropriate section on the auditory-perceptual examination form. These ratings will provide the clinician with an indication of the degree of dyspnea experienced by the client during standard speaking activities. What the clinician learns from these ratings may correspond closely to what the client reported during the case history interview, or it may not. The value of on-line ratings is that they do not rely on the client's long-term memory.

If dyspnea is a salient feature of a client's speech breathing disorder, the clinician may want to go beyond the three speaking activities specified above. For example, it may be important to obtain dyspnea ratings while the client walks and converses simultaneously, if this is one of his major complaints. Or ratings may be obtained immediately after singing, lecturing, or any other vocal performance that is part of the client's daily activities.

Sometimes it is prudent to obtain dyspnea ratings from clients who have denied experiencing dyspnea. Such clients may occasionally exhibit what appear to be signs of dyspnea during speech breathing. For example, a client may show noticeable signs of neck muscle activity indicating a possible increase in physical effort. Or a client may insert nonspeech breaths between spoken breath groups during a reading activity, suggesting that he is attempting to catch his breath. In cases such as these, the clinician may find that if she queries the client immediately after what appears to be a stressful speaking performance, she may uncover previously unreported dyspnea.

PHYSICAL EXAMINATION OF THE BREATHING APPARATUS

Physical examination of the breathing apparatus is an essential component of any comprehensive speech breathing evaluation. It is essential in the same way that visualization of the larynx is essential to the evaluation of laryngeal structure and function and that an oral mechanism examination is essential to the evaluation of upper airway structure and function.

In this section, a protocol is provided for performing a physical examination of the breathing apparatus. The items included in this protocol are designed to provide information about the status and function of the rib cage wall, abdominal wall, and diaphragm. The number of items is limited by design, so that the protocol can be administered with relative ease. There are, however, additional items that may be included in a physical examination of the breathing apparatus, many of which are discussed in a series of articles by Hixon and Hoit (1998, 1999, 2000).

Examination Set-Up

The physical examination should be carried out in a quiet and comfortable room. The environment should be free of distractions and interruptions (e.g., no ringing telephones and a "Do Not Disturb" sign on the door). The room should have adequate, though not bright, lighting. Room temperature should be such that the client can remove clothing without becoming chilled. There should be a minimum number of people in the room, preferably just the client, the speech-language pathologist, and an assistant. Under some circumstances, the inclusion of a family member may also be appropriate.

Before beginning the examination, the clinician should take a few moments to explain to the client why a physical examination of the breathing apparatus is being conducted and generally what it will entail. The client should then be provided with a loose-fitting gown that ties at the back of the neck, such as that used during an examination performed by a physician. Use of the gown makes it possible for the clinician to view the breathing apparatus as needed and allows the client the freedom to move without restriction. The client should then be left alone (or with an attendant if assistance is required) to disrobe and put on the gown. The client should be told to disrobe to the waist, remove any belt, and loosen any waistband on pants. In the case of a female client, she should be instructed to either remove her bra (if wearing one) or loosen its fasteners. During the examination, the gown can be adjusted to reveal structure or function.

It is essential that the speech-language pathologist be completely at ease when examining the breathing apparatus. If the clinician is not comfortable, the client almost certainly will not be comfortable. If the demeanor of the clinician is confident and matter-of-fact, the client will be more apt to relax and be able to concentrate on performing the required tasks. With practice, the speech-language pathologist should become increasingly comfortable and skilled at conducting a physical examination of the breathing apparatus. Eventually, it becomes second nature, like conducting an oral mechanism examination.

The first part of the examination should be conducted with the client in the seated, upright body position. A straight-back chair should be used. It should be comfortable and configured so that the client can sit with minimal effort. The client should sit relatively erect with the back supported, the arms and hands resting on the thighs, and the feet flat on the floor. If the client has difficulty sitting erect, the shoulders should be stabilized in a manner that does not encumber the rib cage wall. This can be done with shoulder straps or with the aid of an assistant standing behind the client and bracing his shoulders by pulling back on them gently.

The second part of the examination should be conducted with the client in the supine body position. The client should be lying on a firm, supporting surface, such as an examining table. The table should be padded for comfort and should be adjustable so that it can be raised or lowered according to the requirements of the examination. A sturdy step should be provided for the client to get up on the table. In some cases it may be easier to have the client transfer to a low table and then raise the table. In cases where the client is severely impaired physically, it may be necessary to enlist the aid of a physical therapist, nurse's aid, or other appropriately trained person to perform the transfer safely. Once the client is in position on the examining table, his head should be slightly elevated with a pillow. The client's arms should be resting at his sides, his legs should be extended comfortably, and his knees should be unlocked.

These standardized upright and supine body positions should be used during the physical examination whenever possible. If they are not, certain observations may be confounded and inappropriate inferences may be drawn.

Examination Protocol

Form 4-3 should be used while conducting the physical examination of the breathing apparatus. The top part of the form provides space to enter comments relevant to the examination. Examples might be: "For the upright parts of the examination, the client was in a wheelchair tilted back toward supine by about 20°," "The client was supported by shoulder straps during the upright parts of the examination," or "The client reported feeling weaker than usual today."

Form 4-3 includes two major sections, one for structural observations and one for functional observations. Structural observations are carried out in the standardized upright body position, whereas functional observations are carried out either in the standardized upright body position (inspiratory rib cage wall, expiratory rib cage wall, and abdominal wall) or in the standardized supine body position (diaphragm). Protocol items on the form are discussed in detail below with respect to recommended performance activities and recommended observations. A single rating scale is suggested for all activities. Rating choices range from normal (0) to profoundly abnormal (-4). Spaces are provided for comments at strategic locations on the form.

Structural Observations

Structural observations should be made first. This is important because certain structural signs (see hernia example below) may contraindicate proceeding with functional observations. Also, structural knowledge may help in interpreting functional observations.

Structural observations are concerned with continuity, composition, alignment,

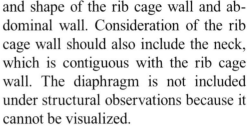

and shape of the rib cage wall and abdominal wall. Consideration of the rib cage wall should also include the neck, which is contiguous with the rib cage wall. The diaphragm is not included under structural observations because it cannot be visualized.

In the structural observations section of Form 4-3, the structures (rib cage wall and abdominal wall) are listed horizontally and the features for consideration (continuity, composition, alignment, and shape) are listed vertically. Rating options are provided for each structure and space is included for comments.

Continuity

The rib cage wall and abdominal wall are relatively smooth and continuous. Normal interruptions to continuity are the nipples (rib cage wall) and the umbilicus (abdominal wall). Other discontinuities reflect abnormal conditions. Scarring, resulting from surgery or trauma, may be a sign of damage to underlying muscles and/or nerves. Extensive scarring may decrease the compliance of one or both structures. Partial or complete breast amputation may also disrupt continuity and alter the mass-loading properties of the rib cage wall. Hernia, the protrusion of a structure through its containment wall, may be seen in the abdominal wall. If a hernia is observed or suspected, the clinician should immediately terminate the physical examination and refer the client to a physician.

An important discontinuity seen occasionally in the neck is a tracheostomy. This is a surgically created opening at the front of the neck between the external neck and trachea. A tracheostomy is found in clients who have had the larynx removed, in clients who are required to use certain types of ventilatory support, and in clients who have life-threatening breathing difficulties due to airway (tracheal, laryngeal, or pharyngeal) obstruction.

Composition

The rib cage wall is composed primarily of bone, cartilage, muscle, and fat, whereas the abdominal wall is composed primarily of muscle and fat. Abnormalities in composition may be seen in the rib cage wall, abdominal wall, or both. Such abnormalities are often in the form of disproportionate amounts of fat relative to muscle. Or there may be fat loss and muscle wasting due to muscle and/or nerve damage. Loss of innervation can also lead to the development of fibrosis (i.e., the replacement of muscle by stiff, stringy tissue) and a concomitant decrease in compliance. The presence of a well-defined muscle group is not considered abnormal and, in fact, may be an indication of fitness, with the possible exception of neck muscle hypertrophy. Large and prominent neck muscles may be a sign of prolonged compensation for a weak diaphragm and/or weak inspiratory rib cage wall muscles.

Usual composition of the rib cage wall may also be altered by breast reduction (removal of breast tissue) or augmentation (addition of new material). Both procedures can change the compliance and mass-loading properties of the rib cage wall.

Alignment

The rib cage wall (including the neck) and abdominal wall should be aligned with the long axis of the trunk. Problems of alignment can be seen in one or both of these parts, and can be caused by separate problems or a common problem. Abnormal alignment can result from skeletal deviations. Abnormal lateral curvature of the spine (i.e., scoliosis) can cause misalignment, as can abnormal curvature of the spine with rearward convexity (i.e., kyphosis). Misalignment can also result from defective closure of the bony encasement of the spinal cord (i.e., spina bifida).

Neuromotor problems can also cause misalignment. Misalignment is particularly apparent when the degree of involvement is different on the two sides of the body. In the case of the abdominal wall, the umbilicus may deviate toward the stronger side and away from the weaker side. If hypercontraction of one side is present, the rib cage wall and/or abdominal wall may be rotated or bent toward that side. If differential involvement between the two sides is substantial, the entire structure may rotate or bend toward the stronger side. Sometimes misalignment can involve only one structure. For example, the neck may be affected exclusively in someone with cervical torticollis (abnormal posturing caused by dystonia). It is more common, however, for misalignment of one structure to influence alignment of other structures. For example, abnormal abdominal wall activity can exert abnormal force on the lower rib cage and cause misalignment of the rib cage wall. In cases such as this, it may be difficult to differentiate primary involvement from compensatory adjustments of adjacent structures.

If misalignment is apparent, the clinician should determine if the client is able to achieve a more normal alignment voluntarily. If the client is unable to do so, the clinician should determine if it is possible to effect a more normal alignment by external adjustments. This might be done, for example, by providing additional trunk support through the use of cushions or arm rests. By making functional observations with and without the aid of such support, it may be possible to determine whether misalignment is a sign of primary involvement, compensatory adjustment, or both.

Shape

The normal shape (configuration) of the breathing apparatus depends on body type. Endomorphic individuals have substantial body fat, often associated with a convex anterior abdominal wall. Mesomorphic individuals have large bones, little fat, and well-developed muscles. They have broad shoulders, a flat anterior abdominal wall, and a muscular neck. Ectomorphic individuals have small bones, little fat, and not much muscle mass. Such individuals have a long and narrow torso with a flat anterior abdominal wall. Although these body shapes are all normal, it is important to realize that they can influence speech breathing behavior (see section on body type and speech breathing in Chapter 3).

An abnormal rib cage wall shape can result from a variety of conditions. One example is pectus excavatum (funnel chest), a congenital disorder in which the sternal portion of the rib cage wall is sunken. Another example is pectus carinatum (pigeon chest), a congenital protrusion deformity of the anterior rib cage wall. And still another example is bifid sternum (split chest), a congenital defect in which the sternum fails to fuse properly at the midline (along part or all of its length). A condition called barrel chest (bulged sides) is often seen in adults with obstructive lung disease. This results from the rib cage wall being maintained in an abnormally expanded state. Finally, a collapsed lung, in which the pleural linkage between the lung and the rib cage wall is disrupted, can cause the affected side of the wall to rest in an outwardly expanded position.

Another cause of abnormal shape is paresis or paralysis. An abnormal shape may be related to uniform weakness of the two sides of the rib cage wall and/or abdominal wall. It may also be caused by weakness of just one side of the wall(s) or both sides of the wall(s), but to different degrees. In cases of differential side-to-side weakness, the structures usually appear to be asymmetrical. Differential involvement may also be seen in the upper and lower regions of the rib cage wall and/or abdominal wall. Weakness of the abdominal wall is often indicated by a protrusion of the anterior wall. Such a protrusion usually is more prominent in lower than upper regions of the wall because the hydrostatic pressure gradient along the long axis of the abdomen shows a pressure increase in the caudal direction (in the upright body position).

Once structural observations have been made, the examination should turn to functional observations. These are concerned mainly with movement and force production capabilities.

Functional Observations

Functional observations focus on prescribed performance activities. These activities are listed in Form 4-3, together with suggested observations and rating options for different structures. Each performance activity has a descriptive label along with proposed verbal instructions. The suggested wording has been found to be effective in eliciting target behaviors. If a client does not make an effort to perform an activity or does not appear to understand an instruction, the examiner may want to demonstrate the activity and/or provide a different instruction.

Inspiratory Rib Cage Wall (Upright)

Activities included in this part of the protocol are designed to evaluate inspiratory rib cage wall function. They are performed in the standardized upright body position and include the following: (a) maximum inspiration and breath hold; and (b) forced inspiration.

Maximum Inspiration and Breath Hold: Maximum inspiration and breath hold (near the total lung capacity) serves to activate the inspiratory rib cage wall muscles to maximum or near-maximum levels. The inspiratory muscles (rib cage wall and diaphragm) must overcome the resistance to inspiratory flow and counteract the relaxation pressure that would otherwise cause the breathing apparatus to expire to its resting level. The maximum inspiration phase of the activity is characterized by extensive outward movement of the rib cage wall and abdominal wall that is relatively slow and smooth. The breath hold phase of the activity is characterized by relatively fixed positions of the same two structures.

Extent of RC Movement. The rib cage wall should move outward substantially during a maximum inspiration. Limited outward movement of the rib cage wall may reflect weakness of its inspiratory muscles, with or without weakness of the diaphragm. Outward movement of the rib cage wall may also be limited by abnormal stiffness of the wall, such as might accompany fibrosis or abnormally high muscle tone. Note that some expansion of the rib cage wall can result from diaphragm contraction and a concomitant rise in abdominal pressure, even when the rib cage wall is significantly impaired.

Smoothness of RC Movement. The rib cage wall should move smoothly during a maximum inspiration. Unsteadiness may reflect various forms of hyperkinesis (e.g., tics, chorea, myoclonus, tremor). The magnitude of hyperkinesis may change as the rib cage wall moves outward and the fibers of its inspiratory muscles change length. What appears to be hyperkinesis of the rib cage wall does not always originate in the rib cage wall itself. That is, actions of the diaphragm and/or abdominal wall may cause the rib cage wall to be unsteady. It is possible to parse out the relative contributions of the rib cage wall, diaphragm, and abdominal wall to suspected hyperkinesis by making observations at a variety of lung volumes and chest wall shapes. For example, at large abdominal wall volumes, the effect of the diaphragm is minimized because it is flatter and its muscle fibers are shorter. For another example, at small abdominal wall volumes, the effect of the abdominal wall muscles is minimized because the abdominal wall is flatter and its muscle fibers are shorter.

Steadiness of RC Position During Breath Hold. The rib cage wall should be maintained in a relatively stable position during the hold period following the maximum inspiration. Inability to hold the rib cage wall in a fixed (fully inspired) position may be a sign of muscle weakness or fatigue. Unsteadiness during the hold phase of the activity may also indicate hyperkinesis.

Firmness of Rib Interspaces During Breath Hold. The rib interspaces should be firm to palpation during the breath hold phase of the activity. If the interspaces are floppy or spongy, the intercostal muscles may be paretic or paralyzed. If the interspaces feel overly stiff, the intercostal muscles may be fibrotic or they may have abnormally high tone.

Forced Inspiration: Forced inspiration calls for a very rapid and extensive intake of air. Usually, it is initiated at or near the resting level of the breathing apparatus and terminated within the inspiratory reserve volume. This activity is associated with very rapid outward movements of the rib cage wall and abdominal wall.

Speed of RC Movement. Outward movement of the rib cage wall should be very rapid. If it is not, there is a strong possibility that the inspiratory rib cage wall muscles are paretic or paralyzed. This may or may not be accompanied by weakness of the diaphragm. Another possibility is that the resistance of the pulmonary airways is abnormally high. If high resistance contributes to a slow inspiration, there is usually an accompanying noise emanating from the pulmonary airways (e.g., wheeze). To eliminate the possibility that the source of high resistance may be in the nasal pathway, it is important to ensure that the client is inspiring with his mouth open. It is also important to consider that noise may emanate from laryngeal structures. For example, high laryngeal airway resistance (and associated noise) may be caused by paradoxical vocal fold dysfunction.

Phase of Left-Right RC Movement. The left and right sides of the rib cage should move outward together at the same rate. If one side lags behind the other, the side that lags should be suspected of being weaker than the side that leads. When one side of the rib cage wall is paralyzed and the other is normal or mildly paretic, the phase difference between the two sides (or of different regions within a side) may be marked. It is even possible that the weaker side may move in the opposite direction (i.e., inward) if the force exerted by the diaphragm is strong enough to lower pleural pressure sufficiently to suck the weaker side of the rib cage wall inward. Another factor that may contribute to a left-right phase difference is a left-right difference in stiffness. If one side is stiffer than the other (e.g., from fibrosis, scarring, or joint disease), the stiffer side may lag behind the more compliant side. In all cases, a phase difference is more likely to be revealed during a rapid inspiration (such as that required when performing a forced inspiration) than during a slow inspiration (such as that used in the previous task involving maximum inspiration and breath hold).

A phase difference between the left and right sides of the rib cage wall may be less striking than between two proportionately involved sides of the abdominal wall. This is because the hinged ribs cause the rib cage wall to operate as a contiguous left-right unit more so than does the abdominal wall without an analogous hinged structure.

Phase of Upper-Lower RC Movement. The upper and lower parts of the rib cage wall should move outward together during forced inspiration. When upper and lower regions move out of phase with one another, it may indicate paresis or paralysis. Inward (i.e., paradoxical) movement of the upper rib cage wall and outward movement of the lower rib cage wall during inspiration is referred to as "reversed breathing." Reversed breathing is commonly seen in cases where the rib cage wall is highly compliant, such as in infants and children with severe cerebral palsy. Inward movement of the upper rib cage wall is caused by negative pleural pressure (resulting from diaphragm contraction), whereas outward movement (or "flaring") of the lower rib cage wall is caused by upward pull exerted directly on the lower ribs by the muscle fibers of the diaphragm. A phase difference between movement of the upper and lower regions of the rib cage wall is more apt to be revealed during a forced inspiration (very rapid and forceful intake of air) than during a slower and less vigorous inspiration.

Phase of RC Movement and Lung Volume Change. The rib cage wall should move outward (i.e., in the inspiratory direction) during forced inspiration. If it does not, but instead lags behind the onset of inspiration, does not move at all, or moves paradoxically (i.e., in the expiratory direction), weakness or paralysis of the inspiratory rib cage wall muscles should be suspected. In this context, paradoxical movement of the rib cage wall means that it is being sucked inward by the lowering of pleural pressure through action of the diaphragm. Paradoxical movement may be more prominent at increasingly larger lung volumes where increasingly negative pleural pressure is developed by contraction of the diaphragm. Paradoxical (inward) movement of the rib cage wall is more likely to occur during a forced inspiration than during a slow inspiration because the force generated by the diaphragm is greater.

Phase of RC Movement and AB Movement. The rib cage wall and abdominal wall should move outward together during forced inspiration. If the rib cage wall moves inward (i.e., paradoxically) and the abdominal wall moves outward, it is likely that rib cage wall muscles are weak, as described above. If the rib cage wall moves outward and the abdominal wall moves inward (i.e., paradoxically), it may be that the rib cage wall is compensating for a weak diaphragm. Such a sign may serve as confirmatory evidence of diaphragm dysfunction in association with observations made during the diaphragm function portion of the examination.

Stability of Rib Interspaces. The rib interspaces should not change substantially in appearance during a forced inspiration. If, however, they are sucked inward and form a series of indentations of the rib cage wall, it is very likely to be indicative of paretic or paralyzed intercostal muscles. It is, in fact, a cardinal sign of rib cage wall muscle paresis or paralysis when such indentations are marked.

Expiratory Rib Cage Wall (Upright)

Two activities are included in this part of the protocol. These are designed to evaluate expiratory rib cage wall function and are performed in the standardized upright body position. They are as follows: (a) maximum expiration and breath hold; and (b) forced expiration.

Maximum Expiration and Breath Hold: Maximum expiration and breath hold (near the residual volume) serves to activate the expiratory rib cage wall muscles increasingly to maximum or near-maximum levels. The expiratory muscles of the rib cage wall and abdominal wall must overcome the resistance to expiratory flow and counteract the relaxation pressure that would otherwise cause the breathing apparatus to inspire to its resting level. The maximum expiration phase of the activity is characterized by extensive inward movements of the rib cage wall and abdominal wall that are relatively slow and smooth. The breath hold phase of the activity is characterized by fixed positions of the same two structures.

Extent of RC Movement. The rib cage wall should move inward substantially during a maximum expiration. If it moves inward only slightly and the abdominal wall moves inward substantially, the expiratory muscles of the rib cage wall may be weak. If both the rib cage wall and abdominal wall move inward only slightly (and very little air is expired), it may be that all expiratory

JAMES C. HARDY (1930-2004)

Hardy spent his entire academic career on the faculty of the University of Iowa and for all that time he had an affiliation with the University Hospital School for Severely Handicapped Children. He spawned a great deal of activity in speech breathing research, including his proposal of an "aerodynamic-mechanical" model of speech breathing that focused on interactions between the breathing apparatus and structures that valve its output during speech performance. Hardy did seminal work on the speech breathing of children with various neuromotor disorders and wrote extensively on the evaluation and management of speech disorders in children with cerebral palsy. He was a meticulous and dedicated teacher and ran an extraordinarily productive laboratory that generated some of the foremost scholars in speech physiology. All who worked with him understood well that his first love was Iowa's children in the Hospital School. He was a mentor to the first of us.

muscles are weak (both in the rib cage wall and abdominal wall). In certain types of disease, limited inward movement of the rib cage wall (and abdominal wall) may also be related to pulmonary airways collapse. Airways collapse prevents the full expiration of air contained within the pulmonary apparatus and mimics the limited volume displacement seen with weakness. Thus, both pulmonary airways collapse and muscle weakness can result in an abnormally small expiratory reserve volume. Obesity and senescence are also variables that may reduce the magnitude of the expiratory reserve volume.

When a small expiratory reserve volume is found (i.e., limited expiratory movement from the resting level of the breathing apparatus), it may be revealing to have the client repeat the expiration and breath hold activity while expiring slowly. If slower expiration results in a larger expiratory reserve volume (i.e., greater expiratory movement from the resting level of the breathing apparatus), it implies collapse of the pulmonary airways. This is because segments of the pulmonary airways tend to collapse sooner when pleural pressure is higher, as it is when expiration is more rapid and forceful.

Smoothness of RC Movement. The rib cage wall should move smoothly during a maximum expiration. Unsteadiness may reflect hyperkinesis. The magnitude of hyperkinesis may change as the rib cage wall moves inward and the fibers of its expiratory muscles change length. It is also possible that what appears to be rib cage wall hyperkinesis does not originate in the rib cage wall itself, but instead reflects actions of the diaphragm and/or abdominal wall. It is possible to parse out the relative contributions of the rib cage wall, diaphragm, and abdominal wall to suspected hyperkinesis by making observations at a variety of lung volumes and chest wall shapes. For example, at small abdominal wall volumes, any hyperkinetic effect of the diaphragm is maximized because the diaphragm is more highly domed and its muscle fibers are longer. For another example, at large abdominal wall volumes, any hyperkinetic effect of the abdominal wall muscles is maximized because the abdominal wall is protruding more and its muscle fibers are longer.

Steadiness of RC Position During Breath Hold. The rib cage wall should be maintained in a stable position during the hold period following the maximum expiration. Inability to hold the rib cage wall in a fixed (fully expired) position can be a sign of expiratory muscle weakness or fatigue. Unsteadiness of the rib cage wall during the hold phase may indicate hyperkinesis.

Firmness of Rib Interspaces During Breath Hold. The rib interspaces should be firm to palpation during the breath hold. If they are floppy or spongy, the intercostal muscles may be paretic or paralyzed. If the interspaces feel overly stiff, it may be that fibrosis is present or that the muscle tone of the intercostal muscles is abnormally high.

Forced Expiration: Forced expiration calls for a very rapid and extensive expulsion of air. Usually it will be initiated following a quick inspiration from the resting level of the breathing apparatus (this is not part of the instruction, but a natural tendency) followed by a substantial expiration that terminates well into the expiratory reserve volume. This activity is associated with very rapid inward movements of the rib cage wall and abdominal wall.

Speed of RC Movement. The inward movement of the rib cage wall should be very rapid. If it is not, there is a strong possibility that the expiratory rib cage wall muscles are paretic or paralyzed. This may or may not be accompanied by weakness of the abdominal wall. Another factor contributing to abnormally slow inward movement of the rib cage wall may be a lower-than-normal compliance (i.e., greater stiffness) of the structure. Still another possibility is that the resistance of the pulmonary airways is high. If resistance is high, there may be an accompanying noise emanating from the pulmonary airways (e.g., wheeze). Noise may also emanate from the larynx if that structure is constricting the airway.

Although the rib cage wall should move inward very rapidly during a forced expiration, it is not unusual for the rate of its movement to decrease somewhat as expiration nears termination. This is partly due to a decrease in the speed of expiration (as expiratory muscle force operates against increasingly higher inspiratory relaxation pressure), and partly due to the tendency to move the abdominal wall inward more than the rib cage wall at very small lung volumes.

Phase of Left-Right RC Movement. The left and right sides of the rib cage wall should move inward together at the same rate. If one side lags behind the other, the side that lags should be suspected of being weaker than the side that leads. When one side of the rib cage wall is paralyzed and the other is normal or mildly paretic, the phase difference between the two sides (or of different regions within a side) may be marked. It is even possible that the weaker side may move in the opposite direction (i.e., outward) if the force exerted by the abdominal wall is strong enough to raise abdominal pressure (and pleural pressure) sufficiently to blow the weaker side of the rib cage wall outward. Another factor that may contribute to a phase difference in inward movement of the two sides of the rib cage wall is any difference between the two sides in structural stiffness. For example, if one side is stiffer than the other because of fibrosis, scarring, or joint disease, that side may lag behind its counterpart. In all cases, a phase difference is more likely to be revealed by a forced expiration than a slow expiration.

A phase difference between the left and right sides of the rib cage wall may not be as striking as that between two proportionately involved sides of the abdominal wall. This is because the movement of the two sides of the rib cage wall is more tightly constrained than the movement of the two sides of the abdominal wall.

Phase of Upper-Lower RC Movement. The upper and lower portions of the rib cage wall should move inward during forced expiration. If upper and lower portions move out of phase with one another, it may indicate paresis or paralysis and/or differential stiffness of those portions. The weaker portion of the structure may remain in position or move outward momentarily during forced expiration as pleural pressure is elevated by the less impaired region of the rib cage wall and by the abdominal wall. As with potential side-to-side differences in movement, upper-lower differences are also more apt to be revealed during a very rapid and forceful expulsion of air (forced expiration) than during a slow and less vigorous expiration.

Phase of RC Movement and Lung Volume Change. The rib cage wall should move inward (i.e., in the expiratory direction) during forced expiration. If it does not, but instead lags behind the onset of expiration, does not move at all, or moves paradoxically (i.e., in the inspiratory direction), paresis or paralysis of the expiratory rib cage wall muscles is likely. Movement of the rib cage wall in the inspiratory direction during forced expiration may indicate that the expiratory rib cage wall muscles are severely or profoundly impaired and that the abdominal wall muscles are overpowering the rib cage wall and lifting it. This sign may be more pronounced at small lung volumes where positive abdominal pressure is high and the lifting force on the rib cage wall is approaching maximum.

Phase of RC Movement and AB Movement. The rib cage wall and abdominal wall should both move inward during forced expiration. If the rib cage wall moves outward (i.e., paradoxically) during expiration, it is likely that the rib cage wall muscles are weak and are being overpowered by the abdominal wall muscles, as described above. If the rib cage wall moves inward and the abdominal wall moves outward (i.e., paradoxically), it may be that the abdominal wall is paretic or paralyzed and is being overpowered by the expiratory rib cage wall muscles. Such an observation can serve as confirmatory to observations made during the abdominal wall function portion of the examination.

Stability of Rib Interspaces. The rib interspaces should not change substantially in appearance during a forced expiration. If, however, they puff out and form a series of bulges along the rib cage wall, it is likely that the intercostal muscles are paretic or paralyzed. Marked bulging is a cardinal sign of rib cage wall paresis or paralysis.

Abdominal Wall (Upright)

Four performance activities are included in this part of the protocol. These are designed to evaluate abdominal wall function and are performed in the standardized upright body position. These activities include the following: (a) maximum abdominal contraction and hold; (b) forced expiration; (c) trunk flexion; and (d) trunk rotation.

Maximum AB Contraction and Hold: Maximum abdominal contraction and hold serves to activate the abdominal wall muscles increasingly to maximum or near-maximum levels. Maximum abdominal contraction is associated with extensive inward movement of the abdominal wall that is usually relatively slow and smooth, whereas the hold phase of the activity is characterized by a fixed position of the abdominal wall. Inward movement and hold are accompanied by an elevated rib cage position, brought about through a passive lifting of the rib cage wall by the abdominal wall (see Chapter 2 for an explanation of the mechanism involved).

Extent of AB Movement. The abdominal wall should move inward substantially during a maximum abdominal contraction. Limited inward movement of the abdominal wall may reflect weakness of the abdominal wall muscles. When judging the extent of abdominal wall movement, it is important to ensure that the abdominal wall is moving inward under its own muscle power and that the inspiratory muscles of the rib cage wall are not being used to suck the abdominal wall inward.

Smoothness of AB Movement. The abdominal wall should move smoothly during a maximum abdominal contraction. Unsteadiness of the abdominal wall may reflect hyperkinesis (e.g., tics, chorea, myoclonus, tremor). The magnitude of hyperkinesis may change as the abdominal wall moves inward and its muscle fibers change length. It is also possible that hyperkinetic signs in the abdominal wall do not originate there, but may be caused by actions of other chest wall components, particularly the diaphragm. It is possible to determine the relative contributions of different chest wall components to abdominal wall hyperkinesis by making observations at different lung volumes and chest wall shapes. For example, at large abdominal wall volumes (outward distentions), the effect of the abdominal wall on hyperkinetic drive is maximized because the muscle fibers of the wall are longer. Simultaneously, at such large abdominal wall volumes, the effect of the diaphragm on hyperkinetic drive is minimized because the muscle fibers of the diaphragm are shorter. Because the abdominal wall and the diaphragm comprise opposite surfaces of the abdominal content, their muscle-fiber length effects are reciprocal.

Steadiness of AB Position During Hold. The abdominal wall should be maintained in a stable position during the hold period following the maximum abdominal contraction. Inability to hold the abdominal wall in a fixed (fully inward) position can be a sign of muscle weakness or fatigue. Unsteadiness of the abdominal wall during the hold phase may indicate hyperkinesis.

Firmness of AB During Hold. The abdominal wall should be firm to palpation during the hold. If it is floppy or spongy, the abdominal wall muscles may be paretic or paralyzed. Regional differences in firmness may reflect regional differences in muscle involvement. When assessing firmness, it is important to take into account the amount of fat covering the abdominal wall.

Forced Expiration: Forced expiration calls for a very rapid and extensive expulsion of air. As noted above, it usually will be initiated with a quick inspiration from the resting level of the breathing apparatus (this is a natural tendency) followed by a substantial expiration that terminates well into the expiratory reserve volume. This performance activity is associated with very rapid inward movements of the rib cage wall and abdominal wall.

Speed of AB Movement. Inward movement of the abdominal wall should be very rapid. If it is not, there is a strong possibility that the abdominal wall muscles are weak (i.e., paretic or paralyzed). Such weakness may or may not be associated with weakness of the rib cage wall. Other factors may slow the speed of abdominal wall movement during forced expiration. One is that the abdominal wall may have a lower-than-normal compliance. Another is that the resistance of the pulmonary airways or larynx may be abnormally high (with concomitant noise generation in either or both). It should be noted that it is normal for the speed of abdominal wall movement to decrease somewhat as expiration proceeds toward termination.

Phase of Left-Right AB Movement. The left and right sides of the abdominal wall should move inward at the same rate. If one side lags behind the other, the side that lags should be suspected of being weaker than the side that leads. When one side of the abdominal wall is paralyzed and the other is normal or mildly paretic, the phase difference between the two sides may be marked. It is possible that the weaker side may move in the opposite direction (i.e., outward) if the force exerted by the abdominal wall is strong enough to raise abdominal pressure sufficiently to force the weaker side of the abdominal wall outward. Another factor that may contribute to a phase difference in inward movement is a difference in structural stiffness. For example, if one side is stiffer because of extensive scarring, that side may lag behind its counterpart. A phase difference is more likely to be revealed by a forced expiration (which is very rapid) than by a maximum abdominal contraction and hold (the maximum contraction part of which may not be rapid).

Phase of Upper-Lower AB Movement. The upper and lower portions of the abdominal wall should move inward during forced expiration. If they move out of phase with one another, it may indicate paresis or paralysis and/or differential stiffness of those portions. The weaker portion of the wall may be seen to remain in position or to move outward momentarily during forced expiration as abdominal pressure is elevated by the less impaired regions of the abdominal wall and rib cage wall. Upper-lower differences are more likely to be observed during a fast and forceful expulsion of air than during a slow and less vigorous expiration.

Phase of AB Movement and Lung Volume Change. The abdominal wall should move inward (i.e., in the expiratory direction) during forced expiration as lung volume decreases. If it does not, but instead lags behind the onset of expiration, does not move at all, or moves paradoxically (i.e., in the inspiratory direction), paresis or paralysis of the abdominal wall muscles is likely. Movement of the abdominal wall in the inspiratory direction during forced expiration may indicate that the abdominal wall muscles are severely or profoundly impaired and that the expiratory rib cage wall muscles are overpowering the abdominal wall and forcing it outward. A sign of this nature may be more pronounced at small lung volumes where increasingly positive pleural and abdominal pressures are operating and the expiratory forces generated by the rib cage wall are approaching maximum.

Phase of AB Movement and RC Movement. The abdominal wall and the rib cage wall should move inward during forced expiration. If the abdominal wall moves outward (i.e., paradoxically) during expiration, it is likely that the abdominal wall muscles are weak and are being overpowered by the expiratory rib cage wall muscles. If the abdominal wall moves inward and the rib cage wall moves outward (i.e., paradoxically), it may be that the rib cage wall is paretic or paralyzed and is being overpowered by the abdominal wall muscles. Such an observation may be confirmatory to observations made during the expiratory rib cage wall portion of the examination.

Trunk Flexion: Trunk flexion is designed to test (to a rough approximation) the force-generating capability of rectus abdominis muscle by the forward thrust delivered by the trunk. Thrust can be sensed by holding the client's shoulders in an erect and fixed position (from the front) while the client attempts to flex the trunk (bend forward) as forcefully as possible. The resultant contraction of rectus abdominis muscle is essentially isometric, and the force being generated is equal to the force required to hold the trunk in a fixed position. Although the rectus abdominis muscles typically are not used during speech production, they may function in a compensatory role for a client with general abdominal wall muscle impairment.

Force of Trunk Movement. Attempted trunk flexion should result in considerable forward thrust. An abnormally weak forward thrust may be a sign of paresis and/or paralysis in one or both of the rectus abdominis muscles.

Force of Left-Side Trunk Movement and Force of Right-Side Trunk Movement. In cases where the rectus abdominis muscles are not equally impaired on the two sides of the abdominal wall, the forward thrust from the two sides may not be equal. Thus, the thrust sensed from the left and right shoulders may feel different in magnitude. Lesser thrust will be produced by the weaker of the two sides. This will include situations in which one side may be paralyzed and the other paretic, or in which both sides are paretic, but one more than the other.

Trunk Rotation: Trunk rotation is designed to test (to a rough approximation) the combined force generating capability of the internal oblique and external oblique muscles of the abdominal wall. During isometric contraction, the external oblique muscle pulls the ipsilateral abdominal wall downward and toward the midline and the internal oblique muscle pulls the contralateral abdominal wall downward and toward the midline. For the purpose of this examination, the functional integrity of the two sides of the abdominal wall can be evaluated under quasi-isometric conditions by determining the manual force needed to hold the shoulders in position. To perform this activity, the client sits in an erect position (without leaning forward) and attempts to rotate the trunk to one side and then the other as the clinician holds his shoulders in place.

Force of Left-Side Trunk Movement and Force of Right-Side Trunk Movement. Attempted trunk rotation should result in considerable torsion thrust in both directions. Weakness of the abdominal wall can cause reduced torsion thrust in one direction or in both directions. Thus, the thrust sensed from the left and the right shoulder may feel different in magnitude. This may be due to paresis or paralysis of the internal oblique and external oblique muscles on the two sides of the abdominal wall. It may also be related to coordinative dysfunction in which the two sides of the abdominal wall fail to engage in reciprocal inhibition (i.e., reduction in neural activation of one side during increased activation of the other side).

Diaphragm (Supine)

Diaphragm function is examined with the client in the standardized supine body position. Performance activities include the following: (a) maximum inspiration and breath hold; (b) forced inspiration; and (c) abdominal thrust against resistance. Because the diaphragm cannot be viewed directly, evaluation of its function focuses on the surface of the abdominal wall, the opposite surface of the diaphragm-abdominal wall unit.

Maximum Inspiration and Breath Hold: Maximum inspiration and breath hold (near the total lung capacity) in the supine body position serves to activate the diaphragm increasingly to maximum or near-maximum levels. The inspiratory muscles (diaphragm and rib cage wall) must overcome the resistance to inspiratory flow and counteract the relaxation pressure that would otherwise cause the breathing apparatus to expire to its resting level. The maximum inspiration phase of the activity is characterized by extensive outward movement of the rib cage wall and abdominal wall that is relatively slow and smooth, whereas the breath hold phase of the activity is characterized by fixed positions of the same two structures.

Extent of AB Movement. The abdominal wall should move outward substantially during a maximum inspiration. This movement is driven by extensive footward displacement of the diaphragm. Limited outward movement of the abdominal wall may reflect weakness of the diaphragm, with or without impairment of the rib cage wall. Limited outward movement of the abdominal wall (and, inferentially, limited displacement of the diaphragm) can also be caused by an abnormally stiff abdominal wall, such as might accompany fibrosis or abnormally high muscle tone within the structure.

Smoothness of AB Movement. The abdominal wall should move smoothly during a maximum inspiration. Unsteadiness of abdominal wall movement (jerkiness or other unevenness) may reflect hyperkinesis. The magnitude of hyperkinesis may change as the abdominal wall moves outward and the fibers of the diaphragm change length. It is also possible that what appears to be diaphragm hyperkinesis actually originates from the rib cage wall muscles and/or abdominal wall muscles. Contributions of the diaphragm, rib cage wall, and abdominal wall to hyperkinesis can be parsed out by making observations at a variety of lung volumes and chest wall shapes. For example, at large lung volumes and abdominal wall volumes, the effect of the diaphragm is minimized because it is flatter and its muscle fibers are shorter. For another example, at large abdominal wall volumes, the effect of the abdominal wall is maximized because of the muscle fiber lengths involved under that condition.

Steadiness of AB Position During Breath Hold. The abdominal wall should be maintained in a stable position during the hold period following the maximum inspiration. Inability to hold the abdominal wall in a fixed (fully inspired) position can be a sign of muscular weakness or fatigue of the diaphragm (one or both sides of the structure). Unsteadiness of the abdominal wall during the hold phase of the activity may indicate hyperkinesis.

Firmness of AB to Palpation During Breath Hold. The abdominal wall should be firm to palpation during the breath hold. If it is floppy or spongy, the diaphragm may be paretic (one or both sides). When assessing firmness, the amount of fat covering the abdominal wall should be taken into account. If the wall feels overly stiff, it may be that fibrosis is present or that the abdominal wall muscles have an abnormally high tone.

Forced Inspiration: Forced inspiration provides a means for examining diaphragm function during a very rapid and extensive intake of air. The inspiration will usually begin at or near the resting level of the breathing apparatus and end within the inspiratory reserve volume. This performance activity is associated with very rapid outward movements of the abdominal wall and rib cage wall.

Speed of AB Movement. The outward movement of the abdominal wall should be very rapid. Slow initiation or execution of abdominal wall movement is likely a sign that the diaphragm is weak (on one or both sides). As with forced inspiration in the upright body position, high resistance in the pulmonary airways or the larynx may contribute to a slower-than-normal forced inspiration. High resistance may be associated with airway noise.

ALEX IN WONDERLAND

"We find ourselves in a dark room or vault with a door in the roof. The floor of this vault, instead of being firm and solid, is a soft membrane or muscle, – not flat like an ordinary floor, but dome-shaped like the top of an open umbrella. The door above is a sort of double trap door set at an angle instead of being flat, and opening upwards. But the most extraordinary thing about this room is, that the floor is in constant motion, heaving upwards and downwards in regular pulsations." Wow! Whoever wrote this seems to have been excited by this stuff. Any idea who it might have been? Maybe you should telephone a friend or two and read it to them and see if they have any ideas. Never mind, we'll tell you. It was written by Alexander Graham Bell (1910, p. 1). Next time you use that cell phone, think about the inventive and fanciful Alex in Wonderland.

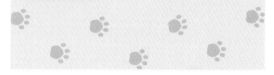

Phase of Left-Right AB Movement. The left and right sides of the abdominal wall should move outward together at the same rate if the diaphragm is fully intact. If they move out of phase, the two sides of the diaphragm may be differentially impaired. This means that one side or the other could be paretic or paralyzed, or that the two sides are both paretic, but differentially so. The side that lags behind the other during the movement is likely to be the more impaired. When one side of the diaphragm is paralyzed and the other is normal or mildly paretic, the phase difference between the two sides of the abdominal wall may be marked. Another factor that may contribute to a left-right phase difference is a left-right difference in the stiffness of either the diaphragm or the abdominal wall. The stiffer side may lag behind the more compliant side under such circumstances.

Because the forced inspiration activity demands rapid contraction of the diaphragm, it is the best of the present activities to reveal differential left-right diaphragm impairment. Left-right comparisons are most easily made if the clinician stands at the head of the client and sights down the long axis of the body. If the forced inspiration activity elicits a slow, rather than a fast, outward movement of the abdominal wall, it is suggestive of major diaphragm impairment. In this case, it may not be possible to determine if there is differential left-right weakness of the diaphragm. This is because a slow contraction of the diaphragm allows time for abdominal pressure to equalize throughout the abdominal content and the surface movements of the abdominal wall to be in phase.

Phase of AB Movement and Lung Volume Change. The abdominal wall should move outward (i.e., in the inspiratory direction) during forced inspiration in the supine body position. If it does not, but instead lags behind the onset of inspiration, does not move at all, or moves paradoxically (i.e., in the expiratory direction), paresis or paralysis of the diaphragm should be suspected. Paradoxical movement of the abdominal wall indicates that it is being sucked inward by the lowering of pleural pressure through inspiratory action of the rib cage wall. Paradoxical movement may be more prominent at increasingly larger lung volumes where increasingly negative pleural pressure (and abdominal pressure) is developed by contraction of the inspiratory muscles of the rib cage wall. The inspiratory force generated by the rib cage wall is greater during a forced inspiration (involving a very rapid and extensive intake of air) than during a slow inspiration so that paradoxical movement of the abdominal wall is more likely to occur.

Phase of AB Movement and RC Movement. The abdominal wall and the rib cage wall should move outward together during forced inspiration. If the abdominal wall moves inward (i.e., paradoxically) and the rib cage wall moves outward, it is likely that the diaphragm is paretic or paralyzed, and that the rib cage wall is compensating for the impaired diaphragm. Such a sign is evidence that the inspiratory function of the chest wall has been shifted from the diaphragm to the rib cage wall and that the abdominal wall is being dragged inward by a lowering of pleural and abdominal pressures.

AB Thrust Against Resistance: This activity is based on the assumption that the ability of the diaphragm to generate force can be determined to a rough approximation by the outward thrust it delivers through the abdominal wall. This thrust can be sensed by placing hands on the client's abdominal wall and holding them in a fixed position while the client contracts the diaphragm (isometrically). It is important that this activity be performed at a constant diaphragm configuration across efforts. A constant configuration is important because the force-generating capability of the diaphragm is influenced by its radius of curvature and the length of its muscle fibers. To standardize diaphragm configuration, the AB-thrust-against-resistance activity should be executed at the resting level of the breathing apparatus. If the client is suspected of using expiratory muscles of the rib cage wall to thrust the abdominal wall outward, this confound can be eliminated by having the client inspire very slowly while performing the abdominal thrust activity.

Force of AB Movement. The thrust of the abdominal wall should be quite forceful. If a lower-than-normal force is required to counteract the force exerted by the client's abdominal wall (being delivered by the diaphragm), diaphragmatic weakness can be inferred. If there is a substantial difference in weakness between the two sides of the diaphragm, this may be possible to detect if the clinician's hands are positioned on the left and right sides of the abdominal wall.

Examination Notes

At the end of Form 4-3 is a section for examination notes where the clinician can provide additional information. This section might be used to document the nature of the paresis or paralysis observed (i.e., flaccid and/or spastic) or to specify the type of hyperkinesis observed (i.e., tics, chorea, myoclonus, tremor, dystonia, among others). This section might also include comments regarding consistency of performance across related activities or on repeated performances of the same activity, the client's apparent motivation, his report of effort or fatigue, and his overall pattern of performance.

INSTRUMENTAL EXAMINATION OF SPEECH BREATHING

Observations of the types suggested in the previous four sections are all essential in the evaluation of speech breathing. The taking of a case history, administration of an auditory-perceptual examination, evaluation of speaking-related dyspnea, and administration of a physical examination go a long way toward determining the existence and nature of a potential speech breathing disorder. Often, however, additional information needs to be obtained through instrumental examination. This section describes instrumental examination of speech breathing as it pertains to the following three areas: (a) mechanical measurements of volume, pressure, and shape; (b) measurements of speech acoustics; and (c) measurements of physiological status.

Mechanical Measurements of Volume, Pressure, and Shape

Mechanical measurements of volume, pressure, and shape can be made during nonspeech activities and speech activities. Although observations of both types of activities can be instructive, it is important to recognize that they provide different information. This is because movements associated with nonspeech activities do not usually involve the precision, speed, and complexity of movements associated with speech activities. Also, the targets in nonspeech activities are not typically acoustic targets, as are the targets for speech activities. And nonspeech activities are under different neural control than are speech activities.

Estimation of Volume Change

The most important volume in speech breathing is lung volume, the volume of air within the pulmonary airways and lungs. This volume reflects the prevailing size of the breathing apparatus.

Volume change can be estimated by measuring volume events at the airway opening or at the body surface. The volume change at these two locations will be the same under certain circumstances, and different under other circumstances. This is because measures obtained at the airway opening and at the body surface do not reflect identical elements of volume change. Measurement at the airway opening "sees" volume displacement, whereas measurement at the body surface "sees" both volume displacement and volume compression/decompression (see sections on volume and pressure variables in Chapter 2).

Measurement at the Airway Opening

Measurement at the airway opening relies on the movement of air to and from the lungs through the oral and/or nasal cavities. When measuring volume at the airway opening, the measurement device is coupled to the client by a mouthpiece (held with the teeth and/or lips) or a mask (placed over the mouth and/or nose). The choice of a mouthpiece or mask depends on the particular application. For example, a mouthpiece (in the form of a large-bore tube) may be adequate for determining a client's vital capacity or the volume he expends during sustained vowel production. By contrast, a facemask is preferred for determining the volume expended during running speech activities. When using a mouthpiece or a mask that fits over the mouth alone, it is necessary to have the client wear a noseclip to ensure that volume is not lost through the nose.

Numerous devices can be used to estimate volume change at the airway opening. Common among these are the following: (a) wet spirometers; (b) dry spirometers; and (c) flow integrators.

Wet Spirometers: Figure 4-1 depicts a wet spirometer. Wet spirometers come in different configurations and sizes, but all include a cylindrical chamber that contains water and a bell that floats inside the chamber. Volume displacement causes air to move into or out of the bell to make it rise or fall, respectively. The height of the bell is directly proportional to the volume of air within the spirometer.

The simplest form of readout for a wet spirometer is a pointer fixed to its floating bell. This pointer moves against the background of a calibrated volume scale. Some wet spirometers have a chain attached to the top of the bell, which extends over an elevated pulley and connects to an ink-writing pen. The pen marks volume change on a rotating drum that is covered with calibrated paper. Some wet spirometers also have a potentiometer attached to the elevated pulley. This device converts volume change into a voltage equivalent that can be processed and displayed in real-time or recorded for subsequent playback.

Certain forms of wet spirometers require that, while in use, their bells be periodically pushed downward to flush them of stale air. Thus, the client coupled

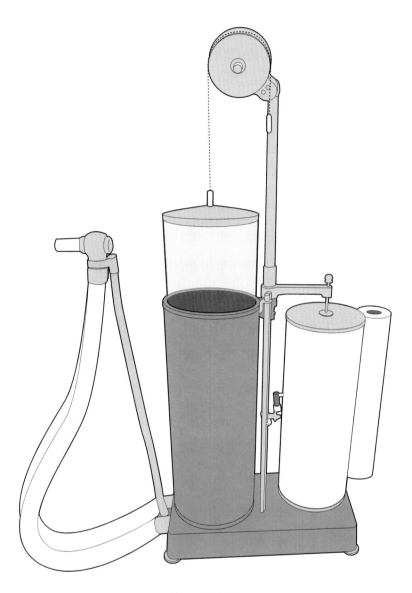

Figure 4-1. Wet spirometer.

to the spirometer must come off the device to allow its renewal with room air (achieved by pulling the bell back up once the system is flushed). Other forms of wet spirometers do not require flushing, but are equipped with systems that remove carbon dioxide with a carbon dioxide-absorber (such as a chamber containing soda lime) and supply oxygen to them with an oxygen wall-line or a tank of compressed oxygen.

Dry Spirometers: Dry spirometers also come in a variety of configurations and sizes. One of the most widely used is the wedge or bellows spirometer. The wedge spirometer is a large, sealed bellows consisting of two flat pans mounted vertically and interconnected by an airtight and flexible plastic membrane. The proximal pan is fixed in position and contains an access port and tubing through which the client can breathe. The distal pan can swing back and forth as air is moved in and out of the bellows chamber.

The simplest form of readout from a wedge spirometer is a pointer fixed to the lower edge of its distal pan. This pointer moves against the background of a calibrated volume scale. Some wedge spirometers have an output that is derived through a linear displacement transducer attached to the distal pan. This transducer senses the position of the distal pan and converts that position into a readout that can be processed and displayed or recorded for later playback. The discussion above on flushing and long-term continuous use of wet spirometers applies to dry spirometers as well.

Flow Integrators (and Pneumotachometers): Flow at the airway opening is a measure of the rate of change of lung volume. Therefore, lung volume change can be estimated by integrating (i.e., accumulating over time) such flow. In this context, flow measurement is like reading the speedometer in an automobile, and volume estimation is like reading the odometer. An odometer reflects an integration of the speedometer reading and indicates how far the automobile has traveled (analogous to lung volume displacement).

Flow measurement at the airway opening can be accomplished with a variety of measurement devices. The most widely used of these are pneumotachometers (i.e., air rate meters). Most pneumotachometers contain a resistive element in a tube. The pressure across this resistive element can be sensed to determine the rate at which air is moving through the tube. Such sensing is usually done with a mechanical-electrical manometer (see section below on the estimation of pressure). As air speeds up, the pressure drop across the resistive element increases and as air slows down the pressure drop across the resistive element decreases (this is true for flow in both directions through the tube). Because the resistance is known, the pressure drop across the element can

---

FULL OF HOT AIR

When measuring volumes, it's important to know temperature differences between where the volumes came from and where they're going. Blow on the back of your hand and you'll notice that the air coming out of you is warmer than room air (unless you're sitting in a sauna bath). Your internal air temperature is somewhere near 37°C, whereas room air temperature is probably more like 15 to 20°C. Thus, the hotter air coming out of you will compress once it encounters the colder air outside your body. Were you to breathe into a spirometer (a volume-measuring device) that was not warmed to your inside air temperature, it would record a smaller volume than you had displaced from your lungs. Be sure to read the instruction manual that comes with your spirometer, especially the section having to do with Body Temperature and Pressure, Saturated (BTPS). Otherwise, your volume data report could be full of hot air.

be converted to a measure of the flow through the element.

Figure 4-2 depicts one form of a commonly encountered pneumotachometer. This form uses a fine-wire mesh as its resistive element, which, when examined end-on, looks much like a view through a screen door. Other pneumotachometers use a cluster of tiny parallel tubes for a resistive element. When examined end-on, their resistive element looks much like a view down a handful of parallel straws. A pneumotachometer will usually have cones on both ends that channel flow toward and away from the resistive element. It will also have pressure taps positioned on each side of its resistive element so that the pressure differential across the element can be sensed. Pneumotachometers that have fine-wire mesh for a resistive element usually have a better frequency response than those that use parallel tubes. This is due to the fact that parallel tubes offer more inertance to the movement of air through them than do the side-by-side holes in a fine-wire mesh (because holes have essentially no length).

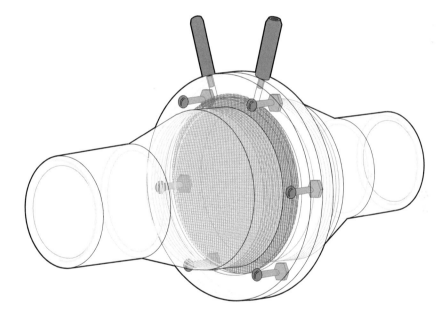

Figure 4-2. Pneumotachometer.

Another type of pneumotachometer consists of a facemask in which the resistive element (fine-wire mesh) is built into the wall of the mask itself. One example of such a device was developed by Mead (1960) and consists of a large mask that is placed over the client's face and secured by a head harness. The front of the mask is formed by a clear plastic plate and contains an opening covered by fine-wire mesh. Pressure within the mask is sensed and taken as a measure of flow through the fine-wire mesh at every instant.

Another form of pneumotachometer in which the resistive element is built into the wall of the mask is a circumferentially vented pneumotachometer often referred to as a Rothenberg mask (Rothenberg, 1973). This device (Glottal Enterprises, Inc., Syracuse, NY) consists of an anesthesia-type facemask containing several relatively large openings in its wall that are covered by fine-wire mesh. These comprise the resistive element of the system, with the pressure differential across them being proportional to the flow into and out of the mask. Pressure sensed inside the mask is used as the measure of flow across the known resistance offered by the collective screens. A handle on the Rothenberg mask can be used to secure it against the face during measurements.

Once a flow signal is obtained by a pneumotachometer, it is then subjected to temporal integration by an electronic integrator to estimate lung volume. A wide range of integrators is available commercially. The quality of an integrator's performance is influenced by the electronic characteristics of the device. For example, the time-constant of an integrator is important in breathing applications because the time-constant determines how well the integrator will resolve rapid flow change and, therefore, how accurately volume change will be estimated.

The readout options for flow integrators are the same as those available electronically on spirometers. They include display in real-time or playback from recorded signals.

Comparison of Devices for Use at the Airway Opening: Spirometers are relatively slow-response devices because of the inertia of their moving parts (i.e., bells and pans). They also present significant resistances in their connecting tubing and, in some cases, in their valves. These factors may not be a problem if volume change is slow. However, if volume change is fast, it may not be followed faithfully by a spirometer.

Spirometers are closed systems. That is, air is exchanged back and forth between the spirometer and the client. Some clients feel claustrophobic when coupled into a closed system, even when carbon dioxide and oxygen levels are appropriate. Clients with dyspnea may become apprehensive when coupled to a spirometer. Even the slight load sensed from the inertia and resistance of the spirometer may trigger client discomfort.

Flow integrators (in association with pneumotachometers) are the devices of choice for applications in which speed of response is important. Thus, they are preferred for measuring most speech breathing events. Their other advantages are that they are open systems that have relatively low resistance, very little dead space, and no moving parts. Clients are less likely to experience claustrophobia or dyspnea when coupled to a pneumotachometer than when coupled to a spirometer. Clients are also breathing room air rather than mixed air, as in a closed spirometer system. Another advantage of a flow integrator (and pneumotachometer) system is that the client has more freedom to move his head and neck compared to when coupled to the tubing of a spirometer. This can be important in clients with certain neuromotor disorders, especially for those who exhibit hyperkinesis.

Measurement at the Body Surface

Measurement at the body surface relies on the sensing of surface movement of the torso and its conversion into an estimate of volume change. Such estimates are most often based on one of three chest wall variables. These include the following: (a) circumferences; (b) anteroposterior diameters; and (c) cross-sectional areas. Measurements of these variables are often made using the following devices: (a) bellows pneumographs; (b) respiratory magnetometers; and (c) respiratory inductance plethysmographs.

Even though these three devices measure different aspects of chest wall function, they share a related measurement framework. In this framework, the chest wall is viewed as a two-part system, consisting of the rib cage wall and abdominal wall. Each part displaces volume as it moves, and together they displace a volume equal to that displaced by the lungs. Surface displacements of the rib cage wall and abdominal wall are approximately linearly related to their respective volume displacements. Thus, they can be used to estimate the volumes displaced by the individual parts (rib cage wall and abdominal wall). And, when the estimated volumes displaced by the individual parts are summed, they provide an estimate of the volume displaced by the lungs (i.e., lung volume change).

The three body surface devices under discussion also share similar calibration procedures. Calibration can be accomplished by having the client perform what is called an isovolume maneuver. This maneuver requires that the client change the shape of his chest wall while holding lung volume constant. For most applications, it is sufficient to perform this maneuver at a single lung volume (usually at the resting level of the breathing apparatus). To perform an isovolume maneuver, the client closes his larynx (to fix lung volume) and slowly displaces volume back and forth between his abdominal wall and rib cage wall (i.e., alternately moves his abdominal wall in and out). The volume exchanged between the two chest wall parts is equal and opposite during this maneuver. To reflect this relationship, the magnitudes of the signals recorded from the two parts are adjusted to be equal and opposite during the maneuver. Thereafter, the adjusted signals represent the volumes of their respective chest wall parts, and their summed signal represents lung volume. Calibration of lung volume change involves having the client inspire and expire known volumes of air while coupled to a device such as a spirometer.

Certain clients may be unable to perform an isovolume maneuver. Most often these are clients with neuromotor impairments who do not have the requisite motor skills or clients with cognitive impairments who cannot conceptualize the task. When obtaining body surface measure from such clients, it is necessary to calibrate in other ways. One option is to mathematically manipulate rib cage wall and abdominal wall data. A common way to do this is to use simultaneous equations to accomplish a least-squares solution (Chada, Watson, Birch, Jenouri, Schneider, Cohn, & Sackner, 1982). This approach can be used if the client is able to change his breathing pattern voluntarily or if his body position can be shifted to bring about change in his breathing pattern. Using this approach, weighted signals are derived for the rib cage wall and abdominal wall that are specific to the client observed.

Another option that can be used for two of the surface measurement devices – respiratory magnetometers and respiratory inductance plethysmographs – is to approximate the calibration by adjusting the signals from the two parts of the chest wall in accordance with their probable weightings, as determined empirically (Banzett, Mahan, Garner, Brughera, & Loring, 1995). For respiratory magnetometers, a scaling of 1:4 (rib cage wall:abominal wall) has been found to be the best approximation for estimating the relationship between rib cage wall and abdominal wall volumes. For respiratory inductance plethysmographs, a scaling of 1:2 (rib cage wall:abdominal wall) has been found to be best. It should be noted, however, that these scale factors were determined on adult subjects and may be different in children.

Another way to calibrate surface measurement signals is to manually adjust a client's chest wall for him. This calibration approach might be used in a client who has severely paretic chest wall muscles and cannot perform an isovolume maneuver independently. This form of assisted isovolume maneuver can be done by having the client hold his breath while the clinician pushes and releases on either the client's rib cage wall or abdominal wall. Manual adjustment must be done carefully, without causing unusual distortion of the structure being displaced. Otherwise, additional degrees of freedom may be induced that can render the calibration invalid.

For any of the body surface devices discussed, the signals for the rib cage wall and abdominal wall can be summed to represent lung volume and can be processed and displayed in real-time or recorded for playback. Displays can include volume-time or volume-volume arrays, the choice depending on the particular clinical application.

Although body surface devices share a conceptual framework and similar procedures for calibration, they differ in their specific functions. The next three sections consider each of the devices individually.

Bellows Pneumographs: Bellows

RUB A DUB DUB, TWO MEN IN A TUB

As told to the first of us by Jere Mead (the subject of a sidetrack in Chapter 3), respiratory magnetometry was born in a boat. Jere, a respiratory physiologist, and his brother John, a geologist, were sailing on a lake in Wisconsin. Talk got around to Jere's problem of trying to find a way to sense anteroposterior diameter changes of the chest wall in breathing studies. Existing methods had required that the subject stand with his back against the wall. John suggested that magnetometry might do the job, a method used in his discipline to track movements of the magnetic poles of Earth. The rest is history. The brothers Mead got out of the boat and went on with colleagues to create respiratory magnetometers (Mead, Peterson, Grimby, & Mead, 1967). And now you know why the first and last author on the seminal respiratory magnetometry article published in *Science* is J. Mead. Rub a dub dub. Two men in a tub.

pneumographs are pneumatic devices used to measure circumferential changes of the chest wall parts to which they are applied. They consist of two stretchable air-filled, rubber, accordian-pleated tubes, one that wraps around the rib cage wall and one that wraps around the abdominal wall. Bellows pneumographs are probably most commonly recognized for their use in lie-detector tests.

As the chest wall moves, the rubber tubes of the bellows pneumograph move with it. When the chest wall moves outward, the tubes stretch and their volumes increase. This causes the air pressure within them to decrease. Conversely, when the chest wall moves inward, the tubes shorten, their volumes decrease, and their internal air pressure increases. Pressure change is sensed by a mechanical-electrical manometer, which converts the pressure sensed into a voltage.

Placement of the bellows pneumograph tubes must be done carefully. Placement of a tube on the rib cage wall needs to be such that the nipples do not interfere with its movement, that it does not encroach on the border between the rib cage wall and abdominal wall, and that it does not roll. Placement of a tube on the abdominal wall also needs to be a reasonable distance from the border where the rib cage wall meets the abdominal wall. And a location should be sought where the tube does not roll. Difficulties may be encountered when attempting to use bellows pneumographs on women (and sometimes men) who have large breasts and on clients of both sexes who have large fat deposits.

It is often helpful to tape the tubes in place at several locations around each of the chest wall parts. Care should be taken to ensure that taping does not interfere with the natural stretching and recoiling of the tubes. When placed on the client, the tubes should be stretched slightly when he is at his resting tidal end-expiratory level. This helps to ensure that the tubes do not uncouple from the chest wall during expirations from that level. Tubes of different lengths are available to accommodate different torso sizes.

Respiratory Magnetometers: Respiratory magnetometers are electromagnetic devices that measure anteroposterior diameter changes of the chest wall parts to which they are applied. A commercial version of the device has been made by GMG Scientific, Inc. (Burlington, MA). Standard respiratory magnetometers consist of two pairs of electromagnetic coils, each of which is encased in plastic. As depicted in Figure 4-3, one pair of coils is designated to measure the anteroposterior diameter change of the rib cage wall and one pair is designated to measure the anteroposterior diameter change of the abdominal wall. For the rib cage wall, one coil is placed on the front at sternal midlength and one is placed on the back at the midline at the same axial level. For the abdominal wall, one coil is placed on the front at the midline just above the umbilicus and one is placed on the back at the midline at the same axial level. The coils are fixed to the skin with double-sided adhesive tape. The long axis of each coil is oriented parallel to the long axis of its mate and perpendicular to the long axis of the torso.

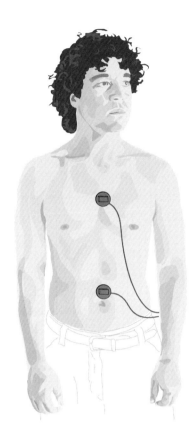

Figure 4-3. Respiratory magnetometers.

Each front coil generates a magnetic field that is sensed by its mate on the back of the torso. The two generating coils operate at different frequencies and each sensor coil responds only to the generating frequency of its mate. The voltage induced in each sensor coil is inversely proportional to the cube of the distance between it and its generator mate. Therefore, as anteroposterior diameter increases and decreases, voltage decreases and increases, respectively. Electronic corrections are built into modern magnetometer systems to linearize the outputs of their sensor coils. This means that a direct measure of absolute diameter change can be obtained from the absolute voltage change for each pair.

Respiratory magnetometers usually come with coils and electronic systems that accommodate measurements in adults. However, customized systems with small coils can be fashioned to make measurements in infants. These systems usually include four coil pairs rather than the two coil pairs used with adults. With four coil pairs, both the anteroposterior and transverse diameters of the rib cage wall and abdominal wall can be measured and cross-products of these diameters can be used to make volume change estimates of the chest wall part to which they are attached. Such a procedure takes into account the extra degrees of freedom encountered in the highly compliant (floppy) chest wall of the infant.

Some respiratory magnetometers for use with adults also have a third coil pair devoted to sensing spinal attitude by monitoring the flexion and extension of the spine. This third coil pair provides a correction for movement artifact that can be introduced by failure of the client to remain in a fixed torso position. More is said below about the problem of movement artifact.

Respiratory Inductance Plethysmographs: Respiratory inductance plethysmographs are designed to measure the average cross-sectional areas of the parts of the chest wall to which they are applied. Two versions of the devices are commercially available: Respitrace (Ambulatory Monitoring, Ardsley, NY) and Respigraph (Non-Invasive Monitoring Systems, Miami Beach, FL). Respiratory inductance plethysmographs are electronic devices. Their sensing elements consist of long electrical wires that are configured in a series of zigzags and are embedded in broad elastic bands. One band is designated to measure the average cross-sectional area of the rib cage wall and one band is designated to measure the average cross-sectional area of the abdominal wall.

As illustrated in Figure 4-4, the upper edge of the rib cage wall band is placed just below the axillae (arm pits). The band itself covers the upper rib cage wall and

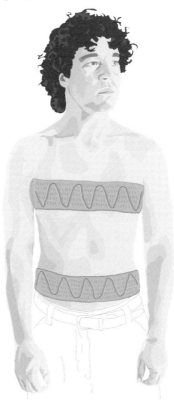

Figure 4-4. Respiratory inductance plethysmographs.

extends downward toward the border between the rib cage wall and abdominal wall. The band for the abdominal wall is positioned low on the wall so it does not cover the lower part of the rib cage wall. Once the two bands are positioned and made relatively secure (perhaps by taping them at a few locations along their edges), they can be further secured, if desired, by an elastic mesh placed over them (i.e., a sort of torso vest).

The expandable wire loop formed within each elastic band is connected to a small oscillator worn on the body. The output of the oscillator is coupled to a circuit that demodulates changes resulting from adjustments of the loop and produces a voltage equivalent of the average cross-sectional area of the portion of the chest wall encircled through the height of the band. Thus, as average cross-sectional area changes, voltage changes proportionately. The elastic transduction bands for respiratory inductance plethysmographs come in a variety of sizes. This makes it possible to use them with infants, children, and adults. The same electronic array can be used with different size bands.

Comparison of Devices for Use at the Body Surface: Compared to measurements made at the airway opening, body surface measurements have two distinct advantages. First, they do not require that the client be coupled to a measurement device through tubing and/or a mask, thus leaving the upper airway unencumbered and free to room atmosphere. Second, they reflect all of the lung volume change, including both volume displacement and volume compression/decompression, under all conditions.

One disadvantage of body surface devices compared to airway opening devices is that they are sensitive to body movements that are not related to breathing (as well as to those that are). For example, flexion and extension of the spinal column can introduce movement artifacts that change the magnitudes of the output signals from the sensing devices (especially that associated with the rib cage wall). An advantage of the three-coil respiratory magnetometer array (discussed above) is that it provides a correction for the flexion/extension variable. However, there are other ways to compensate for the spinal attitude variable and other potential movement artifacts. The easiest way is to videotape the client's performance during breathing measurement and subsequently note when extraneous movement occurs. Those segments noted can then be excluded from analysis.

Devices for making measurements at the body surface may encumber the chest wall somewhat. Those that encircle the chest wall are most restrictive.

Speed of response is generally not a concern when using body surface devices. Very rapid breathing movements can be tracked faithfully, except, perhaps, by bellows pneumographs. Their speed of response has limits imposed by their pneumatic nature. Nonetheless, for most everyday breathing events and many speech breathing events they are perfectly suitable devices.

On occasion there is ambiguity concerning whether the behavior monitored is related solely to the movement of the chest wall part that is targeted. For example, in the case of bellows pneumographs and respiratory inductance plethysmographs, it is sometimes difficult to ensure that the abdominal sensors do not also encircle the lower rib cage wall. This is because the border between the rib cage wall and abdominal wall is not fixed and may shift as breathing movement occurs. For example, during a deep inspiration, the rib cage wall moves up the axis of the torso and drags the abdominal wall with it. Measurement devices that encircle the chest wall, therefore, are prone to measurement artifact if a shifting border comes into play. This is not a problem with respiratory magnetometers because they are essentially point placed and can be positioned well away from the other chest wall part being examined.

If care is not taken, bellows pneumographs and respiratory inductance plethysmographs are subject to sensor rolling or slippage artifact during measurement. This does not occur with respiratory magnetometers. Rolling about the long axes of their electromagnetic coils does not influence their outputs.

Finally, it should be noted that respiratory magnetometers generate low-power electromagnetic fields. The strengths of these fields impose no known dangers for most clients. Nonetheless, it is prudent to avoid using respiratory magnetometers on pregnant women. Also, respiratory magnetometers should not be used on clients who have implanted electronic pacemakers of any type.

> **ONE THING LED TO ANOTHER**
>
> The framework of Konno and Mead (1967) has greatly influenced the study of breathing. As told to the first of us by Jere Mead, a single event got things started. Bouhuys, Proctor, and Mead (1966) were puzzled about the mechanism of inspiratory braking at large lung volumes during singing without recourse to the diaphragm. While trying to elucidate this mechanism, they put pneumobelts around the rib cage and abdomen to record circumference changes. Transduced signals from the pneumobelts were displayed against one another on an oscilloscope. The observation was made that when the abdomen was moved in and out during breath holding, a straight sloping line was formed on the display. Thus, the first isovolume line was serendipitously generated, pondered, and appreciated. Konno and Mead (1967) and Mead, Peterson, Grimby, and Mead (1967) followed and a measurement boom was off and running.

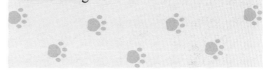

Evaluation of Volume Control

The volume variable can be evaluated by using any of the six devices discussed above. Measurements can be made during nonspeech activities and/or speech activities, depending on the type of information needed.

Measurement During Nonspeech Activities

Volume measurements during nonspeech activities should focus on the following three areas: (a) resting tidal breathing; (b) lung volumes and lung capacities; and (c) selected control of volume change.

Resting tidal breathing should be measured while the client is inattentive to his breathing. Otherwise, he may attempt to guide his breathing and not present his usual spontaneous pattern. Although resting tidal breathing patterns are expected to vary (see section on breathing for life purposes in Chapter 2), normal function should be characterized by smooth inspiratory and expiratory volume excursions, sometimes followed by a brief period of breath holding. Inspiratory duration should be slightly shorter than expiratory duration (a typical ratio might be 1:1.2 for an adult). And the volume excursions should cover about 10% of the predicted vital capacity.

The lung volumes and lung capacities of interest (in addition to the resting tidal volume) are the inspiratory reserve volume, the expiratory reserve volume, the inspiratory capacity, and the vital capacity. These four can be measured from a one-stage vital capacity maneuver (with prior knowledge of the resting tidal volume). For this, the client is instructed to inspire as much as possible from the resting tidal end-expiratory level and then expire as much as possible. It is important that the clinician motivate the client to exert his best effort, usually by cheering him on while he is inspiring and expiring. It may also be important for the client to perform the vital capacity maneuver at a moderate speed. If it is performed too quickly, the airways may collapse in some clients (particularly senescent clients) and the full vital capacity may not be expired.

Selected control of volume change can be measured during a number of activities, depending on what the speech-language pathologist wishes to know about the client's nonspeech control capability. The following examples are used for illustration: (a) breath holding at different lung volumes with the larynx open; and (b) tracking a prescribed volume change pattern.

Having the client breath hold at different lung volumes with the larynx open can be instructive. When breath holding is done at lung volumes that are larger or smaller than the resting level of the breathing apparatus, muscular pressure is required to oppose the relaxation pressure and maintain the apparatus in a fixed position. Breath holding at large lung volumes requires inspiratory muscular pressure, and breath holding at small lung volumes requires expiratory muscular pressure. The magnitude of the muscular pressure required depends on the degree of departure from the resting level. It is important to be certain that the breath is being held by muscles of the breathing apparatus and not by muscles of the larynx or upper airway. This can be verified by a quick but gentle push on the client's abdominal wall. If the breathing apparatus is doing the breath holding (as desired), a puff of air will escape through the client's mouth and/or nose. If the larynx or upper airway is doing the holding, no air will escape.

Tracking is also a useful method for evaluating nonspeech volume control capability. One approach is to have the client attempt to adjust volume continuously in a prescribed pattern. This requires that volume change be sensed by a device with an electronic output that can be monitored in a volume-time display. The clinician begins by drawing a sine wave pattern on the display for the client to track. The pattern should be a large and slowly changing volume excursion, perhaps encompassing as much as 50% of the client's vital capacity, and perhaps covering 10 seconds for a full cycle. The client is instructed to track the pattern as precisely as possible by changing his lung volume. Individuals with normal control of the breathing apparatus will track such a pattern with little difficulty, showing only small deviations from its course.

Measurement During Speech Activities

Volume measurements during speech breathing should include a variety of activities. These are as follows: (a) utterances produced throughout most of the vital capacity; (b) running speech breathing; (c) running speech produced outside the usual lung volume range; and (d) running speech produced at other-than-usual loudness.

Lung volume should be measured for a sustained vowel produced at the client's normal loudness, pitch, and quality, following a maximum inspiration and continuing for as long as possible. A series of syllable repetitions or an activity such as counting aloud may also be used in this context. Individuals with normal control of the breathing apparatus should exhibit large volume excursions for such activities, excursions that approach their vital capacities.

For running speech breathing, lung volume measurements should be made while the client reads aloud, speaks extemporaneously, and engages in conversational speaking. Guidelines for the performance of these activities are provided above in the section on the auditory-perceptual examination. Normal performance of these types of running speech activities usually involves initiation of breath groups at lung volumes that are larger (typically 20 %VC or so) than the resting tidal end-expiratory level. Breath groups usually end in the vicinity of the resting tidal end-expiratory level, with occasional continuation to smaller lung volumes. Lung volume excursions for running speech activities typically encompass about 20 %VC.

The ability to speak outside the usual lung volume range is an indication of the flexibility of speech breathing control. Such flexibility can be evaluated by having the client attempt to generate running speech at lung volumes that are different than usual. The easiest way to accomplish this is to instruct the client to speak at large lung volumes and then to speak at small lung volumes. Allowing the client to see a display of his lung volume can facilitate his performance. For example, delimiting usual, large, and small lung volume ranges on a volume display is often helpful.

Observation of lung volume change during running speech of other-than-usual loudness can also provide insights into a client's speech breathing control. This is most easily tested by having the client read aloud. Specifically, the client is asked to read the same passage at usual loudness, at half-usual loudness, and at twice-usual loudness while his lung volume is being monitored. Half-usual loudness is generally associated with smaller-than-usual volume initiations and twice-usual loudness is generally associated with larger-than-usual volume initiations. The typical strategy is to increase the breath group initiation level for louder speech to take advantage of greater relaxation pressure at larger lung volumes.

Estimation of Pressure

The important pressure for speech breathing is alveolar pressure, the pressure inside the air sacs of the pulmonary apparatus. This pressure represents the net driving pressure for speech production and information about it is relevant to the evaluation of speech breathing.

Alveolar pressure is inaccessible to direct measurement in humans because of the location of the alveoli within the body. Nevertheless, it is possible to estimate alveolar pressure (or closely related tracheal pressure) by measuring oral pressure under specified conditions. These conditions require that the airways between the alveoli and oral cavity are unobstructed and that flow through them is zero (or nearly so).

When estimating alveolar pressure from oral pressure, it is important that the velopharynx and lips be sealed airtight. If velopharyngeal incompetence or insufficiency is known or suspected, the anterior nares should be occluded with a noseclip or gloved fingers. And, if an incompetent or insufficient lip seal is observed or suspected, the lips should be supported with tape or gloved fingers. Leaks at the velopharynx and/or lips will result in a falsely low estimate of alveolar pressure.

It is also important that the oral pressure being generated relates solely to the alveolar pressure being generated. Therefore, care must be taken to ensure that the client does not impound oral pressure through adjustments of the cheeks, tongue, and other structures that can compress or decompress the oral volume.

When making a measurement of oral pressure, the client is coupled to some sort of measurement device by way of a connecting tube. The form of this tube depends on the particular application and may range from a long and large-bore tube to a short and small-bore catheter to a plastic drinking straw.

Measurement in the Oral Cavity

Various instruments can be used to measure oral pressure. Common among these are the following: (a) air-gauge manometers; (b) water-bubble manometers; (c) U-tube water manometers; and (d) mechanical-electrical manometers.

Air-Gauge Manometers: Air-gauge manometers have various presentations, but all have a gauge with a needle that indicates the pressure being generated. The face of the gauge resembles that of a clock, with clockwise rotation of the needle reflecting increases in air pressure. The gauge is calibrated in some unit of pressure relative to atmospheric pressure.

Two common air-gauge manometers are the aneroid-gauge manometer and the Bourdon-gauge manometer. Each has a gear arrangement that drives the deflection of its needle. The aneroid-gauge manometer relies on the expansion and contraction of a sealed-capsule element as pressure changes. This capsule expands and contracts like a sealed bag of potato chips that expands and contracts when pressure around it changes with changes in elevation or altitude. The Bourdon-gauge manometer, by contrast, has a flexible-tube element that uncurls and curls as pressure changes. This element is like a carnival blower that unrolls and rolls up as pressure is applied and withdrawn.

Water-Bubble Manometers: A water-bubble manometer is depicted in Figure 4-5. This device is a bricolage constructed from a drinking glass, masking tape, a paper clip, and a straw. The glass is calibrated by placing a vertical strip of tape on its side and marking it off in centimeter (cm) intervals. The zero level for the calibration tape is placed an inch or so below the rim of the glass and intervals are numbered sequentially downward (1, 2, 3, etc.). Water is placed in the glass up to the zero level on the calibration tape.

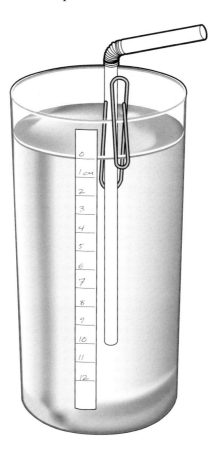

Figure 4-5. Water-bubble manometer. (After Hixon, Hawley, & Wilson, 1982)

The principle underlying the water-bubble manometer is that, to blow a bubble under water, the pressure exerted by the air in the straw must be greater than the pressure exerted by the water at the submerged end of the straw. Thus, if the straw is submerged so that its end is 10 cm below the surface of the water, the air pressure exerted to generate a bubble must be greater than 10 cmH$_2$O. The submerged end of the straw need only be adjusted vertically to change the pressure required to blow a bubble.

U-Tube Water Manometers: Figure 4-6 depicts a U-tube water manometer. Note the term "water" in this context. ***Never use a U-tube mercury manometer for this clinical purpose. Such a manometer poses serious risks if mercury contacts the skin or is aspirated into the pulmonary airways and lungs.***

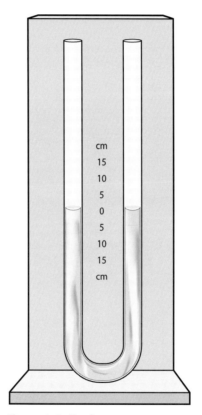

Figure 4-6. U-tube water manometer.

A connecting tube is coupled to one arm of the U-tube water manometer and the other arm of the device is left open to atmosphere. Pressure applied to the manometer through its connecting tube displaces the water in the U-tube, down one side and up the other. A distance scale behind the U-tube, calibrated in cm intervals, reveals the extent to which the water columns in the two arms are displaced. Pressure values are read as the difference in height between the two water columns. For example, a downward displacement of 2.5 cm for one column (the side with the connecting tube) and an accompanying upward displacement of 2.5

cm for the other column is equal to a height difference of 5.0 cm, or a pressure reading of 5.0 cmH$_2$O.

Mechanical-Electrical Manometers: The mechanical-electrical manometer is the most technically sophisticated of the four types of manometers discussed here. Mechanical-electrical manometers are also called air pressure transducers. Such manometers come in several forms, but have in common that they convert the pressure applied to them into an electrical signal (usually a voltage analog). Figure 4-7 shows three mechanical-electrical manometers. Pressure is delivered to one side of the manometer and the other side remains open to atmosphere (the two sides are partitioned by an intervening diaphragm). The output signal of the manometer (which reflects the pressure operating across its diaphragm) is amplified and displayed for monitoring and/or recorded for later playback.

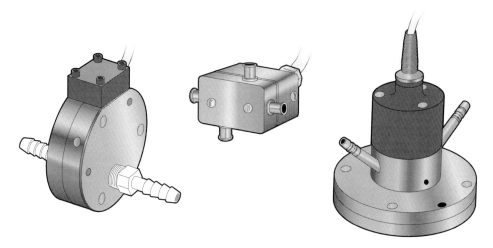

Figure 4-7. Three mechanical-electrical manometers (pressure transducers).

The output signal can be calibrated in pressure units against a known pressure source. The U-tube water manometer is the most common device used for this purpose. Calibration can be carried out so that divisions along the vertical axis on a visual display represent some convenient value. A time-base for displaying the pressure signal can also be set to sweep across the display at some convenient rate.

Comparison of Devices for Use in the Oral Cavity: All four devices discussed above for measuring oral pressure are relatively simple to use. Nevertheless, they have relative advantages and disadvantages.

The air-gauge manometer, water-bubble manometer, and U-tube water manometer are slow-response devices because of the inertia inherent in their moving parts and/or the water they contain. Also, these three devices require that the observer make on-line pressure readings. For the air-gauge manometer and U-tube water manometer, this requires that the observer do a visual determination (perhaps aver-

At the end of a short course presented by the first of us along with two colleagues, our Stockholm hosts held a banquet in our honor. We'd all heard of Swedish hospitality, but none of us was quite prepared. Part of the short course had discussed the clinical uses of the water-bubble manometer introduced in an article in the *Journal of Speech and Hearing Disorders* (Hixon, Hawley, & Wilson, 1982). Each guest entering the banquet hall was given a copy of that article and each setting at the banquet table included a handmade water-bubble manometer. Surely, that many water-bubble manometers had never before been assembled in one place. After the formal dinner, the intent of the planners became clear. The Swedish attendees sang folk songs to us well into the night. Before each song, those about to sing would blow into their water-bubble manometers in mock test of the adequacy of their driving pressure for performance. All passed.

aging) of the pressure magnitude being displayed on the dial face or water-column grid, respectively. For the water-bubble manometer, it requires that the observer make a judgment concerning the nature of bubble generation (e.g., rate and magnitude).

A disadvantage of the air-gauge manometer, water-bubble manometer, and U-tube water manometer is that they do not provide a permanent record of the pressure generated. Thus, it is not possible to check for reading errors. Nor do these three devices provide a time reference. Thus, the duration and variability of pressure generation is not easily documented. An external timing device, such as a stopwatch, can be used as a time reference, but this does not solve the problem of documenting variability.

The mechanical-electrical manometer (air pressure transducer) is the device of choice for estimating alveolar pressure from oral pressure. It provides a permanent record that documents duration and variability of pressure generation. The mechanical-electrical manometer has a fast response time and faithfully follows even the most rapid of pressure changes generated. In addition, there is less chance of reading error on the part of the clinician, because the permanent record can be examined repeatedly and by others. The resulting record can be included as a part of the client's file for future reference and may be of value when examining the client's performance within and across activities.

Evaluation of Pressure Control

The pressure variable can be evaluated through the use of the four measurement devices discussed. All four have potential application for the evaluation of nonspeech activities, whereas only the mechanical-electrical manometer has application for the evaluation of speech activities. A special case exists for the evaluation of pressure control in the client with a tracheostomy.

Measurement During Nonspeech Activities

Pressure measurements during nonspeech activities should focus on the following three areas: (a) pressure screening; (b) maximum inspiratory pressure and maximum expiratory pressure; and (c) selected control of pressure change.

Pressure screening uses pass/fail criteria for magnitude and duration. The task for the client is to generate oral pressure at a prescribed magnitude and to maintain that pressure for a prescribed duration. The most common practice is to ask the client to generate an oral pressure of 5 cmH_2O for 5 seconds. This is sometimes referred to as the 5-for-5 screening criterion and is believed to approximate the minimal demands encountered in running speech production.

To perform a pressure screening, the client is instructed to take a moderately deep breath, perhaps to twice resting tidal breathing depth, and then blow into the measurement device. It is helpful to mark the pressure display on the device with the targeted pressure. When using the water-bubble manometer, the targeted pressure is indicated by the depth of the distal end of the straw. A targeted duration for pressure generation can be indicated for the mechanical-electrical manometer, but not for the other types of manometers. When using another type of manometer, duration of pressure generation can be screened with a stopwatch. There is, of course, the option of counting time to the cadence of one thousand one, one thousand two, one thousand three, etc. This can provide a rough quantification of elapsed time in seconds.

When using water-containing manometers, there is the risk that if a high enough pressure is generated, the water may be blown out of the device. In attempts to avoid this problem, it is good practice to instruct the client to just moderately exceed the targeted pressure. Without such instruction, a client (usually a child or a teenager) may assume that the task is to generate the greatest pressure possible.

When measuring oral pressure, it is important to ensure that the pressure sensed by the device relates solely to the client's alveolar pressure. To eliminate the potential confound of contributions from pressure generated by oral structures, a leak tube can be inserted into the oral cavity at one corner of the mouth. The presence of this tube makes it necessary for the client to continuously re-supply air to the upper airway and interferes with his ability to compress air with oral structures. The leak tube should be 5 cm long with an internal diameter of 2 mm. The resistance offered by such a tube is approximately 75 cmH_2O/LPS (centimeters of water per liter per second) at a flow of 0.1 LPS and serves to simulate laryngeal airway resistance associated with a sustained vowel produced at normal loudness, pitch, and quality (Netsell & Hixon, 1978). Thus, although the site of the resistance is shifted downstream of the larynx to the mouth, the breathing apparatus still "sees" a resistance that is comparable to that associated with a sustained vowel production. The presence of a low flow does not significantly violate assumptions underlying the pressure measurement. When there is free communication under relatively low-flow conditions, the pressure between the alveoli and the oral cavity is likely to be highly similar and to differ only due to the resistive pressure loss between them. This loss is very small under low-flow conditions so that alveolar and oral pressures may be thought of as one and the same. Inducing a leak to prohibit the client from impounding oral pressure is far more important for measurement purposes than is the small error introduced by the use of a leak tube.

Turning to maximum inspiratory pressure and maximum expiratory pressure, the best devices for this application are air-gauge manometers and mechanical-electrical manometers because they can accommodate a large range of pressure. Maximum inspiratory pressure and maximum expiratory pressure are determined by having the client suck as hard as possible and blow as hard as possible, respectively, for a brief period at the resting tidal end-expiratory level while connected to a manometer. Because the relaxation pressure is zero at the resting level, any pressure developed is attributable entirely to the muscular pressure exerted. A normal young adult male might generate in excess of 100 cmH_2O of inspiratory muscular pressure and in excess of 150 cmH_2O of expiratory muscular pressure. Note that often these measures are obtained at lung volume extremes (i.e., near the residual volume for maximum inspiratory pressure and near the total lung capacity for maximum expiratory pressure) so that caution should be exercised when making comparisons to published values.

There are certain clients for whom maximum efforts (such as are required for the generation of maximum inspiratory pressures and maximum expiratory pressures) are contraindicated. These include clients with velopharyngeal incompetence (who might inflate their eustachian tubes and cause pain), those with heart disease, those with abdominal hernias, and those with cardiovascular reflex problems, among others. For such clients, maximum effort tasks may be eliminated altogether or relatively low-effort substitutes may be considered with the approval of the appropriate physician. On the expiratory side, for example, the pressure needed for speech production rarely exceeds 15 cmH_2O. Thus, raising pressure to that level, with medical clearance for certain clients, would provide a good deal of information about expiratory muscular pressure without causing significant risk.

For evaluating nonspeech control of pressure change, two paradigms are suggested. Both of these call for use of the mechanical-electrical manometer because this is the only manometer that provides a record of pressure over time. One paradigm is used to evaluate how well the client can target and maintain a specified pressure (the standard leak tube is used during this test). This is done by showing the client the pressure-time display and having him attempt to maintain a target that is marked on the display. Several target values may be chosen to represent a range of pressures that are characteristic of normal speech production, for example, 5.0, 7.5, and 10 cmH_2O. Individuals with normal pressure control should be able to sustain a pressure quite steadily for a protracted period (perhaps 10 seconds or more) without difficulty.

The second nonspeech pressure control paradigm is similar to that already described for the evaluation of volume control. In this paradigm, the client is asked to adjust pressure continuously in a prescribed pattern. The suggested pattern to trace is a simple sine wave, representing a slowly changing pressure. The pressure excursion might be as large as 10 cmH$_2$O and the cycle might be as long as 10 seconds. The client is instructed to look at the pressure-time display and track the pattern as precisely as possible. It is advisable to use a leak tube to prevent the client from manipulating pressure with his upper airway structures. Individuals with normal control of the breathing apparatus should be able to track such a prescribed pressure pattern, showing only small deviations from its course.

Measurement During Speech Activities

It is not possible to estimate alveolar pressure continuously from oral pressure during speech production. This is because speech production involves frequent obstructions and constrictions of the laryngeal and upper airways. These events cause pressure to vary along these airways, primarily because of resistive losses, so that alveolar pressure and oral pressure are often different. Nevertheless, alveolar pressure can be estimated from oral pressure during speech production by using a method in which discontinuous estimates of alveolar pressure are obtained. This method requires a mechanical-electrical manometer and a particular type of speech sample.

The key to this method is that it capitalizes on the brief period during the production of voiceless stop-plosives when oral pressure and alveolar pressure are identical. This brief period occurs during the closed phase of voiceless stop-plosives, when the oral and velopharyngeal airways are sealed and the laryngeal airway is open. During the latter part of this closed phase, the pressure within the oral cavity behind the site of airway closure equilibrates with the pressure in the alveoli. This equilibration is coincident with the occurrence of the peak (i.e., maximum) oral pressure. Thus, the peak oral pressure measured during the production of a voiceless stop-plosive can be taken as an estimate of the alveolar pressure at that instant. When an utterance sequence includes appropriately interspersed voiceless stop-plosives, it is possible to use measurements of successive oral pressure peaks to infer the alveolar pressure contour underlying the utterance. This can be done by constructing an estimated contour from successive linear interpolations between adjacent pressure peaks.

Any voiceless stop-plosive can be used to estimate alveolar pressure from oral pressure. There are, however, distinct advantages to using /p/ (versus /t/ or /k/) for clinical applications. One is that the place of production for /p/ is the most anterior of the voiceless stop-plosives so that the measurement of oral pressure can be made with the least intrusion on articulation. Another advantage is that the competency of closure of the oral airway around the sensing tube is more easily verified on /p/ than it is at other places of production.

The general method for measuring oral pressure involves the insertion of a small polyethylene sensing tube at one corner of the mouth, perpendicular to the air stream and slightly behind the front teeth. The other end of the tube is connected to a mechanical-electrical manometer (air pressure transducer) and associated instrumentation.

PRESSURE POINTS

Some who have estimated alveolar pressure from oral pressure during speech production have suggested that oral pressure must reach a plateau to be an adequate representation of the estimated pressure. Therefore, they do things that alter usual speech behavior in ways that generate relatively flat oral pressure tracings, things like dramatically slowing and modifying utterances. This is a misguided practice. Pressure equilibration along the airway does not require a prolonged steady pressure plateau within the oral cavity. The only thing required is that there be an "instant" of equilibration at the peak oral pressure. The peak oral pressure during naturally produced voiceless stop-plosives is as close to the truth as one can get without directly measuring alveolar pressure. It's perfectly okay, even desirable, for tracing profiles of oral pressure to be pointed rather than flat.

The most common practice when using this method is to have the client generate a series of consonant-vowel syllables (e.g., /pipipipipi/) on a single expiration initiated from about twice resting tidal breathing depth. Five to seven syllables in a series are typically encouraged, but somewhat shorter strings may be acceptable, depending on the capabilities of the client. The client is first asked to produce the syllable string at his usual loudness, pitch, and quality with equal stress on each syllable. It is standard to have the client attempt to use a repetition rate equal to or greater than 1.5 syllables per second. This is because a slower rate is sometimes accompanied by intermittent velopharyngeal opening between syllables, even in individuals with normal velopharyngeal function. Accurate estimates of alveolar pressure cannot be made in the presence of an open velopharynx.

Application of this method is usually straightforward. However, the method should be modified for clients who present with incompetent velopharyngeal and/or oral valves. Such incompetence causes continuous flow during speech production, and continuous flow makes it impossible to attain equilibration between oral and alveolar pressures. In the case of velopharyngeal incompetence, one solution is to occlude the anterior nares, either with a noseclip or digitially (wearing latex gloves), during the recording of oral pressure. In the case of oral incompetence, one solution is to digitally support the lips (or support the lower lip with tape) to help the client form a seal between the lips and the pressure sensing tube. Velopharyngeal and/or oral incompetence (or insufficiency) occurs most often in clients who demonstrate neuromotor or craniofacial disorders. Oral incompetence is also sometimes encountered in healthy senescent individuals.

Although it might seem that data gathered in the presence of a leak would be of no value, this is not true. Because flow is continuous in the presence of a leak, the pressure sensed by the oral pressure probe will always be falsely lower than the corresponding alveolar pressure (for air to flow outward there must be a decreasing pressure gradient between the alveoli and atmosphere). Thus, if a client generates a given pressure in the presence of a leak, the clinician can assume that the client has the capability to generate at least that much pressure and maybe more. This is a useful principle to keep in mind even when a precise determination cannot be made about the presence or absence of a leak.

Control of pressure during speech production can be evaluated during syllable productions such as those just described. A simple approach is to have the client produce a string of syllables at usual, half-usual, and twice-usual loudness. Or the client can be instructed to produce a string with increasing loudness on successive syllables or decreasing loudness on successive syllables. Or the client might be asked to place increased linguistic stress on selected syllables in a string. Individuals with normal speech breathing control have no difficulty effecting such patterns of alveolar pressure change.

It is possible and often desirable to estimate alveolar pressure from oral pressure during speech samples other than syllable repetitions. For example, it may be instructive to estimate alveolar pressure during the client's production of the voiceless stop-plosive /p/ when it is strategically imbedded with a carrier phrase, such as "Say /ipi/ again." As another example, alveolar pressure can be estimated while reading aloud a paragraph that is heavily loaded with /p/ segments to gain insight into pressure control during more continual forms of speech production. As with series of syllables, running speech samples can be varied in loudness and linguistic stress to determine the pressure control capability of the client.

Measurement in the Client with a Tracheostomy

The client with a tracheostomy presents a special case when it comes to the estimation of alveolar pressure. Such a client offers the opportunity to estimate alveolar pressure from the measurement of tracheal pressure. The coupling of the client to the measurement device should be done with care and under the supervision of a physician. The client must be able to inspire through his upper airway with his tracheostomy occluded. If he cannot, he is not a candidate for the pressure evaluation procedures described below.

The approach used to sense tracheal pressure depends, in part, on whether or not the client has a tracheostomy tube (i.e., a tube situated within the tracheostomy). If he does not have a tracheostomy tube, a small rubber cork can be used to couple the client to a measurement device. The cork is prepared by boring a center hole throughout its length. One end of a connecting tube is inserted into the cork and its other end is coupled to an appropriate measurement device. Selection of the size of the cork is dictated by the size of the client's tracheostomy and the need to ensure that the cork fits airtight. If the client has a tracheostomy tube, a cork can be sized to fit the tracheostomy tube. Another option is to use a commercially available adapter that fits tightly into the tracheostomy tube and has a membrane through which a small hole can be bored. One end of a polyethylene connecting tube is inserted through the cork (or through the membrane of a tracheostomy tube adapter) far enough to reach the other end of the cork, but not so far as to contact the posterior tracheal wall. The other end of the connecting tube is attached to a pressure measurement device.

One advantage of estimating alveolar pressure from tracheal pressure is that there is no need to be concerned about incompetent or insufficient velopharyngeal and/or lip closure invalidating the measurement. Nevertheless, if a client presents with a known or suspected velopharyngeal leak, it is instructive to estimate alveolar pressure (from tracheal pressure) with the anterior nares unoccluded and occluded. This allows the clinician to gain insight into breathing strategies used by the client to compensate for the velopharyngeal leak. The same principle could apply to a problematic lip seal. The other major advantage of estimating alveolar pressure from tracheal pressure is that estimates can be sampled continuously during both nonspeech and speech activities.

Two of the measurement devices discussed can be used to estimate alveolar pressure from tracheal pressure for nonspeech activities – the air-gauge manometer and the mechanical-electrical manometer. The mechanical-electrical manometer is the only device appropriate for use for speech activities. *The U-tube water manometer and the water-bubble manometer should never be used to make measurements at the tracheostomy because of the danger of water aspiration into the pulmonary airways and lungs.*

The evaluation procedures for the client with a tracheostomy differ somewhat from those for the client without a tracheostomy. For the nonspeech pressure screening procedure, the client should be instructed to inspire to about twice resting tidal breathing depth and blow through an appropriate leak tube inserted between the lips while tracheal pressure is being measured. The 5-for-5 criterion (i.e., 5 cmH$_2$O for 5 seconds) is appropriate here. For the other nonspeech procedures (maximum inspiratory pressure, maximum expiratory pressure, and control of pressure change), the larynx or upper airway should be closed. To ensure closure, it may be necessary to occlude the client's anterior nares with a noseclip or gloved fingers. For speech procedures, no special modifications are required. In fact, because tracheal pressure measurement during speech production is made upstream of the laryngeal and upper airway valves, there is no need to be restricted to the use of voiceless stop-plosives to obtain a valid estimate of alveolar pressure. The same types of variables can be tested (e.g., ability to increase or decrease pressure by manipulating loudness or linguistic stress), but the phonetic content of the speech sample is much less important.

Estimation of Shape

The shape of interest in the present context is that of the chest wall, a structure that derives its shape from the combined positioning of the rib cage wall and abdominal wall. Shape is important because it influences the prevailing mechanical advantages of different parts of the chest wall and allows inferences to be made concerning underlying muscular mechanisms.

Shape can be estimated during both nonspeech activities and speech activities by monitoring surface movements of the rib cage wall and abdominal wall. Such movements can be quantified using measurements of circumferences, anteroposterior diameters, and average cross-sectional areas. These are the same measurements discussed for estimating lung volume change from the body surface. Thus, exactly the same measurement issues considered there also apply here.

Measurement of Shape

Shape can only be measured at the body surface. Common measurement devices for monitoring surface movements include bellows pneumographs, respiratory magnetometers, and respiratory inductance plethysmographs, the same devices used to measure lung volume change at the body surface. What is different, however, is that the signals from the rib cage wall and abdominal wall are not summed electronically to create a lung volume signal, but are considered in their own right in a different form of graphic display. The standard for such a display is a diagram of rib cage wall volume against abdominal wall volume, with rib cage wall volume increasing upward on the vertical axis and abdominal wall volume increasing rightward on the horizontal axis.

Comparison of Devices for Use at the Body Surface: The relative advantages and disadvantages of the three measurement devices have been discussed above in relation to the measurement of lung volume change. The same relative advantages and disadvantages apply here to shape measurements.

Evaluation of Shape Control

The shape variable can be evaluated with any of the three devices. All that is needed is a display of a surface movement variable for the rib cage wall against one similar in kind for the abdominal wall.

Measurement During Nonspeech Activities

Shape measurements during nonspeech activities should focus on the following: (a) resting tidal breathing; (b) prescribed control of shape under an isovolume condition; and (c) prescribed altering of shape toward its extremes.

Shape during resting tidal breathing should be characterized by a slight inward positioning of the abdominal wall and a slight outward positioning of the rib cage wall from their respective relaxation positions when seated or standing (upright). By contrast, when lying down (supine), the rib cage wall would be expected to be positioned inward slightly and the abdominal wall to be positioned outward slightly from their respective relaxation positions.

Shape control can be evaluated under an isovolume condition by having the client close his larynx and alternately shift volume back and forth between the abdominal wall and rib cage wall. This can usually be effected by asking the client to "hold your breath and then slowly move your belly in and out as far as you can." This maneuver, if performed at or near the resting end-expiratory level, should elicit extensive and reciprocal movements of the rib cage wall and abdominal wall.

Prescribed shape changes can be evaluated by having the client attempt to assume disparate shapes while monitoring the rib cage wall-abdominal wall display and adjusting his shape to move from quadrant to quadrant in the display. A simple paradigm is to have the client attempt to change his shape to manifest the following four combinations: (a) expanded rib cage wall and expanded abdominal wall; (b) expanded rib cage wall and contracted abdominal wall; (c) contracted rib cage wall and expanded abdominal wall; and (d) contracted rib cage wall and contracted abdominal wall. These adjustments approach the four polar coordinates of the display of rib cage wall volume versus abdominal wall volume. Normal individuals can accomplish these adjustments relatively easily.

Measurement During Speech Activities

Shape measurements should also be made during speech activities. Suggested speech activities include the following: (a) utterances produced throughout most of the vital capacity; and (b) running speech activities.

Shape control should first be evaluated by having the client attempt to adjust shape during the production of a sustained vowel. The client is instructed to inspire maximally and then sustain a vowel at his usual loudness, pitch, and quality for as long as he can while "alternately moving his belly in and out as far as possible." Performance of this activity should elicit a wide range of rib cage wall and abdominal wall movements.

When producing running speech in the upright body position, the abdominal wall volume should be smaller and the rib cage wall volume should be larger than they are during relaxation. By contrast, in the supine body position, the rib cage wall volume should be smaller and the abdominal wall volume should be larger than they are during relaxation. Shape should be monitored while the client reads aloud, speaks extemporaneously, and engages in conversational speaking.

Shape control during running speech activities can be evaluated by having the client speak at other than his usual shape. The easiest way to do this is to instruct the client to speak with his abdominal wall markedly inward and then markedly outward. Individuals with good shape control can accomplish these tasks with little difficulty.

Measurements of Speech Acoustics

Most readers probably have experience with recording speech (acoustic) signals. The purpose here is not to provide a tour de force about measurements of speech acoustics. Rather, it is merely to offer suggestions related to the use of microphones for sensing and transducing speech associated with breathing events.

Some clients with speech breathing disorders have hyperkinesis and are subject to either predictable or unpredictable extraneous movements of the torso, head, and neck. For these clients, a head-mounted microphone is recommended. This type of microphone helps to ensure that a constant mouth-to-microphone distance is maintained throughout the evaluation. Another way to ensure a constant mouth-to-microphone distance is to tape a small microphone to the client's forehead.

While head-mounted microphones are the best choice for most clients, some clients may be hypersensitive to devices placed on the head and face. With these clients, other types of microphones may be considered, such as lapel microphones or stand-mounted microphones.

Whatever microphone is being used, an attempt should be made to maximize the sensing of the client's speech while minimizing background noise, so that the signal-to-noise ratio is as favorable as possible. Also, it is essential that mouth-to-microphone distance remains constant if sound pressure level measurements or loudness judgments are planned. If comparisons in sound pressure level or loudness are to be made across recording sessions, the precise placement of the microphone (e.g., distance from mouth, angle relative to lips) should be documented so that the same placement can be used across sessions.

Measurements of Physiological Status

Measurements of physiological status are safety-related measurements. They are critically important when evaluating and managing certain clients, but may not be necessary for others. Whether or not such measurements need to be made should be determined by the client's pulmonologist or other appropriate physician, and some of these measurements should be made in consultation with the client's respiratory therapist. Measurements of physiological status are essential when managing clients who require ventilatory support (see Chapter 6).

There are many measurements of physiological status. The four discussed here – heart rate, blood pressure, oxygen saturation, and partial pressure of carbon dioxide – are strong indicators of cardiopulmonary status and are relatively easy to obtain. The physician may require that additional safety-related measurements be made for certain clients.

Heart Rate

Heart rate can be measured by sensing the client's pulse (e.g., on the wrist or neck) and counting the number of beats over the course of a minute (or some fraction). A better procedure is to monitor moment-to-moment heart rate by using a device such as a pulse oximeter. A pulse oximeter (also used to estimate oxygen saturation, as described below) often provides a continual display of heart rate.

Heart rate should be monitored and noted during a baseline period to determine the natural heart rate fluctuations for that particular client. The baseline period should include both resting tidal breathing and speaking because heart rate usually differs for these two activities (i.e., it is usually higher during speaking). It is important to remember that heart rate can vary from moment-to-moment and from day-to-day, so that baseline monitoring should be done within the same session and on different days as evaluation or management activities are carried out. When there are concerns regarding a client's heart rate, his pulmonologist or cardiologist should set the heart-rate limits within which it is safe for him to participate in evaluation or management activities involving speech production.

Blood Pressure

Blood pressure, like heart rate, is subject to change and can be influenced by evaluation and management activities. Blood pressure can be measured noninvasively through the use of a sphygmomanometer. The sphygmomanometer can be inflated by hand or automatically with the press of a button. The blood pressure cuff is usually secured around the upper arm. However, if this is a difficult placement (e.g., because of the presence of bulky clothing or because the arm is too small), it is acceptable to secure the cuff around the leg. It should be recognized, however, that the placement of the blood pressure cuff relative to the heart determines the average blood pressure. Thus, blood pressure will vary across cuff placements.

As with heart rate, blood pressure should be monitored and noted during a baseline period of both resting tidal breathing and speaking to determine the natural fluctuations for a particular client. Also, as with heart rate, blood pressure can be expected to vary from time-to-time and day-to-day, so that baseline monitoring should be done during each evaluation or management session. The physician should set the blood pressure limits within which it is safe for a particular client to participate in speech breathing evaluation and management protocols.

Oxygen Saturation

Oxygen saturation (usually abbreviated SaO_2) is defined as the percent of hemoglobin in arterial blood that is saturated with oxygen. Oxygen saturation can be measured directly from arterial blood or it can be estimated noninvasively using a pulse oximeter (in which case, it is abbreviated SpO_2). The pulse oximeter transmits light pulses through a region of the body containing a highly arterialized capillary bed. The degree of light absorption is related to the degree to which hemoglobin is saturated with oxygen. The light-emitting and sensing part of the pulse oximeter is called a probe and is configured to fit over a finger or an earlobe. The SpO_2 value is usually displayed digitally on the pulse oximeter unit. The values obtained using pulse oximetry are close to those measured directly from arterial blood.

Normal values for SpO_2 are 95 to 100%. If SpO_2 falls below 90%, supplemental oxygen may be indicated. The client's pulmonologist should set a minimum SpO_2

below which a client should not be allowed to fall. This will be especially important when evaluating or managing clients who tend to desaturate when speaking. In some clients, such as those who have poor circulation in the extremities, it may not be possible to obtain valid measures of SpO_2. In such cases, the pulmonologist may require additional safety measures if the client is at risk for desaturation.

Pulse oximetry is simple to use and does not require special technical expertise. Clients can, in fact, be trained to monitor their own SpO_2. Nevertheless, the speech-language pathologist should be instructed in its application by the respiratory therapist. The monitoring of SpO_2 is the single most important safety procedure that a clinician can follow for clients with ventilation or gas exchange impairments. As long as the SpO_2 minimum is maintained, the client is not at risk for hypoxemia (i.e., not enough oxygen in the blood).

Partial Pressure of Carbon Dioxide

The partial pressure of carbon dioxide (PCO_2) is that part of the pressure (expressed in mmHg) in blood or gas that is exerted by carbon dioxide. PCO_2 is the primary indicator of ventilation. Ventilation is considered adequate if arterial PCO_2 is in the normal range (i.e., 35 to 45 mmHg). A higher-than-normal arterial PCO_2 is a sign of hypoventilation and a lower-than-normal arterial PCO_2 is a sign of hyperventilation.

Arterial PCO_2 is measured directly from arterial blood, but it can also be estimated using noninvasive measures. One noninvasive estimate of arterial PCO_2 comes from measures of PCO_2 obtained with a transcutaneous gas-monitoring device. This device includes heated electrodes that are fixed to the skin, usually on the anterior rib cage wall (where arterial perfusion is good and fat deposits are minimal). Transcutaneous PCO_2 can provide a close estimate of arterial PCO_2.

Another noninvasive estimate of arterial PCO_2 can be obtained from measures of end-tidal PCO_2. End-tidal PCO_2 is the PCO_2 in expired gas at the end of a tidal breath. In most clients, end-tidal PCO_2 is measured from gas expired through the nose. In this case, the client wears nasal cannulae, which are connected to a gas analyzer. End-tidal PCO_2 is measured at the end of a resting tidal (nonspeech) expiration while the client's mouth is closed. End-tidal PCO_2 is measured with a capnometer (a device that measures carbon dioxide) that uses one of several available gas sensing techniques (e.g., infrared, mass spectrometry). A capnometer usually provides a digital display of the calculated value for end-tidal PCO_2 along with the analog waveform of the expired PCO_2 (called a capnogram). End-tidal PCO_2 can provide a close estimate of arterial PCO_2 in healthy individuals (i.e., usually 1 to 4 mmHg lower than arterial PCO_2). However, end-tidal PCO_2 can be a poor estimate of arterial PCO_2 in clients with pulmonary disease.

Although both transcutaneous PCO_2 and end-tidal PCO_2 measures provide estimates of arterial PCO_2, they do so in different ways. Transcutaneous PCO_2 changes relatively slowly, reflecting arterial PCO_2 status over the course of minutes. It is valid to use transcutaneous PCO_2 as an estimate of arterial PCO_2 during speech production (or any other activity) as long as a sufficient amount of time has elapsed so that the new level of ventilation (if there is one) can be reflected accurately. This may take as long as 5 to 10 minutes. By contrast, end-tidal PCO_2 provides a breath-by-breath estimate of arterial PCO_2. However, it does not necessarily provide a valid estimate of arterial PCO_2 during speech production. Accordingly, measurements of end-tidal PCO_2 should be made during resting tidal breathing before and immediately after a period of speaking to check for speaking-related changes in end-tidal PCO_2 (and presumably ventilation). Measures of transcutaneous PCO_2 are most useful for assessing long-term changes in ventilatory status and measures of end-tidal PCO_2 are useful for assessing both long-term and short-term changes in ventilatory status.

BEDSIDE SCREENING OF SPEECH BREATHING

There are times when a quick screening procedure for speech breathing may be needed. At such times, it is important that the speech-language pathologist be prepared with a concise screening battery that maximizes the possibility of detecting a speech breathing problem, if there is one. The discussion below, along with Form 4-4, offers one set of screening options. These options take into account the following realities: (a) the time available to see the client may be very limited; (b) the client may fatigue quickly; (c) instrumentation may not be available; and (d) the screening may have to occur with limited privacy.

Case History Interview

The screening should begin with a very brief case history interview that focuses on breathing. The following open-ended questions are suggested to initiate this portion of the screening: "Do you ever have difficulty with your breathing? If so, can you tell me about it?" Additional questions can be posed to gain possible insight into disease processes and client compensations. Suggested questions regarding disease processes are: "Has a doctor ever told you that you have a breathing problem? If so, what is it and what do you know about it?" Suggested questions regarding compensations are: "Do you do anything to relieve the breathing problem you just told me about? If so, what do you do and how does it help you?" To determine the effects of breathing problems on speaking, if any, the following questions can be posed: "Does your breathing affect the way you speak? If so, can you tell me about it?"

Auditory-Perceptual Observations

Auditory-perceptual observations of the client's speech breathing comprise the next part of the screening. These observations can be made while the client responds to the case history queries just discussed. However, it is often difficult for the clinician to judge the client's speech breathing at the same time she is trying to listen to and transcribe what he is saying. Therefore, auditory-perceptual observations of speech breathing are usually best made while the client speaks on an unrelated topic. For this purpose, various "Tell me about" probes are recommended. Examples are "Tell me about your family," "Tell me about your pets," "Tell me about your job or hobbies." The client should be encouraged to speak as continuously as possible and keep speaking for a minute or two. As he does, the clinician should make a global judgment about the client's speech breathing and indicate whether it is normal or abnormal by checking the appropriate box on the form. If it is judged to be abnormal, the clinician should then go on to judge whether breath group length, average loudness, loudness variability, and inspiratory duration are normal or abnormal. These judgments are recorded on Form 4-4, along with explanatory comments. For example, the clinician might note that breath group length was very short and only involved the production of 2 to 3 syllables per breath group.

Client Perceptions

The client's perceptions of his speech breathing should be probed as soon as he has finished speaking (and the clinician has completed her auditory-perceptual judgments). The first two questions are meant to determine how the client perceives the present state of his speech and breathing in comparison to his usual state. They are: "Do you think your speech is better than usual, worse than usual, or the same as usual today?" and "Do you think your breathing is better than usual, worse than usual, or the same as usual today?" If the client responds that his speech or breathing is "better" or "worse" than usual, the clinician should ask for more information ("In what way?")

The next four questions are aimed at determining if the client experienced dyspnea while he was speaking, and, if so, the quality of his dyspnea. These questions are: "Did you feel breathless or hungry for air while you were speaking?" "Did your breathing require noticeable physical work or effort while you were speaking?" and "Did you have to think about your breathing while you were speaking?" Finally, an open-ended question, such as "Is there anything else you want to tell me about your speaking or breathing?," allows the client to offer any additional information that may not have been elicited by the previous questions (e.g., a feeling of chest tightness, anxiety about breathing).

Physical Structure and Function

A physical structure and function screening is the final focus of the bedside screening of speech breathing. Because such screening is meant to be brief, it is conducted in only one body position (i.e., that in which the client presents). Interpretation of certain performance activities will differ somewhat depending upon whether the client is in upright, supine, or some other body position.

This part of the screening should begin by asking the client: "Do you have any physical problems with your chest, belly, or back? For example, have you had any surgeries or injuries? Or do you have any hernias or muscle weakness? If so, please tell me about them." Answers to these questions should help direct the clinician to salient structural features of the client's breathing apparatus. If the client responds affirmatively, the clinician should ask the client to show her the scar, hernia, area of weakness, or other abnormality. The clinician should look at the breathing apparatus directly if possible. If there are privacy concerns (and the client is not wearing a gown), the clinician should view the breathing apparatus by lifting the clothing in sections (e.g., in the front, then in the back). The clinician should judge whether the chest wall (i.e., combined rib cage wall and abdominal wall) is normal or abnormal with respect to continuity, composition, alignment, and shape. These judgments are recorded on Form 4-4 along with explanatory comments. For example, the clinician might note that continuity is "abnormal" and comment that there is a "large scar on the anterior rib cage wall from cardiac surgery."

Next, the client is asked to perform several simple maneuvers. These are designed to determine selected functional capabilities. The clinician should view the breathing apparatus (directly or through the client's clothing) while the client performs such maneuvers. Visual observations should be combined with auditory-perceptual observations, especially of the duration and loudness of the sounds associated with inspiration and expiration.

The first maneuver is elicited by instructing the client to "Take in all the air you can and then blow out all the way." This is essentially a vital capacity maneuver. This maneuver provides information about the extent to which the client can displace lung volume in both the inspiratory and the expiratory directions. By watching the client's movements and listening to accompanying flow-related sounds, the clinician should be able to judge whether the client is able to inspire and expire relatively appropriate amounts of air and, thereby, estimate the adequacy of his inspiratory capacity, expiratory reserve volume, and vital capacity.

The next maneuver is to "Sniff as fast as you can." This maneuver tests

THE POWER OF THE OLD BRAIN

The first of us was asked to go on grand rounds in a regional medical facility that specialized in traumatic brain injury. It was in a far northern clime and a young female client had suffered severe facial and brain injury from a cable strung across a snowmobile trail. She was having great difficulty speaking and demonstrated control problems throughout her body. There was something vaguely familiar about the smile she struggled to present. Her eyes also seemed to beg for recognition. A glance at her chart revealed the name of a former undergraduate student from a very far southern clime. All clinical skills were rendered useless at that moment of understanding. The limbic system won out in a struggle against years of clinical inoculation against emotion. Only the host was puzzled by the tearful breach of immunity. Grand rounds moved on while the first of us talked about old and new times with his student.

the speed with which the client can inspire. If this maneuver is performed in a supine body position, it can be considered a test of diaphragm function. If performed in an upright body position, it is likely to reflect a combination of diaphragm and inspiratory rib cage wall function. If flow appears to be limited by high nasal-pathway resistance or the client complains of nasal congestion, the instruction should be changed to "Gasp as though you were just startled by something" so that the client will inspire through the mouth.

The client is then instructed to "Pretend you're blowing out a candle as fast as you can." This tests the speed with which the client can expire. This maneuver can be accomplished with expiratory rib cage wall muscles, abdominal wall muscles, or a combination of the two.

The final maneuver is elicited by the instruction "Pant like a puppy." This maneuver tests the client's ability to produce rapid, alternating inspirations and expirations. It requires muscle strength and coordination. This maneuver may be particularly challenging for the client with impaired neuromotor control.

REVIEW

A speech breathing evaluation should enable the speech-language pathologist to offer a reasonable diagnosis when appropriate, develop a rational, effective, and efficient management plan, monitor the client's progress over the course of management, and provide a reasonable prognosis as to the extent and speed of improvement that can be expected.

Clients with speech breathing disorders come in many forms and present with a variety of bases for their disorders, the latter ranging from functional causation that can be managed behaviorally to profound neuromotor causation that is managed with ventilatory support.

The speech breathing case history is designed to gain information about alerting signs and symptoms, airway risk factors, medical evaluations, diagnoses, and treatments, breathing and speaking experiences, and client perceptions of speech breathing.

The auditory-perceptual examination is intended to gain a global impression of the degree of speech breathing abnormality, gain insight into how individual breathing control variables may be contributing to speech breathing abnormality, and gain information concerning a client's adjustment capabilities through the use of prescribed speech activities.

Speaking-related dyspnea (breathing discomfort) can be a salient feature of a client's speech breathing disorder and needs to be both qualitatively (through verbal description) and quantitatively (through scale ratings) documented prior to the development of a management plan.

Physical examination of the breathing apparatus entails a comprehensive analysis that includes structural observations regarding continuity, composition, alignment, and shape, and functional observations regarding performance capabilities of the rib cage wall, abdominal wall, and diaphragm.

Many aspects of speech breathing performance are best evaluated through instrumental examination, especially those features related to mechanical measurements of volume, pressure, and shape, measurements of speech acoustics, and measurements of physiological status.

The speech-language pathologist should be prepared to administer a quick and concise screening battery for speech breathing that includes a very brief case history interview, a set of auditory-perceptual observations, selected probes of the client's perceptions of his problems, and a set of structural and functional observations designed to elucidate the status of the breathing apparatus.

REFERENCES

Bailey, E., & Hoit, J. (2002). Speaking and breathing in high respiratory drive. *Journal of Speech, Language, and Hearing Research, 45*, 89-99.

Banzett, R., Mahan, S., Garner, M., Brughera, A., & Loring, S. (1995). A simple and reliable method to calibrate respiratory magnetometers and Respitrace. *Journal of Applied Physiology, 79*, 2169-2176.

Banzett, R., Lansing, R., Brown, R., Topulos, G., Yager, D., Steele, S., Londono, B., Loring, S., Reid, M., Adams, L., & Nations, C. (1990). 'Air hunger' from increased PCO_2 persists after complete neuromuscular block in humans. *Respiration Physiology, 81*, 1-17.

Banzett, R., Lansing, R., Reid, M., Adams, L., & Brown, R. (1989). 'Air hunger' arising from increased PCO_2 in mechanically ventilated quadriplegics. *Respiration Physiology, 76, 53-67.*

Bass, C. Kartsounis, L., & Lelliott, P. (1987). Hyperventilation and its relationship to anxiety and panic. *Integrative Psychology, 5*, 274-291.

Bell, A. (1910). *The mechanism of speech.* New York, NY: Funk and Wagnalls Company.

Bouhuys, A., Proctor, D., & Mead, J. (1966). Kinetic aspects of singing. *Journal of Applied Physiology, 21*, 483-496.

Braun, N., Abd, A., Baer, J., Blitzer, A., Stewart, C., & Brin, M. (1995). Dyspnea in dystonia: A functional evaluation. *Chest, 107*, 1309-1316.

Campbell, E., Gandevia, S., Killian, K., Mahutte, C., & Rigg, J. (1980). Changes in the perception of inspiratory resistive loads during partial curarization. *Journal of Physiology (London), 309*, 93-100.

Chada, T., Watson, H., Birch, S., Jenouri, G., Schneider, A., Cohn, M., & Sackner, M. (1982). Validation of respiratory inductive plethysmography using different calibration procedures. *American Journal of Respiratory Disease, 125*,

644-649.

Gandevia, S., Killian, K., & Campbell, E. (1981). The effect of respiratory muscle fatigue on respiratory sensations. *Clinical Science, 60,* 463-466.

Gardner, W. (1996). The pathophysiology of hyperventilation disorders. *Chest, 109,* 516-534.

Hixon, T., Hawley, J., & Wilson, K. (1982). An around-the-house device for the clinical determination of respiratory driving pressure: A note on making simple even simpler. *Journal of Speech and Hearing Disorders, 47,* 413-415.

Hixon, T., & Hoit, J. (1998). Physical examination of the diaphragm by the speech-language pathologist. *American Journal of Speech-Language Pathology, 7,* 37-45.

Hixon, T., & Hoit, J. (1999). Physical examination of the abdominal wall by the speech-language pathologist. *American Journal of Speech-Language Pathology, 8,* 335-346.

Hixon, T., & Hoit, J. (2000). Physical examination of the rib cage wall by the speech-language pathologist. *American Journal of Speech-Language Pathology, 9,* 179-196.

Hoit, J., & Hixon, T. (1987). Age and speech breathing. *Journal of Speech and Hearing Research, 30,* 351-366.

Kersten, L. (1989). *Comprehensive respiratory nursing: A decision making approach.* Philadelphia, PA: W. B. Saunders.

Konno, K., & Mead, J. (1967). Measurement of the separate volume changes of rib cage and abdomen during breathing. *Journal of Applied Physiology, 22,* 407-422.

Lansing, R., Im, B., Thwing, J., Legedza, A., & Banzett, R. (2000). The perception of respiratory work and effort can be independent of the perception of air hunger. *American Journal of Respiratory and Critical Care Medicine, 162,* 1690-1696.

Lee, L., Loudon, R., Jacobson, B., & Stuebing, R. (1993). Speech breathing in patients with lung disease. *American Review of Respiratory Disease, 147,* 1199-1206.

Manning, H., Shea, S., Schwartzstein, R., Lansing, R., Brown, R., & Banzett, R. (1992). Reduced tidal volume increases 'air hunger' at fixed PCO_2 in ventilated quadriplegics. *Respiration Physiology, 90,* 19-30.

Martinez, F. (2001). The coming-of-age of the hygiene hypothesis. *Respiratory Research, 2,* 129-132.

Maschka, D., Bauman, N., McCray, P., Hoffman, H., Karnell, M., & Smith, R. (1997). A classification scheme for paradoxical vocal cord motion. *The Laryngoscope, 107,* 1429-1435.

Mead, J. (1960). Control of respiratory frequency. *Journal of Applied Physiology, 15,* 325-336.

Mead, J., Peterson, N., Grimby, G., & Mead, J. (1967). Pulmonary ventilation measured from body surface movements. *Science, 156,* 1383-1384.

Moosavi, S., Topulos, G., Hafer, A., Lansing, R., Adams, L., Brown, R., & Banzett, R. (2000). Acute partial paralysis alters perceptions of air hunger, work and effort at constant PCO_2 and $\dot{V}_E$. *Respiration Physiology, 122,* 45-60.

Netsell, R., & Hixon, T. (1978). A noninvasive method for clinically estimating subglottal air pressure. *Journal of Speech and Hearing Disorders, 43,* 326-330.

Newman, K., Mason, U., & Schmaling, K. (1995). Clinical features of vocal cord dysfunction. *American Journal of Respiratory and Critical Care Medicine, 152,* 1382-1386.

Rothenberg, M. (1973). A new inverse-filtering technique for deriving the glottal airflow waveform during voicing. *Journal of the Acoustical Society of America, 53,* 1632-1645.

Schwartzstein, R., & Cristiano, L. (1996). Qualities of respiratory sensation. In L. Adams & A. Guz (Eds.), *Lung biology in health and disease*: *Respiratory sensation* (pp. 35-62). New York, NY: Marcel Dekker.

Simon, P., Schwartzstein, R., Weiss, J., Fencl, V., Teghtsoonian, M., & Weinberger, S. (1990). Distinguishable types of dyspnea in patients with shortness of breath. *American Review of Respiratory Disease, 142,* 1009-1014.

FORM 4-1
SPEECH BREATHING CASE HISTORY

Client: _____   Date: _____

Date of Birth: _____   Examiner: _____

Sex: _____

"I'm interested in finding out as much as I can about your speech and any problems you may be experiencing with your speech. I'm going to spend a few minutes asking you about your breathing because breathing is an important part of speaking. Your breathing may or may not have anything to do with your speech problems. I'm just trying to get as complete a picture as I can."

ALERTING SIGNS AND SYMPTOMS

Have you recently experienced any of the following?

_____ frequent coughing
_____ persistent hoarse voice
_____ coughing up mucus
_____ coughing up blood
_____ wheezing in the chest
_____ difficulty breathing
_____ chest pain or chest ache
_____ numbness, weakness, coordination problems, or involuntary movements

If so, please explain.

AIRWAY RISK FACTORS

Have you ever smoked?
    If so, when did you start smoking?

Do you smoke now?
    If not, when did you quit?

How much do/did you smoke per day?

Are you, or have you been, exposed to "side smoke" on a regular basis?
    If so, please explain.

Have you had long-term exposure to dust or chemical fumes?
    If so, please explain.

MEDICAL EVALUATIONS, DIAGNOSES, AND TREATMENTS

Have you ever been seen by any of the following?

_____ pulmonologist (breathing doctor)
_____ laryngologist (throat doctor)
_____ cardiologist (heart doctor)
_____ neurologist (nervous system doctor)
_____ respiratory therapist (breathing therapist)
_____ physical therapist (walking therapist)
_____ speech-language pathologist (speech therapist)

If so, please explain.

Has a doctor ever diagnosed you with any of the following?

_____ hay fever/allergies
_____ asthma
_____ chronic bronchitis
_____ emphysema
_____ chronic obstructive pulmonary disease (COPD)
_____ cystic fibrosis
_____ pneumothorax
_____ arthritis (in shoulders, spine, or hips)
_____ scoliosis or kyphosis
_____ pneumonia
_____ fibrosis
_____ coccidioidomycosis (valley fever)
_____ tuberculosis (TB)
_____ tumor in the lung or chest cavity
_____ pulmonary edema
_____ congestive heart failure
_____ adult respiratory distress syndrome (ARDS)
_____ pulmonary embolism
_____ muscular dystrophy
_____ myasthenia gravis
_____ amyotrophic lateral sclerosis (ALS, or Lou Gehrig's disease)
_____ post-polio syndrome
_____ multiple sclerosis
_____ Parkinson disease
_____ dystonia
_____ tremor
_____ stroke
_____ spinal cord injury
_____ other breathing disease (specify)
_____ other heart disease (specify)
_____ other nervous system disease (specify)

If so, please explain.

Do you have any other medical problems that might affect the way you breathe?
    If so, please explain.

Do you have any psychological conditions that might affect the way you breathe?
    If so, please explain.

Do you take medications for breathing problems, heart problems, nervous system problems, or psychological problems?
    If so, what are they?

Have you ever had surgery involving your stomach, chest, back, or neck?
    If so, please explain.

Do you have a tracheostomy?
    If so, do you ever occlude your tracheostomy? (specify finger, plug, or one-way valve)

Do you have a tracheostomy tube?
    If so, does your tracheostomy tube have a fenestration (hole)?

Does your tracheostomy tube have a cuff?
    If so, when is the cuff inflated?

Do you use oxygen or have you ever used oxygen?
    If so, please explain.

Do you wear an abdominal binder or back support?
    If so, please explain.

BREATHING AND SPEAKING EXPERIENCES

Do you ever have problems with your breathing?
    If so, what sort of problems?

When did you first experience problems with your breathing?

How often do you experience problems with your breathing?

Under what circumstances do you have problems with your breathing?

Do you have problems with your breathing when you lie down?

Do you have problems with your breathing when you walk on level ground?

Do you have problems with your breathing when you walk up stairs?

Do you have problems with your breathing when you eat?

Do your breathing problems limit your participation in activities?
  If so, in what way?

What do you do when you have problems with your breathing?

Are you having problems with your breathing today?

Do you ever have problems with your breathing while speaking?
  If so, what sort of problems?

When did you first experience problems with your breathing while speaking?

How often do you experience problems with your breathing while speaking?

Under what circumstances do you have problems with your breathing while speaking?

Do you have problems with your breathing when you speak loudly?

Do you have problems with your breathing when you speak for a long time?

If asked to speak continuously, how long do you suppose you could continue speaking comfortably?

Do you have problems with your breathing when you sing?

Do you have problems with your breathing when you speak and walk at the same time?

What activities do you participate in routinely that involve speaking?

Do your breathing problems limit your participation in speaking activities?
  If so, in what way?

What do you do when you have problems with your breathing while speaking?

Are you having problems with your speech breathing today?

Have you had any special training in breathing, speaking, singing, or wind instrument playing?
  If so, please explain.

How well do people understand you when you speak?

How well do they understand you on the telephone?

Do you use a speech recognition system?
  If so, how well does it work for you?

Is there anything else you would like to tell me about your breathing or your speech?

What do you hope I can do for you?

CLIENT PERCEPTIONS OF SPEECH BREATHING				

For each item, ask: *"Do you ever experience (percept) while speaking? If so, in what situation(s) do you experience it? How strong is the (percept): mild (m), moderate (M), severe (S), or intolerable (I)?"*

Percept	**Situation(s)**	**Strength**			
		m	M	S	I
☐ Frequent awareness of breathing					
☐ Hunger for air					
☐ Uncomfortable urge to breathe					
☐ Breathlessness					
☐ Shortness of breath					
☐ Hard work to breathe					
☐ High effort to breathe					
☐ Weak breathing muscles					
☐ Tired breathing muscles					
☐ Difficulty breathing in					
☐ Difficulty breathing out					
☐ Tightness in chest					

Percept	Situation(s)	Strength			
		m	M	S	I
☐ Difficulty coordinating breathing movements					
☐ Need to think about breathing					
☐ Feelings of distress with breathing					
☐ Feelings of panic with breathing					
☐ Other breathing-related feelings (specify)					

Which of the words or phrases just discussed (*list percepts selected*) best describes your breathing discomfort while you are speaking?

FORM 4-2
SPEECH BREATHING AUDITORY-PERCEPTUAL EXAMINATION

Client: _____   Date: _____

Date of Birth: _____   Examiner: _____

Sex: _____

Auditory-Perceptual Key: 0 = normal; -1 = mildly abnormal; -2 = moderately abnormal; -3 = severely abnormal; -4 = profoundly abnormal.

Dyspnea Key: N = none; m = mild; M = moderate; S = severe; I = intolerable.

RUNNING SPEECH ACTIVITIES

	Reading Aloud

	0	-1	-2	-3	-4
Global Rating					

Comments:

Variable-Based Ratings

	Abnormally Short					Abnormally Long			
	-4	-3	-2	-1	0	-1	-2	-3	-4
Breath Group Length									

Comments:

	Abnormally Soft					Abnormally Loud			
	-4	-3	-2	-1	0	-1	-2	-3	-4
Average Loudness									

Comments:

	Abnormally Even					Abnormally Variable			
	-4	-3	-2	-1	0	-1	-2	-3	-4
Loudness Variability									

Comments:

	Abnormally Short					Abnormally Long			
	-4	-3	-2	-1	0	-1	-2	-3	-4
Inspiratory Duration									

Comments:

Dyspnea Rating

		N	m	M	S	I
Term:						
Rating						

Extemporaneous Speaking

	0	-1	-2	-3	-4

Global Rating

Comments:

Variable-Based Ratings

	Abnormally Short					Abnormally Long			
	-4	-3	-2	-1	0	-1	-2	-3	-4
Breath Group Length									

Comments:

	Abnormally Soft					Abnormally Loud			
	-4	-3	-2	-1	0	-1	-2	-3	-4
Average Loudness									

Comments:

	Abnormally Even					Abnormally Variable			
	-4	-3	-2	-1	0	-1	-2	-3	-4
Loudness Variability									

Comments:

	Abnormally Short					Abnormally Long			
	-4	-3	-2	-1	0	-1	-2	-3	-4
Inspiratory Duration									

Comments:

Dyspnea Rating

		N	m	M	S	I
Term:						
Rating						

| Conversational Speaking |

	0	-1	-2	-3	-4

Global Rating

Comments:

Variable-Based Ratings

	Abnormally Short					Abnormally Long			
	-4	-3	-2	-1	0	-1	-2	-3	-4
Breath Group Length									

Comments:

	Abnormally Soft					Abnormally Loud			
	-4	-3	-2	-1	0	-1	-2	-3	-4
Average Loudness									

Comments:

	Abnormally Even					Abnormally Variable			
	-4	-3	-2	-1	0	-1	-2	-3	-4
Loudness Variability									

Comments:

	Abnormally Short					Abnormally Long			
	-4	-3	-2	-1	0	-1	-2	-3	-4
Inspiratory Duration									

Comments:

Dyspnea Rating

Term:					N	m	M	S	I
Rating									

PRESCRIBED SPEECH ACTIVITIES

Volume (Breath Group Length)

"Take in a deep breath and go as long as you can before taking in another breath."

	0	-1	-2	-3	-4
Breathing Out Through Pursed Lips					

Comments:

	0	-1	-2	-3	-4
Sustaining a Vowel					

Comments:

	0	-1	-2	-3	-4
Counting Aloud					

Comments:

Pressure (Loudness)

"Use your loudest possible comfortable voice."

	0	-1	-2	-3	-4
Sustaining a Vowel					

Comments:

	0	-1	-2	-3	-4
Counting Aloud					

Comments:

"Use your softest possible voice."

	0	-1	-2	-3	-4
Sustaining a Vowel					

Comments:

	0	-1	-2	-3	-4
Counting Aloud					

Comments:

"Begin with your usual loudness, then gradually make your voice louder and louder."

	0	-1	-2	-3	-4
Sustaining a Vowel					

Comments:

"Begin with your usual loudness, then gradually make your voice softer and softer."

	0	-1	-2	-3	-4
Sustaining a Vowel					

Comments:

"Begin with your usual loudness, then abruptly make your voice louder."

	0	-1	-2	-3	-4
Sustaining a Vowel					

Comments:

"Begin with your usual loudness, then abruptly make your voice softer."

	0	-1	-2	-3	-4
Sustaining a Vowel					

Comments:

"Use your usual loudness and hold it as steady as you can."

	0	-1	-2	-3	-4
Sustaining a Vowel					

Comments:

Shape (Inspiratory Duration)

"Count as quickly as you can until I tell you to stop. You may take as many breaths as you need."

	0	-1	-2	-3	-4
Counting Aloud					

Comments:

"Once again, count as quickly as you can until I tell you to stop. You may take as many breaths as you need." (Clinician applies pressure to client's anterior abdominal wall with hands.)

	0	-1	-2	-3	-4
Counting Aloud					

Comments:

FORM 4-3
PHYSICAL EXAMINATION OF THE BREATHING APPARATUS

Client: _____   Date: _____

Date of Birth: _____   Examiner: _____

Sex: _____

Comments:

Key: 0 = normal; -1 = mildly abnormal; -2 = moderately abnormal; -3 = severely abnormal; -4 = profoundly abnormal.

STRUCTURAL OBSERVATIONS

	Rib Cage Wall						Abdominal Wall				
	0	-1	-2	-3	-4		0	-1	-2	-3	-4
Continuity											
Composition											
Alignment											
Shape											

Comments:

FUNCTIONAL OBSERVATIONS

Inspiratory Rib Cage Wall (Upright)

Maximum Inspiration and Breath Hold
"Take in all the air you can and then hold your breath for several seconds."

	0	-1	-2	-3	-4
Extent of RC Movement					
Smoothness of RC Movement					
Steadiness of RC Position During Breath Hold					
Firmness of Rib Interspaces During Breath Hold					

Forced Inspiration
"Take in a big breath as fast as you can."

	0	-1	-2	-3	-4
Speed of RC Movement					
Phase of Left-Right RC Movement					
Phase of Upper-Lower RC Movement					
Phase of RC Movement and Lung Volume Change					
Phase of RC Movement and AB Movement					
Stability of Rib Interspaces					

Comments:

Expiratory Rib Cage Wall (Upright)

Maximum Expiration and Breath Hold
"Blow out all the air you can and then hold your breath for several seconds."

	0	-1	-2	-3	-4
Extent of RC Movement					
Smoothness of RC Movement					
Steadiness of RC Position During Breath Hold					
Firmness of Rib Interspaces During Breath Hold					

Forced Expiration
"Blow out a big breath as fast as you can."

	0	-1	-2	-3	-4
Speed of RC Movement					
Phase of Left-Right RC Movement					
Phase of Upper-Lower RC Movement					
Phase of RC Movement and Lung Volume Change					
Phase of RC Movement and AB Movement					
Stability of Rib Interspaces					

Comments:

Abdominal Wall (Upright)

Maximum AB Contraction and Hold
"Pull in your belly as far as you can and hold it there for several seconds."

	0	-1	-2	-3	-4
Extent of AB Movement					
Smoothness of AB Movement					
Steadiness of AB Position During Hold					
Firmness of AB During Hold					

Forced Expiration
"Blow out a big breath as fast as you can."

	0	-1	-2	-3	-4
Speed of AB Movement					
Phase of Left-Right AB Movement					
Phase of Upper-Lower AB Movement					
Phase of AB Movement and Lung Volume Change					
Phase of AB Movement and RC Movement					

Trunk Flexion

"Try to lean your trunk forward as hard as you can against my hands."

	0	-1	-2	-3	-4
Force of Trunk Movement					
Force of Left-Side Trunk Movement					
Force of Right-Side Trunk Movement					

Trunk Rotation

"Try to twist your trunk back and forth from left to right as hard as you can against my hands."

	0	-1	-2	-3	-4
Force of Left-Side Trunk Movement					
Force of Right-Side Trunk Movement					

Comments:

Diaphragm (Supine)

Maximum Inspiration and Breath Hold

"Take in all the air you can and then hold your breath for several seconds."

	0	-1	-2	-3	-4
Extent of AB Movement					
Smoothness of AB Movement					
Steadiness of AB Position During Breath Hold					
Firmness of AB to Palpation During Breath Hold					

Forced Inspiration

"Take in a big breath as fast as you can."

	0	-1	-2	-3	-4
Speed of AB Movement					
Phase of Left-Right AB Movement					
Phase of AB Movement and Lung Volume Change					
Phase of AB Movement and RC Movement					

AB Thrust Against Resistance

"Push your belly out as hard as you can against my hands."

	0	-1	-2	-3	-4
Force of AB Movement					

Comments:

Examination Notes:

FORM 4-4
BEDSIDE SCREENING OF SPEECH BREATHING

Client: _____   Date: _____
Date of Birth: _____   Examiner: _____
Sex: _____

CASE HISTORY INTERVIEW

Do you ever have difficulty with your breathing? If so, can you tell me about it?

Has a doctor ever told you that you have a breathing problem? If so, what is it and what do you know about it?

Do you do anything to relieve the breathing problem you just told me about? If so, what do you do and how does it help you?

Does your breathing affect the way you speak? If so, can you tell me about it?

AUDITORY-PERCEPTUAL OBSERVATIONS

Extemporaneous speaking (*"Tell me about . . ."*)

	Normal	Abnormal
Speech Breathing (Global)		
Breath Group Length		
Average Loudness		
Loudness Variability		
Inspiratory Duration		

Comments:

CLIENT PERCEPTIONS

Do you think your speech is better than usual, worse than usual, or the same as usual today? (In what way?)

Do you think your breathing is better than usual, worse than usual, or the same as usual today? (In what way?)

Did you feel breathless or hungry for air while you were speaking?

Did your breathing require noticeable physical work or effort while you were speaking?

Did you have to think about your breathing while you were speaking?

Is there anything else you want to tell me about your speaking or breathing?

PHYSICAL STRUCTURE AND FUNCTION

Do you have any physical problems with your chest, belly, or back? For example, have you had any surgeries or injuries? Or do you have any hernias or muscle weakness? If so, please tell me about them.

Structural Observations:

	Normal	Abnormal
Continuity		
Composition		
Alignment		
Shape		

Comments:

Functional Observations:

	Normal	Abnormal
"Take in all the air you can and then blow out all the way."		
"Sniff as fast as you can."		
"Pretend you're blowing out a candle as fast as you can."		
"Pant like a puppy."		

Comments:

chapter five

Management of Speech Breathing

INTRODUCTION

This chapter addresses the management of speech breathing. For many clients, speech breathing management can pay off handsomely, especially when approached in a systematic and comprehensive fashion. The management approaches considered in this chapter have been chosen for emphasis because of past successes achieved through their application. Some of these approaches are familiar to speech-language pathologists, whereas others are relatively novel. Some are supported by literature, whereas others have yet to be subjected to formal study. Presented here is a blend of the clinical science and the clinical art of speech breathing management.

RONALD W. NETSELL

Netsell is among the world's foremost leaders in the study of neurogenic speech disorders. His credentials include an enviable blend of speech physiologist and speech-language pathologist. A good deal of his work has focused on the neurobiological underpinnings of speech disorders in children. He has also masterfully applied aeromechanical principles to the noninvasive evaluation of speech disorders. This has included the development and use of methods for monitoring several aspects of breathing behavior. A hallmark of his work has been his skill in translating research findings into clinical applications. A photograph of Raymond H. Stetson hangs on his laboratory wall and in some ways Netsell's career bears similarity to Stetson's. He plays outstanding piano. He also loves to play basketball, although the first of us can attest to the fact that he moves only moderately well to his left.

This chapter begins by addressing the nature of the task involved in the management of speech breathing and continues with a discussion of how such management should be staged. The remainder of the chapter is devoted to the description of individual management approaches. Application of these approaches in various combinations is considered in a series of clinical scenarios in Chapter 7.

NATURE OF THE TASK

When developing a management plan for a client with a speech breathing disorder, the speech-language pathologist must integrate substantial and diverse information. This information comes from the case history interview, the auditory-perceptual examination of the client's speech, reports of his perceptions about his speech breathing, the physical examination of the breathing apparatus, and the instrumental examination of speech breathing. In addition, information must be considered from reports of other professionals, such as physicians, physical therapists, respiratory therapists, orthotists, and counselors, among others.

Many clients come to the speech-language pathologist without having been seen by other healthcare professionals for conditions related to their speech breathing disorder. In some cases, it will not be necessary for the client to be seen by other professionals. For example, if a client presents with a speech breathing disorder caused by functional misuse of the breathing apparatus, the speech-language pathologist may be the only professional to manage him. In other cases, it may be critical that the client also be managed by other professionals. For example, if a client exhibits signs and reports symptoms of pulmonary disease, he should be referred to a pulmonologist. When a client is under the care of a pulmonologist, the pulmonologist has the responsibility of overseeing the client's management as it relates to his breathing (i.e., ventilation, gas exchange, comfort). In such cases, it is critical that the speech-language pathologist keep the pulmonologist informed regarding the nature and severity of the client's speech breathing disorder and obtain approval for any management procedures that might affect the client's general breathing status.

Although the pulmonologist oversees the client's breathing, the speech-language pathologist has the role of directing those aspects of management that pertain to speech breathing. Most pulmonologists and other respiratory care professionals, although knowledgeable about general breathing problems, are not well-informed about the speech-specific features of such problems. Nor are they usually aware of modern developments in speech breathing habilitation and rehabilitation. Accordingly, it is the responsibility of the speech-language pathologist to ensure that such information is considered and incorporated into a client's overall management program. The speech-language pathologist is the most qualified member of the management team to make judgments about speech breathing behavior and she must be an assertive advocate for the client in such matters.

Much of this chapter is devoted to describing management approaches that are exclusively designed to improve a client's speech breathing. Nevertheless, it is important to not lose sight of the fact that the ultimate goal of management is to improve the client's quality of life. This means that, although a particular management approach may be highly effective for improving speech breathing, it may be contraindicated for other reasons. For example, consider the situation in which a client's speech breathing improves when he assumes a supine body position. His speech may become louder, his inspirations shorter, and his speech breathing less effortful. However, if the client would rather speak in an upright seated body position, then management would be better focused on approaches designed to maximize speech breathing in his preferred position.

Management goals should be realistic. For one client, the acquisition of normal function or a return to normal function is a reasonable expectation. For another client, normal function cannot be acquired or restored, but function can be improved. For still another client, no amount of work can overcome his profound disabilities, a fact that must be faced squarely by the clinician, the client, and the client's family so that realistic alternatives can be found. It is also important for all concerned to recognize that management goals may need to change. Sometimes goals must change because progress is faster or slower than expected. Sometimes they must change because the client's medical condition changes (such as rapid developmental alterations in a child with cerebral palsy, or sudden deterioration in an adult with a degenerative neural disease). Finally, for management to reach its full potential for success, the client must be an active participant in the process. Most of the management approaches discussed in this chapter cannot be implemented unless the client is willing and able to make certain behavioral adjustments.

Management is, of course, tailor-made to meet the needs and capabilities of the individual client. Clients demonstrate a wide variety of speech breathing disorders and the solutions to their problems require a wide variety of management approaches. For some clients, the management process is unidimensional, involving only a single variable, and is simple and straightforward. For other clients, the process is multidimensional, involving a complicated set of variables, and entailing a great deal of clinical creativity. This chapter contains many suggestions as to how to manage the vast array of potential speech breathing disorders, but it is not a cookbook. It is up to the clinician with her insight, skill, and ingenuity to use these suggestions to weave a unique management plan for each of her clients.

STAGING MANAGEMENT

Some speech breathing disorders occur in isolation and are the only manifestations of dysfunction within the speech production apparatus. Disorders caused by spinal cord injury or emphysema are examples. Other speech breathing disorders occur in conjunction with disorders of the larynx and/or upper airway, such as those associated with cerebral palsy or amyotrophic lateral sclerosis.

A speech breathing disorder, as defined in this book, is restricted to abnormal function of the breathing apparatus proper (i.e., the pulmonary-chest wall unit) and does not include abnormal function of the larynx and/or upper airway under its rubric. Nevertheless, abnormal function of the larynx and/or upper airway, such as might cause abnormal constrictions and obstructions of the air stream, can influence the load (i.e., mechanical opposition) "seen" by the breathing apparatus during speech production. When staging management, it is often advisable to manage such load disorders before managing the breathing apparatus proper.

The following discussion considers downstream load disorders as the initial stage of the management process for clients with speech breathing disorders. Discussion then centers on the staging of management within the breathing apparatus proper. Finally, consideration is given to implementing a comprehensive management plan for speech breathing disorders.

Considering Downstream Load Disorders

Downstream load disorders result from dysfunction of the larynx, upper airway, or both. Downstream in this context means downstream of the breathing apparatus during speech production, when air flows from the breathing apparatus through the larynx and upper airway. Admittedly, dysfunction of the larynx and upper airway can also cause upstream load disorders, if the inspiratory phase of the speech breathing cycle is affected. For example, an upstream load disorder occurs with paradoxical vocal fold dysfunction (in which the vocal folds tend to adduct during inspiration). Nevertheless, most load disorders of interest when managing speech breathing disorders occur during the expiratory phase of the speech breathing cycle and are the focus of discussion here.

Downstream load disorders can be caused by primary dysfunction of the larynx and/or upper airway, such as might occur with Parkinson disease, amyotrophic lateral sclerosis, traumatic brain injury, or other neuromotor conditions that can affect all subsystems of the speech production apparatus. Downstream load disorders may also reflect attempts of a normal larynx and upper airway to "come to the rescue" of the breathing apparatus. For example, downstream load compensations are often observed in clients with spinal cord injury, spinal muscular atrophy (without bulbar signs), poliomyelitis (without bulbar signs), or chronic obstructive pulmonary disease. Although these conditions cause dysfunction that is limited to the breathing apparatus proper, abnormal valving by the larynx and upper airway may be part of a client's overall coping strategy for producing speech.

When a downstream load disorder is identified, it is important to determine whether it is the result of a primary disease process, compensation for changes caused by a primary disease process, or both. Its status should be re-evaluated periodically during the course of management, because the relative contributions of the primary disease and compensation for it may change over time, especially in a child undergoing development or in a child or adult with progressive disease. Although detailed consideration of downstream load disorders is beyond the scope of this book, evaluation and management of such disorders are recognized as essential to any rational management plan and their importance cannot be overstated.

Downstream load disorders can come in several forms. Often they present as lower-than-normal resistive loads. This means that laryngeal and/or upper airway (i.e., velopharynx, jaw, tongue, or lips) valving for speech production is "leaky," and the client may have difficulty impounding oral pressure or restricting oral flow. Clients with flaccid paresis or paralysis of the larynx and/or upper airway often present with such problems. When downstream loads are lower-than-normal, breath groups may be initiated from larger-than-normal lung volumes, fewer-than-normal syllables may be uttered per breath group, and higher-than-normal flow may be associated with the speech produced. Colloquially, the challenge faced by the breathing apparatus is not unlike that of a person trying to pump up a tire with a hole in it. The person operating the pump has a far more demanding task in the presence of a leak than if he were to patch the tire first. The lesson is obvious. The behavior of the breathing apparatus, whether itself normal or impaired, is conditioned by the behavior of downstream structures.

Downstream loads can also be higher-than-normal when higher-than-normal resistances are generated by the larynx and/or upper airway. When the breathing apparatus "sees" an abnormally high load, it must work through that load to produce speech. This can cause speech production to feel effortful. Clients with spasticity, such as those with spastic cerebral palsy or traumatic brain injury, often present with such problems. Clients with high downstream loads will usually generate lower-than-normal flows, even when they use high pressure in an attempt to overcome the high load. Higher-than-normal downstream loads are not always caused by a primary impairment, but may instead reflect a compensatory strategy. An example is the client with a severely limited vital capacity who attempts to valve the air stream as economically as possible. The goal, in this case, is to conserve a limited air supply. This compensatory strategy is, in fact, one of the management approaches suggested in this chapter.

An essential component of the clinical process is to determine the degree to which abnormal speech breathing signs and symptoms are attributable to impairment of the breathing apparatus proper and the degree to which they are attributable to compensatory behaviors of the breathing apparatus in response to downstream load disorders. For example, a client with a normal breathing apparatus and a relatively small velopharyngeal opening during oralized speech production may be able to easily compensate for his velopharyngeal leak by driving higher flow into the oral cavity to raise his oral pressure to normal. By contrast, a client with a weak breathing apparatus and an equivalent velopharyngeal leak may not be able to drive a high enough flow to normalize oral pressure. Or, if he can, he may operate at the extremes of his capabilities, and in so doing, may be plagued by effortful breathing and fatigue. In short, the same leak in the client with the impaired breathing apparatus could overwhelm his ability to compensate.

Ideally, downstream load disorders should be managed before attempting to manage an accompanying speech breathing disorder. The previous example illustrates why. Until his velopharyngeal function is managed, the client with the impaired breathing apparatus has little hope of achieving normal speech breathing because he will always have to "fight" the velopharyngeal leak. The aim of managing downstream load disorders is to minimize taxation of the breathing apparatus. Once this is done, management of the breathing apparatus can be more effective.

Although it is preferable from the perspective of the breathing apparatus to manage downstream load disorders first, this is not always possible, nor is it always the most reasonable management scheme. Sometimes downstream load disorders need not be managed at all, sometimes they should be managed first, sometimes they should be addressed at the same time the speech breathing disorder is managed, and sometimes they should be addressed at key times during the management process.

Figure 5-1 presents five sample management programs. These have been time-normalized for illustrative purposes (the left-hand and right-hand bars bound the duration for each program). Medical diagnosis for each "client" is indicated at the right. Dark arrows indicate times when the direct management of speech breathing is

ADJECTIVAL CLIENTS

We have a devotion to the elimination of adjectival references to clients. Examples are stroke patients, cerebral-palsied children, brain-damaged teenagers, dysarthric individuals, Parkinson patients, cleft-palate speakers, aphasic patients, and dysphonic clients. There's nothing grammatically wrong with such designations, but they place emphasis on the disorder or disease rather than on the person who has the disorder or disease. For example, "cerebral-palsied children" focuses on the disease, as compared to "children with cerebral palsy," which focuses on the children who also happen to have cerebral palsy. The same is true of "Parkinson patients" compared to "patients who have Parkinson disease" or "cleft-palate speakers" compared with "speakers with clefts of the palate." We believe it's demeaning to label people adjectivally. Decide for yourself. We only ask that you think about it. We have.

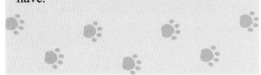

in progress. Light arrows indicate times when the direct management of downstream load disorders is occurring. The nature of the downstream load intervention is described by phrases below the light arrows.

Program (a) schematizes a management program for an adult with a spinal cord injury. Impairment in this case is confined to the breathing apparatus and the program of management is focused continuously on the apparatus proper.

Program (b) schematizes a management program for an adult with spinal muscular atrophy (without bulbar signs). Impairment is confined to the breathing apparatus and management is focused entirely on the apparatus proper. Disease progression includes periods of remission or slow deterioration, during which management is discontinued.

Program (c) schematizes a management program for an adult who has had a cerebral vascular accident (stroke). Impairment in this case is distributed across the breathing apparatus and other downstream subsystems, including severe flaccid involvement of the velopharynx. Management begins with the restoration of velopharyngeal competence through the use of a velar-lift prosthesis (including a period of adaptation and instruction), and is followed by work on the breathing apparatus proper. In this case, attention to the speech breathing disorder follows downstream load management.

Program (d) schematizes a management program for a young child with spastic cerebral palsy. Impairment in this case is distributed across the breathing apparatus and all downstream subsystems. Function of the larynx, jaw, tongue, and lips is moderately impaired and function of the velopharynx is mildly impaired. Management is focused on the concurrent alteration of laryngeal and upper airway loads (using behavioral strategies) and breathing behavior (using a combination of behavioral strategies and body positioning). In this case, habilitation concentrates on all impaired subsystems simultaneously.

Program (e) schematizes a management program for a teenager with Friedreich's ataxia. Impairment in this case is distributed across all downstream subsystems, with severe paresis of the velopharynx and moderate paresis and dyscoordination of the jaw, tongue, and lips. Management is focused initially on the breathing apparatus

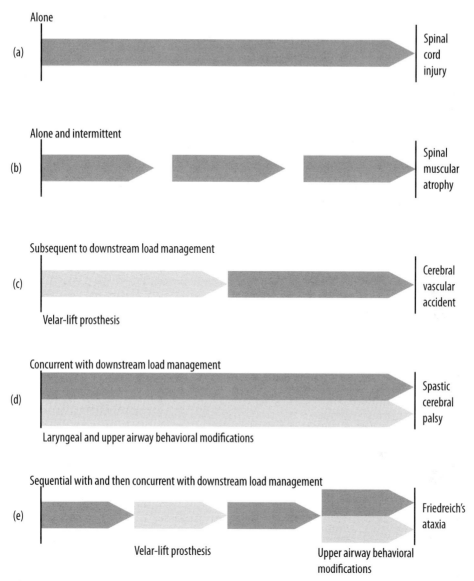

Figure 5-1. Five sample management programs.

alone (to bring the apparatus to a minimum functional level for speech production), followed by intervention with a velar-lift prosthesis to improve velopharyngeal function (including a period of adaptation and instruction). This is followed by a period of work on the breathing apparatus alone. Finally, work on the breathing apparatus is carried out concurrently with work on altering downstream loads (using behavioral strategies to modify valving competencies of the jaw, tongue, and lips). Thus, rehabilitation is focused on impaired subsystems both sequentially and concurrently.

Considering the Breathing Apparatus Proper

There are staging considerations for speech breathing management, even when speech breathing disorders present without co-occurring downstream load disorders. That is, there are staging considerations within the breathing apparatus proper.

The first step in the management of the breathing apparatus proper is to address the client's medical status, if necessary. Abnormalities in medical status are of foremost importance and always take precedence over a speech breathing disorder. Usually, it is the pulmonologist who manages the client's medical status. However, depending on the nature of the problem, medical status may also be managed primarily by a neurologist, a cardiologist, or other specialty physician. Medical management can take many forms, including pharmacological treatments or surgical interventions. It might also include oxygen therapy, humidification treatments, nocturnal ventilatory support, back bracing, or postural drainage. Appropriate medical management helps to form a stable base from which the speech-language pathologist can plan management for a client's speech breathing disorder.

Once the client's medical status has been optimized, direct management of the speech breathing disorder may begin. The speech breathing management program is usually organized around the three speech breathing variables – volume, pressure, and shape. These variables may have different relative priorities in the management of different clients. Nevertheless, management is usually most effective and efficient when the sequence of focus is pressure, volume, and shape.

Pressure is usually targeted first because a minimum drive is required to produce voice and to articulate high-pressure consonants. It makes little difference if a client has an adequate volume swing and an appropriate chest wall shape if pressure is too low. Accordingly, the first priority of management is almost always pressure generation and control.

Volume change is most often the next priority. This is because volume is a critical factor in generating a desirable quantity of speech. So, just as pressure enables the client to be "heard," delivering the requisite pressure over a larger volume excursion enables the client to be "heard longer." Pressure and volume are the key elements to speech breathing performance and the production of functional speech.

The importance of shape is largely in its potential to improve the mechanical advantage of certain chest wall muscles. Use of an appropriate shape can increase speed and magnitude of inspiration (because inward displacement of the abdominal wall tunes the diaphragm) and, thereby, improve the fluency of running speech. Shape can also be manipulated to enhance pressure and volume control for speech production (because inward displacement of the abdominal wall places expiratory rib cage wall muscles at a mechanical advantage).

Considering a Comprehensive Management Plan

A comprehensive management plan for a client with a speech breathing disorder includes the goals of optimizing speech breathing, optimizing spoken communication, and optimizing overall communication. Many of the management approaches described in the remainder of this chapter are designed to optimize speech breathing. These approaches include direct behavioral modification of the three breathing variables (see section on adjusting breathing variables), which can be facilitated by the use of certain forms of feedback (see section on exteroceptive feedback). Other approaches include a variety of behavioral and mechanical interventions that are designed to address the three breathing variables and increase client comfort (see sections on economical valving, body positioning, mechanical aids, muscle training, glossopharyngeal breathing, relieving speaking-related dyspnea, and monitoring gas exchange). These approaches constitute the "core" of a speech breathing management program.

Another goal of speech breathing management is to optimize spoken communication. This calls for additional management strategies to be brought into play, especially those that enhance the quality of conversational interchange (see sections on mouthing and buccal speaking, conversational strategies, and optimizing the environment). Counseling is also an essential component of successful speech breathing management (see section on counseling). Counseling enhances communication by providing the client with emotional support and education that are meant to help him deal positively with his speech breathing disorder. Counseling should begin immediately and continue throughout management.

Some clients require technological support to achieve the goal of optimizing overall communication (see sections on assistive speech devices, augmentative communication, and alternative communication). These are clients whose breathing apparatus is not able to provide the requisite drive to produce intelligible or otherwise functional speech. In such cases, communication may be enhanced through the use of assistive, augmentative, and alternative strategies. Sometimes these strategies provide communication solutions while other aspects of management are in progress. At other times, the decision to use alternative communication signals the end of speech breathing management, and speech management in general.

ADJUSTING BREATHING VARIABLES

In most cases, the best place to begin management is with direct attempts to adjust the breathing variable(s) judged (during the evaluation) to be contributing to the speech breathing disorder. This section focuses on an auditory-perceptual approach to adjusting the breathing variables (see next section on exteroceptive feedback for an instrumental approach to adjusting breathing variables). When more than one breathing variable is judged to be abnormal, the sequence in which they are managed is usually pressure, volume, and shape.

Behaviors related to pressure, volume, and shape are usually not modified instantly, given that learning or relearning any behavior requires practice. Because speech breathing behaviors are motor behaviors, their learning or relearning may be best implemented according to principles of motor learning (Schmidt & Lee, 1996).

Although few such principles have been tested as they apply to speech breathing, they offer a rational approach to maximizing the retention of new motor behaviors. Examples of these principles are as follows: (a) include many practice trials (so that the targeted behavior is performed many times within a practice session); (b) include variability of practice (so that the targeted behavior varies from trial to trial); and (c) include appropriate feedback (so that clinician-provided feedback and, in some cases, instrumental forms of feedback are meaningful to the client and scheduled so as to move the client toward independence). Underlying these principles is the idea that a new motor behavior is better retained if the learning process includes substantial practice, demands motor flexibility, and requires self-evaluation.

In general, behaviors related to pressure, volume, and shape are better modified through the use of speech activities than they are through the use of nonspeech activities. As mentioned in the context of the speech breathing evaluation, nonspeech activities differ from speech activities in significant ways. They generally have lower precision, speed, and complexity demands compared to speech activities and their goals are usually not acoustic, as they are in speech activities. And, perhaps most importantly, they are under different neural control than speech activities. Thus, when adjusting breathing variables, the emphasis should be on speech activities whenever possible.

When using speech activities to modify pressure, volume, and shape, it is generally preferable to move through a hierarchy of simple to complex. This form of hierarchy is well-known to speech-language pathologists and represents the usual approach to management. In the present context, a hierarchy of speech activities might appear as follows: (a) sustaining vowels; (b) counting or reciting the alphabet; (c) reading aloud; (d) speaking extemporaneously; and (e) speaking conversationally. Such a hierarchy is generally characterized by increasing motor control demands and cognitive-linguistic demands. Although this would be an appropriate management hierarchy for most clients, there may be special cases in which this hierarchy should be modified. For example, a client with an abnormally high drive-to-breathe might experience his greatest difficulty when reading aloud, because the continual speaking demands associated with this task may compete with his ventilation needs. In this case, reading aloud would be the last task in the hierarchy. As another example, a client who is concerned about his breathing during singing would require that a singing hierarchy be developed as part of his management plan.

The following sections describe management activities that address abnormalities in pressure, volume, and shape by modifying their associated auditory-perceptual features. For present purposes, the assumption is made that the speech disorder is caused by abnormal function of the breathing apparatus, and not by abnormal function of the larynx and/or upper airway. The speech breathing management activities described here are not all-inclusive, but are meant to serve as examples of some of the more effective strategies. Many of these activities should be familiar to the speech-language pathologist because they resemble those found in textbooks on neuromotor speech disorders and voice disorders. What may be novel is that they are organized according to the present breathing variables framework.

Pressure

Pressure is nearly always the first breathing variable to be addressed in management. Without adequate pressure, there can be no speech. Pressure can be adjusted by targeting speech loudness, the closest auditory-perceptual correlate of pressure. Problems with pressure control come in many forms, including abnormally low pressure, abnormally high pressure, abnormally even pressure, and abnormally variable pressure.

Abnormally Low Pressure

Abnormally low pressure is associated with abnormally low loudness. Pressure and loudness may be consistently low throughout the breath group. Clients with Parkinson disease often exhibit this low-loudness pattern. Pressure may also decrease over the course of the breath group, causing loudness to trail off as the breath group proceeds. Clients with cervical spinal cord injury may show this fading loudness pattern. In its most extreme form, abnormally low pressure makes it impossible to produce voiced speech, because the pressure difference across the larynx is too small to oscillate the vocal folds. This is seen in some clients with severe paresis of the breathing muscles.

One way to increase pressure is to merely ask the client to "speak louder." This simple instruction may be all that is needed to elicit the targeted speech breathing behavior. If the client is able to speak louder without any specific instruction as to how to do so, his natural strategies for increasing loudness will be revealed. These strategies might include increasing the depth of inspiration before speaking, increasing his muscular driving pressure, increasing his laryngeal opposing pressure, increasing his mouth opening, and/or adjusting his posture, among other strategies. This unifying concept of "loud" is the basis of a management program developed for clients with Parkinson disease (Ramig, Pawlas, & Countryman, 1995).

If the client does not increase loudness with the general instruction to "speak louder," he may need more specific guidance. Thus, the next step might be to offer instructions designed to increase pressure by targeting either muscular driving pressure or relaxation pressure. For example, the clinician might instruct the client to "squeeze hard with your belly and chest while you speak." This instruction is designed to increase the muscular pressure generated during speech production. As another example, the clinician might instruct the client to "take a deeper breath before speaking." This instruction is designed to increase the prevailing relaxation pressure, at least at the beginning of the breath group. If the client is able to carry out either or both of these instructions, he should be able to produce louder speech and/or produce speech when it might not have been possible before.

There is an additional strategy that may be helpful for the client who attempts to speak in long breath groups, despite the fact that his loudness trails off (or, in extreme cases, voicing ceases). When this behavior is observed, the client should be instructed to "put just a few words on a breath" (or the clinician may specify the targeted number of words or syllables). The goal is for the client to speak only during that part of the breath group in which pressure is adequately high to produce adequately loud speech. This strategy can improve intelligibility without increasing pressure-generation demands.

The behavioral strategies described here are often more effective if they are used in combination. For example, if the client is able to increase both muscular pressure and relaxation pressure, his speech will be louder than if he increases just one or the other. Also, additional gains may be made if these strategies are combined with other management approaches, such as those that incorporate changes in body position, the use of mechanical aids, and/or the implementation of a muscle training program (all of which are described in this chapter).

Abnormally High Pressure

Abnormally high pressure is associated with abnormally loud speech. High pressure might be generated throughout the breath group or it may occur near the beginning of the breath group. An example of a client who generates consistently high pressure might be someone with an aggressive personality who uses an excessively loud voice as a means of establishing and maintaining social dominance. An example of a client who generates especially high pressure near the beginning of breath groups might be someone who initiates breath groups at relatively large lung volumes, but does not engage appropriate inspiratory muscular effort to counteract (i.e., brake) the high relaxation pressure.

One strategy for managing abnormally high pressure is to instruct the client to speak more softly. If the client was not previously aware that his speech was too loud, this may be all that is required to modify his behavior. Or more explicit instructions may be necessary. If excessive muscular pressure is suspected, the client might be instructed to "try not to push so hard when speaking." For the client who exhibits bursts of loudness at the beginning of breath groups, it may be helpful to instruct him to "hold back the air" (i.e., brake with his inspiratory muscles) or "let the air out slowly" while speaking (Netsell, 1995). Another way to reduce excessive relaxation pressure at the beginning of the breath group is to instruct the client to "take smaller breaths before speaking."

Abnormally Even Pressure

Abnormally even (i.e., steady) pressure is associated with abnormally limited loudness variability (sometimes called monoloudness). Generally, when loudness is abnormally even, this indicates that the quick pressure changes usually associated with linguistic stress and vocal expressiveness are reduced or absent. Clients with

Parkinson disease or other forms of parkinsonism often exhibit this speech breathing sign.

One way to manage abnormally even pressure is to ask the client to produce a syllable train and "punch" a given syllable. For example, the clinician might instruct a client to "say TA-ta-ta and punch the first syllable" and then "say ta-ta-TA and punch the last syllable." Another commonly used behavioral approach to increasing loudness variation is through the use of contrastive stress drills with meaningful speech, such as those described by Fairbanks (1960) and elaborated by Rosenbek and LaPointe (1985) among others. These drills are constructed so that the client emphasizes a targeted syllable within a phrase, and the targeted syllable changes across productions. Of course, linguistic stress can be signaled by increases in loudness, pitch, duration, or some combination of these percepts. For the present purpose, the goal is to signal stress primarily by manipulating loudness.

Another way to manage abnormally even pressure is to ask the client to express selected emotions with his voice, while emphasizing loudness variability in doing so. For example, the clinician might instruct the client to hum sentences (to focus the client on his vocal, rather than his articulatory, expressiveness) such as "I'm so angry!" and "I'm completely content." The first of these should be produced with substantial loudness variability (and high overall loudness) and the second should be produced with much less loudness variability (and low overall loudness). Although pitch and pitch variability may also differ between these types of productions, the clinician should emphasize manipulation of the loudness component in her instructions and in her demonstrations. After the client has reached his target performance level with the humming task, he can move on to running speech activities. When managing abnormally even pressure, whether it be from a linguistic stress or a vocal expressiveness perspective, it is often helpful to incorporate pressure feedback or sound-pressure-level feedback into management (see section below on exteroceptive feedback).

Abnormally Variable Pressure

Abnormally variable pressure is associated with abnormally variable loudness. Pressure (and loudness) variability

---

LUNGUISTIC STRESS

You're right. It is a typographical error. Actually, it's a typographical error made while writing a portion of this text. But, once it was there on the computer screen it was transfixing. It seemed a wonderful new word, coined by a quick right middle finger in a hurry to get to a meeting and flying around the keyboard at break-finger speed, trying with its nine siblings to complete a paragraph. But now this new word is there for all to see and ponder. It's powerful because it emphasizes the importance of the breathing apparatus in the production of linguistic stress. There are other ways to stress, but this one has primacy, especially for heavy stress, and now it can be immortalized (well, maybe that's a bit dramatic) for all to see as a reminder that linguistic stress usually has its roots in an alveolar pressure adjustment. Lunguistic stress. Now that really has a ring to it.

can be rhythmic (such as in tremor or myoclonus), irregular (such as in chorea), and even explosive (such as in dyskinetic cerebral palsy). When loudness is too variable, this generally indicates that pressure is too variable, laryngeal opposing pressure is too variable, or a combination of the two. Therefore, it is essential to sort out the relative contributions of the breathing apparatus and the larynx before proceeding with management. Upper airway contributions to loudness change can usually be identified or ruled out by monitoring the upper airway visually.

A strategy for reducing loudness variability, when pressure variation is the source, is to have the client increase the overall loudness of his speech, as long as his loudness is not already excessive. The rationale for increasing loudness to manage loudness variability can be illustrated with the example of a breathing-based voice tremor. If the loudness variability reflects a pressure change of 2.5 cmH_2O peak-to-peak, and the average pressure across the breath group is 5 cmH_2O, then the pressure change represents 50% of the average pressure. However, if the average pressure is increased to 10 cmH_2O, then a 2.5 cmH_2O peak-to-peak change represents only 25% of the average pressure. The perceptual consequence of this increase in average pressure (translated perceptually to an increase in average loudness) should render the pressure variability (translated perceptually to the loudness variability) less salient and, therefore, less noticeable to the listener. How much to increase the average loudness is determined by noting when the variability is minimized.

Volume

Volume control problems come in different forms. The most common are abnormally positioned volume excursions (i.e., where they are located within the vital capacity), abnormally small volume excursions, and abnormally large volume excursions.

Abnormally Positioned Volume Excursions

Volume excursions for speech breathing are usually positioned within the midrange of the vital capacity. The advantage of using the midrange is that the muscular pressure for speech breathing is generally minimized. Nevertheless, there are clients who tend to position volume events outside of the midrange.

A client may position his volume excursions for speech breathing at abnormally small lung volumes. For example, a client with a functional voice disorder who complains of vocal fatigue may produce most of his speech breathing at lung volumes that are much smaller than the resting tidal end-expiratory level. When this occurs, voice quality may be pressed, especially near the ends of breath groups. Conversely, a client may position volume excursions for speech breathing at abnormally large lung volumes. For example, a client with a psychogenic disorder characterized by feelings of "not being able to breathe" might exhibit this latter type of speech breathing pattern.

To help a client change the position of his lung volume excursions for speech breathing, it is usually necessary to enhance his awareness of how his breathing apparatus feels when it is functioning within the volume midrange. This might be done by asking him to note that the breathing apparatus is "most relaxed at the bottom of a breath." He might then be instructed to inspire from that relaxed position and speak until he feels he has reached that position again. In other words, his inspirations should begin and his expirations (speaking) should end near the resting tidal end-expiratory level. If the client is able to modify his speech breathing behavior as instructed, he should experience a reduction in effort. If he is not successful at modifying his speech breathing behavior, it may be necessary to incorporate feedback into management that enables him to monitor his lung volume directly (see section below on exteroceptive feedback).

THE CHOIR CONSPIRACY

A colleague of ours worked with a client who had Friedreich's ataxia, a progressive spinocerebellar disease. The client was a young man who was having difficulties with both his balance and his speech. He was also having difficulty with his singing. He sang in a church choir and reported that he would often run out of air in the middle of musical phrases. His disease had robbed him of the sensations he would normally use to feel the impending depletion of his air supply. Our colleague offered up a very ingenuous solution for his problem. She instructed the client to look down at the movement of his shirt and belt buckle to determine where he was in his volume stroke. With practice, his perfectly intact visual system provided a substitute means for guiding performance. He and the church choir were breathing together (i.e., conspiring) again.

Abnormally Small Volume Excursions

Abnormally small volume excursions are associated with abnormally short breath groups. Clients with diaphragm paresis, for example, usually exhibit abnormally short breath groups. To identify this speech breathing problem, it is important to take into account the client's behavior during the entire breath group (i.e., expiratory phase of the speech breathing cycle). In some cases, it is easy to be misled into thinking that a client is using abnormally small lung volume excursions when, in fact, he is not. For example, if a client produces just a few syllables per breath group, it might seem that his lung volume excursions are small. However, his lung volume excursions may actually be normal. They may only seem abnormally small because he is speaking during the initial part of the breath group, and then expiring (without speaking) during the latter part of the breath group. Clients with certain types of pulmonary disease may demonstrate this pattern.

Abnormally short breath groups are usually best addressed by instructing the client to "take a deeper-than-usual breath before starting to speak." If the client is able to do this, it should be relatively easy to coach him to extend breath group length. Nevertheless, it is important to recognize that larger-than-usual inspirations require greater-than-usual inspiratory work. For clients with impaired inspiratory muscle function, this strategy may cost too much energy to be a reasonable management approach. In such cases, other approaches such as body positioning, mechanical aids, and/or muscle training may be more useful.

Abnormally Large Volume Excursions

Abnormally large volume excursions are associated with abnormally long breath groups. Clients who have prolonged inspirations (due to inspiratory muscle impairment) might use long breath groups so as to produce as much speech as possible before having to pause for the next inspiration. Even clients without muscle impairments may feel driven to produce as much speech as possible on each breath to avoid inspiratory pauses. To modify this speech breathing behavior, the client is instructed to "put fewer words on a breath," while being guided through an appropriately sequenced set of practice trials. When a client shortens his breath groups to make them of more normal length, he typically experiences a reduction in speech breathing effort.

Shape

In upright body positions, such as standing or sitting, the normal chest wall shape for speech breathing is a smaller-than-relaxed abdominal wall and a larger-than-relaxed rib cage wall. When chest wall shape is abnormal, the opposite is usually true – the abdominal wall is displaced outward (from relaxation) and the rib cage wall is displaced inward (from relaxation). This shape is often seen in clients with paralyzed abdominal wall muscles. Abnormal shape may be associated with the auditory-perceptual correlates of abnormally long inspirations (because the diaphragm is at a mechanical disadvantage for generating inspiratory pressure change) and abnormally reduced loudness variation for producing linguistic stress (because the expiratory muscles of the rib cage wall are at a mechanical disadvantage for generating rapid expiratory pressure change).

To adjust chest wall shape, the client is asked to "pull your belly in while you speak." If he is able to do this, then it may be possible to train this into a habitual behavior. However, in clients with abdominal wall muscle impairment, it may not be possible to adjust chest wall shape by instruction alone. In such cases, management of abnormal chest wall shape will require some form of external adjustment, such as a change in body position or the use of a mechanical aid.

EXTEROCEPTIVE FEEDBACK

Exteroceptive feedback is sensory information that comes from stimuli outside the body. Several forms of exteroceptive feedback are relevant to the management of speech breathing disorders. Perhaps the most common is what has been called clinician-provided feedback (Duffy, 1995). This is the feedback that the speech-language pathologist offers the client, sometimes verbally (e.g., "That breath wasn't quite deep enough.") and sometimes nonverbally (e.g., head shake and hand gesture indicating that inspiration should be deeper). The client receives clinician-provided feedback primarily via auditory input (by listening to the clinician's comments), visual input (by watching the clinician's body language and facial expression), and occasionally by tactile input (by feeling the clinician's hands on his breathing apparatus). Clinician-provided feedback is delivered intermittently and on a variety of schedules. For example, when the client is first acquiring a new speech breathing behavior, the clinician might offer feedback throughout the client's performance and immediately after he has completed it. As the client shows evidence of learning the behavior, the clinician might cease offering feedback during his performance and momentarily delay her feedback about his completed performance so that the client can begin self-evaluation. Finally, when the client's skill nears the target level, the clinician might withhold her feedback and ask the client to evaluate his own performance. Clinician-provided feedback is a natural part of the therapeutic interaction between clinician and client and one of the core elements of effective speech breathing management.

Other forms of exteroceptive feedback can be provided through the use of instrumentation. Such exteroceptive feedback can offer the client information about aspects of his behavior that are not usually available to him, and it can offer such information continuously. In this way, instrumentally provided exteroceptive feedback can enable the client to gain control over his behavior in ways that might not otherwise be possible (Yates, 1980). In the context of speech breathing, exteroceptive information can come from analog representations of the positions and movements of the breathing apparatus, aeromechanical events associated with speech breathing, activities of the muscles of the breathing apparatus, and the acoustic signal that results from the act of speech production (i.e., speech). The idea behind providing a client with instrumental exteroceptive feedback is to help him bring his speech breathing behavior under conscious control. Once he is able to control such behavior consciously, the goal is to use the principles of motor learning to help bring it under more automatic control so that it becomes a natural part of his everyday speech breathing performance.

The instrumentation used for exteroceptive feedback in the management of speech breathing is the same as that described for the evaluation of speech breathing (see section on instrumental examination in Chapter 4), with the addition of myoelectric instrumentation (described below). The nature of the feedback depends somewhat on whether the instrumentation is mechanical or electronic. With mechanical instrumentation, the variable of interest can usually be read directly from the instrument. Thus, visual feedback is an inherent feature of the instrument itself. An example is an air-gauge manometer, in which the needle points to the pressure produced, or a wet spirometer, in which the excursion of the pen reflects the change in volume. With electronic types of instrumentation, several components are usually required to make feedback available to the client. To begin, there needs to be a sensor that can detect the biological or acoustic phenomenon of interest. Next, the signal detected by the sensor must be changed into another form through use of a transduction system. This transduced signal is then often amplified and sometimes conditioned (e.g., filtered) before being routed to an output device. The output device offers a visual display or an auditory presentation. An example of a visual display might be a dot moving across an oscilloscope or computer screen (i.e., time-motion display), and an example of an auditory presentation might be a pure tone played through loudspeakers or earphones. As the variable changes, the dot might move up and down on the visual display and the pitch of the tone might increase and decrease. When using a visual display, the clinician often marks a target level for the client. For example, she might use a grease pencil to mark a target on an oscilloscope, or she might use a computer-generated line to mark a target on a computer screen. As the client's performance improves, the clinician can change the target accordingly. When using an auditory presentation, the target is usually to alter the signal in a given way (e.g., raise its pitch, increase its loudness).

It is often convenient to begin feedback management in the context of nonspeech activities. By using nonspeech activities, the client can be introduced to the instrumental set-up and to the visual or auditory feedback without the added complication of achieving a given speech-related performance level. Nevertheless, the move to speech activities should be made as soon as possible. Selection of the specific nonspeech and speech activities and the choice of feedback depend on the client and the nature of his speech breathing control problem.

Instrumentally provided exteroceptive feedback must be accompanied by clinician-provided guidance and feedback, at least initially. That is, the clinician must instruct the client in the use of the instrumental set-up, help him interpret the feedback signals, provide him with targets, and help calibrate his self-evaluation. As the client becomes accustomed to the instrumentation, learns the behavioral tasks, and demonstrates that he can evaluate his own performance, he can be allowed more independence in his own management. As he gains independence, clinician-provided guidance and feedback can be faded. And, eventually, as the client acquires the new speech breathing behavior, the instrumentally provided exteroceptive feedback can be eliminated. By this stage, the client should have created an association between the exteroceptive feedback and his own internally generated sensations of position, movement, and force (i.e., proprioception). The ultimate goal of management is retention of the newly learned behavior, and retention requires that the client rely on his own body sensations and cognitive system to incorporate the new behavior into his repertoire of automatic behaviors.

The use of exteroceptive feedback can be a powerful tool for managing speech breathing behavior, and a number of variables can be used for feedback. Perhaps the most obvious are outputs of the three control variables of speech breathing. Another type of feedback can come from the muscles of the breathing apparatus in the form of myoelectric (i.e., electromyographic) activity. Finally, acoustic feedback can be used to modify selected aspects of speech breathing behavior. Applications of these types of exteroceptive feedback are discussed below.

Feedback of Control Variable Outputs

This section focuses on feedback for speech breathing management that incorporates the outputs of the three speech breathing control variables – pressure, volume, and shape. Principles and methods are discussed for each, and examples are offered for how each might be used in management.

Pressure

When providing pressure feedback, the pressure of interest is alveolar pressure. Alveolar pressure can be estimated from oral pressure using an air-gauge manometer, a water-bubble manometer, a U-tube water manometer, or a mechanical-electrical manometer. In special cases (i.e., when the client has a tracheostomy), alveolar pressure can be estimated from tracheal pressure.

The goals of pressure-feedback management are to help the client generate pressure that is of appropriate magnitude, adequate duration, and/or adequate steadiness, but sufficiently variable for producing linguistic stress and vocal expression. Several nonspeech activities can be employed to meet these goals. To begin, the client might be asked to target a given pressure for a given duration. The pressure and duration targets can be increased as his performance improves. Once this is achieved, the client might be asked to produce the same target pressure for the same duration, but to do so as steadily as possible. For the client who exhibits abnormally reduced pressure variability (i.e., monoloudness), pressure-feedback management might include having the client generate quick pressure increases of given magnitudes. When using pressure feedback during speech activities, a mechanical-electrical manometer is the instrument of choice and the speech materials must contain voiceless stop-plosives (preferably /p/). The client's task for speech activities is to monitor his peak oral pressure during voiceless stop-plosive productions and attempt to match a predetermined pressure target with each production. As with nonspeech activities, the pressure targets can be set to address pressure magnitude and/or variability goals.

Pressure feedback has been used successfully to modify nonspeech pressure control of clients with speech breathing disorders. For example, Netsell and Daniel (1979) described a subject with flaccid dysarthria who could generate only 2 to 3 cmH_2O for a maximum of 3 seconds. Feedback management involved having the subject blow into a water manometer (with a leak tube in place) while attempting to increase pressure magnitude and duration. After several management sessions, the subject was able to generate 10 cmH$_2$O for 10 seconds, thereby far exceeding the 5 cmH$_2$O for 5 seconds minimum suggested by Netsell and Hixon (1978). Others have reported similar success with nonspeech pressure feedback using a water manometer (Netsell & Hixon, 1978) and a mechanical-electrical manometer (Rubow, 1984; Yorkston, Beukelman, Strand, & Bell, 1999).

Pressure feedback can also be provided during speech activities. For example, pressure feedback might be used with a client whose pressure decreases rapidly near the end of breath groups. In this case, the pressure feedback system would be a mechanical-electrical manometer attached to a small catheter, the other end of which would be positioned just behind the client's lips. The client would monitor his peak oral pressure during /p/ productions on an oscilloscope or computer screen and attempt to match a predetermined pressure target (e.g., 5 cmH$_2$O) with each production. As the client became more proficient with the task, the clinician could encourage him to pay attention to his effort level and his loudness during on-target productions. In this way, the client can begin to depend on self-generated cues to maintain the desired pressure profile.

Volume

When providing volume feedback, the volume of interest is usually lung volume. Lung volume can be estimated from measurements made at the airway opening using wet spirometers, dry spirometers, or flow integrators. It can also be estimated from measurements made at the body surface using bellows pneumographs, respiratory magnetometers, or respiratory inductance plethysmographs. When body surface measurement instruments are used, the signals from the rib cage wall and abdominal wall are summed to reflect lung volume. Body surface measurement is the best approach for providing volume feedback during speech activities because body surface instrumentation does not encumber the upper airway as do instruments that require the use of a mouthpiece or mask.

The specific goals of volume-feedback management depend on the nature of the client's volume-control problem. In general, volume-feedback goals include helping the client generate volumes that are appropriately positioned within the vital capacity and/or of appropriate extent (i.e., excursion). To address the first of these goals, the client should be oriented to his resting tidal end-expiratory level so that he can begin to use it as an "anchor" for volume events. He should then be instructed to inspire a moderate volume and expire to the tidal end-expiratory level. To address the second volume goal, the client should be given a targeted lung volume excursion for his inspirations and expirations. The targeted excursion will be either larger or smaller than his usual volume excursions. Even when volume excursions are the only focus of feedback management, it is important to ensure that the client's volume events are also appropriately positioned within the vital capacity. Both nonspeech and speech activities can be used to help achieve these goals, although performance during speech activities is more important.

The successful application of volume feedback was illustrated in a case report of an adult female with mixed ataxic and flaccid neuromotor impairment who tended to initiate utterances at low lung volumes (Yorkston, Beukelman, Strand, & Bell, 1999). It was hypothesized that, if the client were able to monitor her lung volume change, she might learn to speak using more appropriate lung volumes. Toward this end, outputs of respiratory inductance plethysmographs on the rib cage wall and abdominal wall were summed and routed to an oscilloscope to provide a real-time display of lung volume. The client was guided by the clinician to watch the signal during resting tidal breathing to become familiar with its rising-and-falling pattern. She was then asked to initiate sustained phonation at her resting tidal end-inspiratory level and to terminate it near her resting tidal end-expiratory level. Management progressed to more complicated speech activities and eventually the client was able to speak at larger lung volumes (i.e., at a more appropriate position within her vital capacity) by inspiring before she began a new utterance. This shift in lung volume events was accompanied by an improvement in voice quality. The client was able to wean herself from the feedback and transfer her newly learned skill to essentially all communication situations (except when she laughed).

Volume feedback was also used in the speech breathing management of a child with traumatic brain injury (Murdoch, Pitt, Theodoros, & Ward, 1999). Feedback consisted of a time-motion display reflecting rib cage wall movement obtained with a respiratory inductance plethysmograph (abdominal wall movement was also recorded, but not used in the feedback protocol). The intervention called for the subject to match a target trace during performance of nonspeech and speech activities. One of the outcomes of this intervention was that the subject was able to increase inspiratory (rib cage wall) volume.

Shape

Feedback regarding shape can only be provided using instruments that reflect movements of both the rib cage wall and abdominal wall. These are body surface measurement devices (bellows pneumographs, respiratory magnetometers, and respiratory inductance plethysmographs). Although shape feedback can be visualized using individual time-motion displays of the rib cage wall and abdominal wall, the most powerful means of providing shape feedback is by displaying the rib cage wall signal against the abdominal wall signal (see Chapters 2 and 4).

The goals of shape-feedback management for speech breathing are usually to help the client assume a background shape that is mechanically advantageous for speech breathing, minimize exaggerated chest wall movements, and/or eliminate abnormal paradoxing of the rib cage wall or abdominal wall. To address the goal of normalizing background shape, it is often useful to orient the client to his relaxed chest wall shape at the resting tidal end-expiratory level. This can be seen as a point on the rib cage wall-abdominal wall display. From this, the clinician can estimate what his relaxed shapes might be at other lung volumes and draw a predicted relaxation characteristic on the display. Using the characteristic as a reference, the clinician can show the client where on the display his speech breathing should occur. In upright body positions, this should be to the left of the characteristic, such that the rib cage wall is slightly larger and the abdominal wall is slightly smaller than relaxation at the prevailing lung volume. The client can then use visual feedback to achieve this targeted chest wall shape. To address the latter two goals, the clinician can point out shape abnormalities in the client's rib cage wall-abdominal wall tracings and then draw for him how the tracing should appear in smoothness and slope. The client can then take advantage of shape feedback to modify this aspect of his speech breathing behavior.

Modification of abnormal shape using shape feedback can be illustrated with an example of an adult with profound hearing impairment (Forner & Hixon, 1977). This subject exhibited two speech-related shape problems. First, his background chest wall shape was abnormal in that the abdominal wall was displaced too far inward. Second, his speech production was accompanied by frequent and rapid changes in shape. These abrupt shape changes appeared to be caused by the subject's belief that he should emphasize each syllable with a quick inward movement of his abdominal wall. To determine if his speech breathing behavior could be modified, a session of shape feedback was offered. This involved placing respiratory magnetometers on his chest wall and routing the signals to a storage oscilloscope where the rib cage wall signal was displayed on the vertical axis and the abdominal wall signal was displayed on the horizontal axis. To orient the subject to the rib cage wall-abdominal wall display, the signals from each of the two channels were grounded temporarily so that he could see the effect of rib cage wall movement and abdominal wall movement separately. Once he understood the meaning of the display, he was asked to produce a long string of discrete syllables. During his first performance, the oscilloscopic tracing was characterized by his usual frequent and abrupt inward abdominal displacements. Prior to the second trial, he was instructed to smooth out the tracing as he produced the same syllable string. By his third attempt, the subject had generated a smooth tracing. Interestingly, he had also repositioned his abdominal wall so that his background shape was normal. He did this without direct instruction, apparently as a consequence of eliminating his abdominal pulsing behavior.

Myoelectric Feedback

Myoelectric feedback is feedback that reflects the activity of selected muscles. When applied to the management of speech breathing, such activity is best obtained through the use of surface electromyography. Surface electromyography is a non-invasive method for detecting electrical activity in skeletal (i.e., voluntary) muscle, which involves fixing surface electrodes (small metal disks) to the skin that overlies the muscle(s) of interest. The voltage signal sensed by the electrodes reflects the combined electrical activity of multiple motor units in the region of the electrodes. The magnitude of such activity is generally seen as being related to the magnitude of the force exerted by the muscle, although there are several contingencies that must be satisfied for this to hold true (Farina, Merletti, & Enoka, 2004). Fortunately, signals obtained with electromyography for the purpose of speech breathing management are viewed as only gross indicators of muscle activation, and, therefore, many of the problematic details associated with this type of measurement and interpretation are of little concern. When used for feedback, myoelectric activity (hereinafter called muscle activity) is amplified, and sometimes conditioned (e.g., filtered, rectified, and integrated). The resultant signal can be displayed on an oscilloscope or computer screen in either its raw form or in a conditioned form. As muscle activity increases, the amplitude of the visual signal increases. Another, sometimes more motivating, way to provide muscle activity feedback is to present it auditorily through loudspeakers or earphones. This signal sounds something like a combination of crackles and white noise, the loudness of which increases and decreases as muscle activity increases and decreases, respectively.

Although muscle activity can be recorded from any part of the surface of the breathing apparatus, the interpretation of such activity is clearer at some sites than others. The two sites that provide the most easily interpreted signals are the neck and abdominal wall. Neck muscles can only inspire the breathing apparatus, and abdominal wall muscles can only expire the apparatus. Thus, when muscle activity is detected in either of these structures, it is relatively easy to determine the nature of the effect of that activity, as long as the muscles are acting as prime movers. Activity sensed from the rib cage wall is less easily interpreted because the rib cage wall contains both inspiratory and expiratory muscles. Thus, when activity is detected, it may be difficult to know if it originates from inspiratory muscles, expiratory muscles, or both. However, there are placements on the rib cage wall that can provide relatively unambiguous information. Rib cage wall muscle activity can also be instructive when the primary interest is whether or not muscle activity exists, rather than what type of muscle actions are being reflected. Finally, the diaphragm is generally inaccessible from the surface (although it is accessible by swallowing a special electrode). Nevertheless, it is possible to detect diaphragm activity indirectly using surface electromyography, especially if the muscles of the rib cage wall and abdominal wall are paretic or paralyzed and exhibit little or no activity.

Feedback of neck muscle activity can be used to enhance the inspiratory phase of the speech breathing cycle in certain clients. Because neck muscle contraction places inspiratory force on the rib cage wall, targeting neck muscle activity for feedback can encourage the use of neck muscle activity for producing speech inspirations. This management approach might be appropriate for a client who has paretic or paralyzed rib cage wall muscles and/or diaphragm, but whose neck muscles are still quite strong. Often clients spontaneously learn to use neck muscles to compensate for impaired inspiratory muscle function, but feedback may be an appropriate management approach for those who do not or for those who appear to not be using them to their maximum capacity. When sensing neck muscle activity, electrodes

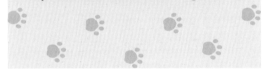

are generally placed along the long axis of the sternocleidomastoid and scalenus muscles either bilaterally or unilaterally. If the client's neck muscle function appears to be symmetrical, unilateral placement should be sufficient. The first task might be for the client to attempt to generate the loudest muscle-activity noise possible (if auditory feedback of muscle activity is presented). To do this he must activate his neck muscles as strongly as he can and continue to do so while attempting to increase the noise level. Under certain circumstances, it may be that this task represents the entire management protocol (see section below on muscle training). The next step might be to incorporate this feedback task into a simple speech task, such as creating the loudest noise possible (i.e., activating neck muscles maximally) prior to sustaining a vowel or counting. Eventually, as the client demonstrates that he is using neck muscle activation consistently during running speech inspirations, the exteroceptive feedback can be removed and the client encouraged to rely on his own internal cues to determine if he is activating his neck muscles appropriately.

Feedback of abdominal muscle activity can be useful for managing the expiratory phase of the speech breathing cycle. The same general approach as was described above for feedback of neck muscle activity can be followed, except that the electrodes are placed on the abdominal wall and the client is instructed to concentrate on activating his abdominal muscles. The best site for recording from abdominal wall muscles is on the skin overlying the lower aspect of the lateral abdominal muscles (external oblique, internal oblique, and transversus abdominis). The electrodes can be placed unilaterally if abdominal wall muscle function appears to be similar on the two sides. Feedback intervention can begin with nonspeech maximum activation of abdominal muscles and move to activation during speech breathing tasks of increasing complexity.

Acoustic Feedback

When the acoustic speech signal is used in the management of speech breathing disorders, there are two general applications. One is to provide feedback of the sound pressure level of speech as a correlate of alveolar pressure and the other is to provide feedback regarding the timing of speech events relative to speech breathing events. Only speech activities are used with this form of feedback.

Sound Pressure Level

The sound pressure level of speech is related to alveolar pressure. As alveolar pressure increases, sound pressure level increases, assuming that laryngeal opposing pressure and mouth opening remain constant. Thus, sound pressure level can be used as indirect feedback regarding alveolar pressure generation during speech production. With this application, the sound pressure level is sensed continuously with a measurement device, such as a sound pressure level meter, and displayed visually for the client to monitor. The resultant signal can be shown on an oscilloscope, computer screen, or volume unit (VU) meter that uses a needle indicator. Digital displays may also be used, or even a bank of lights that illuminates, to reflect the prevailing sound pressure level.

When using sound-pressure-level feedback, a magnitude target is designated for the client. This can be done by marking a target level on the sound-pressure-level display (on the oscilloscope or computer screen) or a target point on the volume unit meter display. Speech activities may begin with sustained vowels and move on to conversational speech. During management, the clinician should take note of any changes in voice quality or mouth opening that might accompany changes in sound pressure level so that she can judge the relative contributions of laryngeal and upper airway behavior to the output. If the client appears to be emphasizing laryngeal and upper airway strategies to increase sound pressure level, the clinician may want to coach the client to modify his behavior in ways that target alveolar pressure (e.g., "Take a deeper breath and squeeze your belly and chest as you speak."). Sound-pressure-level feedback is a commonly used approach in speech management.

Speech Timing

Perhaps the most valuable use of acoustic feedback to speech breathing management is in its application to speech timing. When acoustic feedback is used for this purpose, the speech signal is displayed on an oscilloscope or computer screen as a function of time. This signal is displayed along with, and is time-locked with, the other speech breathing signal(s) of interest. In the present context, the best application of this feedback approach is to combine acoustic feedback with lung volume feedback. A special application that combines acoustic feedback with pressure feedback is described in Chapter 6 for ventilator-supported speech.

The combination of acoustic feedback and volume feedback can be used to manage speech timing in clients who tend to speak at inappropriate lung volumes or who "waste" lung volume during speech production. Specifically, the goals of this form of feedback management might include helping the client to speak in the midrange of the vital capacity and minimize nonspeech expirations. To address the goal of speaking in the midrange of the vital capacity, similar procedures to those described under volume feedback are employed. That is, the client is oriented to his resting tidal end-expiratory level and then instructed where to initiate and terminate speech breathing relative to this level. In this context, the client is asked to notice where speech begins and ends in relation to where lung volume events begin and end. To address the goal of helping the client minimize nonspeech expirations, management focuses on certain features of the combined acoustic and volume feedback display. Specifically, nonspeech expirations are characterized by a cessation of the speech signal (although some expiration-related noise may be visible) and a sudden increase in the slope of the volume tracing. Once the client can recognize these features, he can become aware of where in the breath group he is producing nonspeech expirations and begin to consciously minimize their occurrence. Although this approach should be successful for most clients who demonstrate this speech breathing behavior, it is important to realize that some clients use this as a dyspnea-relieving strategy. In such cases, attempting to eliminate nonspeech expirations may exacerbate speaking-related dyspnea and is, thus, contraindicated.

Combined acoustic and volume feedback can also be applicable to the management of the rare client who speaks during inspiration. This combined feedback offers the client a particularly clear representation of speech events as they relate to inspiration and expiration. It is easy to imagine how such feedback could be used to help such a client produce speech during the appropriate phase of his speech breathing cycle.

ECONOMICAL VALVING

Economical valving refers to the maintenance of a relatively high resistance along the downstream airways (i.e., laryngeal airway and upper airway) during speech production. When downstream resistance is high, air leaves the lungs slowly and more speech can be produced than when downstream resistance is lower. Thus, economical valving can benefit clients whose lung volume excursions are so limited that they produce only a few syllables per breath group. These are usually clients who have profoundly impaired inspiratory and expiratory muscle function.

When attempting to teach a client to use an economical valving strategy, it is often useful to instruct him to "try to use less air when you speak." In many cases, the client will respond by increasing his downstream resistance. However, if the client does not increase his resistance, the clinician may need to provide more specific guidance. For example, she might instruct the client to use a more pressed voice quality, while demonstrating the difference between a normal voice quality and a pressed voice quality. Or she might instruct him to "tighten the throat and/or mouth when speaking so that only a small amount of air leaks out." An effective way to teach these voice quality and articulatory strategies is to offer the client feedback about rate of lung volume change to help guide his performance (see section above on exteroceptive feedback).

Use of an economical valving strategy could pose risks to the health of the larynx. If high laryngeal airway resistance is accompanied by excessive vocal fold collision forces, it is possible for laryngeal pathology to develop (e.g., vocal nodules). Therefore, it is essential that a laryngologist inspect the client's larynx before management begins and again later, after the client has used the economical valving strategy consistently for several weeks, to ensure that no tissue damage has occurred. The development of laryngeal pathology is considered to be an unlikely occurrence, as long as the speech-language pathologist monitors the client's vocal behavior and modifies it, when necessary.

Although direct instruction has been emphasized to this point, it is interesting to note that clients often adopt an economical valving strategy spontaneously, without any instruction. Two published case studies illustrate this point. One case study focused on an adult male with paralysis of the rib cage wall, diaphragm, and abdominal wall caused by poliomyelitis (Hixon, Putnam, & Sharp, 1983). Most of the time, this subject breathed with the aid of a mechanical ventilator. However, at times he "free breathed" using special inspiratory strategies (see section below on glossopharyngeal breathing for a detailed description of this subject's inspiratory behavior). His inspiratory strategies, although successful, were costly in terms of energy and time. Because he had no functional expiratory muscle, pressure for speech production depended entirely on his relaxation pressure. Thus, this subject had a situation in which it was relatively effortful and time-consuming to inspire and in which volume and pressure for speech production were limited. This made an economical valving strategy an excellent compensation for his speech breathing needs. Objective evidence for his successful use of this strategy was obtained in the form of measures of volume expenditure per syllable. During running speech production, he expended less than a third of the volume expended by normal men of his age. Auditory-perceptual judgments of his speech also revealed features that were consistent with an economical valving strategy. These features included strained-strangled voice quality, occasional substitutions of glottal stops for oral fricatives, shortened fricatives, and intrusions of glottal stops.

The second case study was also an adult male with paralysis of the rib cage wall, diaphragm, and abdominal wall (Hoit & Shea, 1996). In this case, the cause of paralysis was traumatic injury to the spinal cord at the C2 level. The subject's ventilation was in the form of neural prostheses that stimulated his phrenic nerves for inspiration (i.e., phrenic nerve pacers, as described in Chapter 6). This subject, like the subject of Hixon et al. (1983), relied solely on relaxation pressure to drive the larynx and upper airway for speech production. His expiratory volume displacement was determined solely by his inspiratory volume displacement, because he was unable to generate any active expiratory muscular pressure to extend his expiration to volumes smaller than the resting level of his breathing apparatus. Perceptual judgments of his speech revealed a mild-to-moderate strained-strangled voice quality and occasionally shortened fricatives. In addition, estimates of his laryngeal airway resistance (determined by dividing tracheal pressure by airway-opening flow) were higher-than-normal for running speech production. This subject's use of an economical valving strategy allowed him to produce an average of 20 syllables per breath group. He also employed a buccal speaking strategy to augment utterance length (see section below on mouthing and buccal speaking).

BODY POSITIONING

Body position refers to the orientation of the body (i.e., the torso) in relation to the pull of gravity. For certain clients with speech breathing disorders, especially those with neuromotor impairment, changes in body position can alter the function of the breathing apparatus significantly. Considered here are management options related to body positioning and their potential effects on speech breathing (management options related to postural adjustments are discussed elsewhere – see sections below on mechanical aids and relieving speaking-related dyspnea).

Each time the body is reoriented within a gravity field, speech breathing requires a different mechanical solution. This means that an impaired breathing apparatus can be placed at relative advantage or disadvantage, depending on the body position assumed. The larger the body, the greater these gravitational effects can be. Thus, the breathing apparatus of an adult is influenced more by a change in body position than is the breathing apparatus of an infant.

Although changing body position is a common management approach, it can carry risks to the client's safety and comfort. To begin, body position change can influence blood pressure, venus return to the heart, and other aspects of cardiovascular function. Associated symptoms and signs can include dizziness, light headedness, and fainting. In clients with spinal cord injury, vasomotor reflexes may be impaired, which can further exacerbate cardiovascular problems. Clients with known or suspected cardiovascular disease or severe neuromotor disorders should not be repositioned, even for management probes, without the approval of a physician.

Another risk of repositioning is that the client may experience physical and/or breathing discomfort. One way to help avoid this is to query the client first and, if he reports discomfort with a certain body position, that position should be avoided in management. Another way to help minimize the possibility of causing the client unnecessary discomfort is to ask him to report his perceptions about physical comfort and breathing comfort as soon as a new body position is assumed. If he reports discomfort, he should be returned to his usual position immediately. Alternatively, it might be possible to relieve his discomfort with additional positional or postural adjustments. Of course, infants as well as certain children and adults are not able to report on their comfort levels. For those clients, attention should be paid to any signs of discomfort (e.g., facial grimacing, struggle to breathe). It may also be helpful to monitor physiological status (e.g., heart rate, blood pressure) to identify potential correlates of discomfort. Physical discomfort or breathing discomfort, either reported or suspected, will exclude that body position as a management option.

A final risk relates to the process of repositioning. Repositioning a client can be tricky and, if done improperly, can cause injury to the client or the clinician. A speech-language pathologist should never attempt to reposition a client without his physician's permission and without the aid of a physical therapist or another appropriately trained person.

Despite the cautions just noted, body position can be altered safely in most clients and may be beneficial to many. The benefits (or drawbacks) associated with a change in body position result from adjustments in the mechanical operation of the breathing apparatus. These are relatively predictable in able-bodied individuals and are reflected in changes in the relaxation pressure, resting level of the breathing apparatus, and lung volumes and capacities.

Shifts in body position can have consequences for relaxation pressure. For example, when a client is shifted from upright through semi-recumbent to supine (i.e., tipped backward and downward) while he holds his breath, the relaxation pressure of the breathing apparatus will progressively increase. From this observation, one might conclude that higher alveolar pressure and louder speech could be achieved by simply repositioning a client toward more downright body positions. This is not true, however, because the resting level of the breathing apparatus also changes with body position and speech breathing is tied to the resting level.

Figure 3-4 (see Chapter 3) shows how the resting level of the breathing apparatus changes across widely different body positions. This change in resting level is due mainly to whether the abdominal content is driven headward or footward as a result of the pull of gravity. For example, as the body moves from upright to supine, the abdominal content pushes air out through the open larynx and the resting level decreases from about 40 to about 20 %VC. Another way to say this is that the expiratory reserve volume gets smaller and the inspiratory capacity gets larger (while the vital capacity remains essentially the same) when moving from the upright body position to the supine body position. Figure 3-4 also shows that lung volume events for speech breathing follow the resting level of the breathing apparatus. Thus, it turns out that the relaxation pressure at the smaller volumes used in the supine body position (approximately 40 to 20 %VC) is about the same as the relaxation pressure at the larger volumes used in the upright body position (approximately 60 to 40 %VC). Only if the client spoke through the same lung volume range in the supine body position as in the upright body position would a relaxation pressure gain be realized. However, this would be unlikely to occur.

Changes in body position can have a substantial effect on lung volumes and capacities, especially in clients with neuromotor-based speech breathing disorders. For example, in clients with rib cage wall weakness who inspire mainly with the diaphragm, vital capacity may increase somewhat when the client is shifted from the upright body position to the supine body position. This is because moving to the supine position improves the mechanical advantage of the diaphragm. By contrast, the vital capacity may decrease in clients with diaphragm weakness who inspire using primarily neck muscles. The smaller vital capacity in the supine body position is due to the fact that their neck muscles are less effective in changing lung volume in that position. As another example, the reduction in the expiratory reserve volume that accompanies a move from the upright body position to the supine body position may cause speech breathing problems for certain clients. These are clients with severe inspiratory muscle impairment who attempt to lengthen breath groups by speaking through lung volumes that are smaller than the resting level of the breathing apparatus. A smaller expiratory reserve volume limits their ability to lengthen breath groups in this way.

What then is to be gained by changing body position, especially from the perspective of speech breathing performance? The answer lies in mechanical changes that occur in different parts of the chest wall with different body positions. For able-bodied individuals, such mechanical changes are relatively insignificant and they are dealt with unconsciously and automatically (see sections on adaptive control and body position in Chapter 3). However, when the breathing apparatus is impaired, mechanical changes can have a strong influence on the function of different parts of the chest wall. Such influence can be either positive or negative for a given chest wall part, depending on its status and the nature of the mechanical change. In general, changes that result in lengthening of a muscle increase its ability to generate muscular pressure, whereas changes that result in shortening of a muscle decrease its ability to generate muscular pressure.

The precise nature of a client's speech breathing dysfunction depends on the pattern and severity of impairment within his breathing apparatus, the nature of his compensatory behavior, and the body position in which he is observed. With these considerations in mind, the clinician must systematically work through how a given change in body position influences the function of different parts of the chest wall, and how the parts of the chest wall are mechanically advantaged or disadvantaged, both individually and in relation to one another. This means that she will need to make judgments about the relative importance of improving the function of one part over another. For example, she may be faced with a question such as "Is a modest gain in diaphragm function a reasonable exchange for a modest loss in abdominal wall function?" The effects of selected downright body positions and some of their clinical implications are offered below. The semi-recumbent, supine, and side-lying body positions are chosen for description because clients with speech breathing disorders often present in these positions or may be repositioned to one or more of them during management.

Shifting from an upright body position toward a semi-recumbent body position is an adjustment that is often made for clients who have neuromotor impairment of the chest wall and spend much of their waking time in wheelchairs. Such an adjustment provides support to the torso and stabilizes it to facilitate breathing. The adjustment also results in fewer postural demands and allows a larger allocation of muscular resources to breathing activities. The magnitude of the angle of tilt toward semi-recumbent has an important influence on the mechanical condition of the chest wall. When shifting from upright to about 30° off-vertical, function is not significantly altered. However, once the angle of tilt reaches 45° off-vertical and beyond, the rib cage wall, diaphragm, and abdominal wall tend to operate like they do in the supine body position.

For the more downright body positions (i.e., more than 45° off-vertical and supine), the inspiratory muscles of the chest wall are placed at opposing mechanical advantages, with the diaphragm being more favorably positioned and the inspiratory rib cage wall muscles being less favorably positioned. The expiratory muscles of the chest wall are also placed at opposing mechanical advantages, with the expiratory rib cage wall muscles being more favorably positioned and the abdominal wall muscles being less favorably positioned. Therefore, the consequences of tilting a client will depend on the relative impairment of different parts of the chest wall. For example, tilting a client with an impaired diaphragm might aid diaphragm function so that deeper inspirations could be taken prior to speech production. At the same time, tilting might also place his expiratory rib cage wall muscles on more favorable portions of their length-tension characteristics and enhance their capability to generate muscular pressure. These two effects, deeper breaths and enhanced expiratory muscular pressure capability, might combine to enable the client to produce longer breath groups and louder utterances. However, if he had been using inspiratory rib cage wall muscles to compensate for his weak diaphragm, then the change in body position might reduce the effectiveness of this compensatory strategy. Also, even if tilting enhances the ability of the rib cage wall to generate expiratory muscular pressure, this benefit might not be manifested if the abdominal wall remains too impaired. That is, if the client attempts to produce loud speech, but his abdominal wall is too weak to resist the expiratory push of the rib cage wall, the result might be unwanted abdominal wall paradoxing. The message to be conveyed here is that clinical compromises may need to be made.

The side-lying body position (left and right lateral) differs from the supine body position in certain important ways. To begin, the resting level of the breathing apparatus is at a slightly larger lung volume for side-lying body positions than for the supine body position because the abdominal mass "hangs out and down" toward the supporting surface. Also, the side-lying body position, compared to the supine body position, is accompanied by more outward positioning of the abdominal wall, less headward positioning of the abdominal mass, less headward positioning of the diaphragm, and a less elevated rib cage wall position. It is also relevant to note that speech breathing function may differ for left lateral and right lateral side-lying positions, depending on degrees of impairment in the two sides of the rib cage wall, diaphragm, and/or abdominal wall. For example, lying on the left side might lead to more severe expiratory dysfunction than lying on the right side if abdominal wall impairment is greater on the left side (lower side). For another example, lying on the right side might result in more severe inspiratory dysfunction than lying on the left side if diaphragm impairment is greater on the right side (lower side). Both of these effects are associated with the greater hydrostatic pressure operating on the lower side.

General guidelines notwithstanding, the best approach for determining the effects of different body positions on speech breathing is simply to try them. The report of the client, the wisdom of the attending physician, and the judgment of the speech-language pathologist all are a part of the data that need to go into decisions related to changing body position as a management strategy. Ultimately, the outcome of a change in body position will depend on the client's neuromotor viability, the mechanical advantages and/or disadvantages effected, and the performance demands of the speech breathing activity (e.g., breath group length, loudness). Currently, there is no precise clinical algorithm for weighting these factors or understanding how they interact. Finally, it is also critical to note that, when using body position as a management strategy, the mechanical state of the breathing apparatus, and, therefore, the neural control solutions for speech breathing, are specific to that position. Because of this, any speech breathing behaviors learned in one body position should not necessarily be expected to generalize to another body position (Hoit, 1995). Thus, the client may need a somewhat different management strategy for each body position in which he plans to speak.

MECHANICAL AIDS

Many clients, especially those with neuromotor impairments of the breathing apparatus, may benefit significantly from the use of mechanical aids. Mechanical aids come in several forms and have in common that they provide structural support and/or movement assistance to the breathing apparatus. This chapter focuses on the use of mechanical aids for clients who breathe on their own. Chapter 6 covers the use of ventilators as mechanical aids for clients who do not usually breathe on their own. The mechanical aids of interest here can be categorized under general postural support, abdominal wall support, and elective noninvasive positive pressure ventilation.

General Postural Support

Clients with torso weakness often manifest improvement in speech breathing when provided with general postural support. General postural support is designed to help position the torso, anchor it, and increase its stability as the platform for speech breathing execution. This support can come in a variety of forms. Some of the more common include the following: (a) shoulder straps that hold the client in an upright body position; (b) trussing devices that hold the torso in a relatively straight orientation; (c) pillows and other compliant objects that can be "stuffed around" the torso to maintain a desired mechanical attitude; and (d) self-bracing with the arms and hands (e.g., by supporting the forearms in elevated slings or gripping the chair). These forms of general postural support can be used alone or in selected combinations. The stability offered by such support relieves the client of taxing postural demands and allows him to allocate more muscular resources to the control of speech breathing.

Abdominal Wall Support

Clients with abdominal muscle impairment are often candidates for abdominal wall support in the upright body position (Goldman, Rose, Williams, Silver, & Denison, 1986). Those with flaccid weakness of the abdominal wall are especially good candidates because of the mechanical circumstances they face. Such circumstances include the following: (a) the rib cage wall is positioned lower than usual, so that its ability to generate expiratory muscular pressure is compromised; (b) the diaphragm is flatter than usual, so that its ability to generate inspiratory muscular pressure is reduced; and (c) the abdominal wall is distended and does not provide a firm base for either the rib cage wall or the diaphragm to work against. These mechanical problems can often be minimized or eliminated by positioning the abdominal wall inward and fixing it in the position used during normal (upright) speech breathing. By providing such abdominal wall support, the following mechanical adjustments can be effected: (a) the rib cage wall can be raised; (b) the diaphragm can take on a more domed configuration; and (c) the impedance of the abdominal wall can be increased so that the abdominal wall is less apt to paradox (i.e., move outward) during speech production. These adjustments have the potential to benefit speech breathing in several ways. To begin, they may increase inspiratory flow (and decrease inspiratory time) by mechanically tuning the diaphragm to produce faster and more forceful inspirations. Mechanical tuning of the diaphragm may also increase inspiratory volume and breath group length. Adjustments resulting from abdominal wall support may increase overall loudness and improve the ability to make quick loudness changes for linguistic stress production. And the mechanical advantages effected by such adjustments may reduce the client's perception of effort during speech breathing.

How and when abdominal wall support should be applied depends largely on a given client's degree of impairment and his medical condition. When external devices are used to provide abdominal wall support, they require a prescription by a physician. Management probes using such devices should take place only with a physician's approval and usually with the assistance of a physical therapist. And, when external devices are already being used by a client, they should never be adjusted or removed without physician consent. These cautions are necessary because application of abdominal wall support can cause significant medical complications. One potential complication may occur when the support device restricts the movement of the lower rib cage wall. Inadequate expansion and ventilation of those portions of the lungs that lie beneath the restricted area may result in atelectasis (regional collapse of lung spaces) and pneumonia (inflammation of the lungs with exudation of fluid into the lung spaces and resultant solidification of lung tissue). Another complication of prolonged use of abdominal wall support can be a further weakening and wasting of abdominal wall muscles due to inactivity. This potential for so-called disuse atrophy needs to be considered whenever any type of external support is a management consideration.

Despite these risks, abdominal wall support can be used safely with many clients. The most convenient and quickest way to determine if such support will improve a client's speech breathing is for the clinician to place her hands on the client's anterior abdominal wall. Her fingers should be spread to maximize the surface area covered, while avoiding contact with the rib cage wall. She should press firmly against the wall so that it moves inward somewhat, but not so far as to cause the client discomfort. To test whether this temporary form of abdominal wall support influences speech breathing, the clinician should have the client perform standardized speech activities with relatively low cognitive-linguistic demands. These might include sustained vowels, counting, and reading aloud. These activities should be performed with and without the clinician-provided abdominal wall support so that comparisons can be made of inspiratory depth and speed, breath group length, speech loudness, linguistic stress, and client effort level. The client should also be queried regarding his breathing comfort while not speaking.

Abdominal wall support can come in the form of binders, trusses, and support surfaces. Abdominal wall binders are elastic and wrap around the abdominal wall. Because binders are often used for purposes other than speech breathing (e.g., blood pressure control in clients with spinal cord injury), they are usually available in clinical settings and are relatively inexpensive. Usually the easiest way to apply this type of binder is to do so with the client in a downright-toward-supine body position. A critical feature of the application is that the binder does not restrict the rib cage. This means that the binder must overlie the abdominal wall only.

Abdominal wall trusses, sometimes called corsets, are more rigid than abdominal wall binders. Trusses may have straps that wrap around the client's abdominal wall and are secured with fasteners. It is usually easier to displace the abdominal wall inward with a truss than a binder because the straps allow the clinician to tighten the truss to the desired size. However, if the lateral and/or posterior aspects of the truss are too wide, it may impinge on the rib cage wall and have the undesirable effect of restricting its movement. The best type of truss for the present application would be one that is custom-made to cover just the abdominal wall, such as that shown in Figure 5-2.

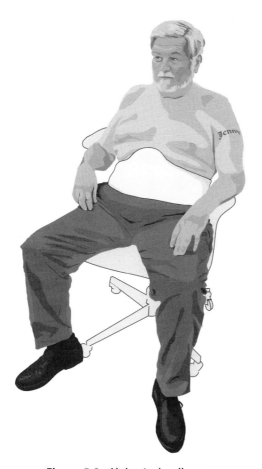

Figure 5-2. Abdominal wall truss.

Support surfaces for the abdominal wall might consist of paddles or other de-vices that the client can lean into when support is desired. The client's arms and hands might be used as an abdominal wall support surface, if the client is able to manipulate them sufficiently. For example, arms and hands might be used to hold the abdominal wall in a fixed inward position or to hold a lap-supported styrofoam block configured to fit the contour of the anterolateral abdominal wall. Arms and hands can also be used to provide surrogate muscular pressure by squeezing the abdominal wall at various times during speech production (e.g., during heavy lin-guistic stress). Combinations of these approaches can also be used. For example, Sataloff, Heur, and O'Connor (1984) reported on an abdominal wall truss that was designed and constructed for a client with a cervical spinal cord injury. The truss had levers extending from it that could be manipulated by the client's lower arms. When the client pulled on the levers, the truss exerted force on the abdominal wall. Several improvements were noted when the client used this device. They included the following: (a) increased vital capacity, primarily due to an increased expiratory reserve volume; (b) absence of paradoxical (outward) abdominal wall movement during expiration; (c) increased alveolar pressure (estimated); and (d) more "forceful" vocalization as judged by the client and listeners.

Where the abdominal wall is positioned when being supported may have an influence on speech breathing behavior, on the client's perceived effort to produce speech, and on the client's perception of breathing comfort. Optimal positioning is determined empirically by making a series of adjustments and noting which abdominal wall position provides the best result. For many clients, this will be a position that is approximately midway along the range of positions that can be assumed by the normally functioning abdominal wall (Watson & Hixon, 2001). This corresponds to the approximate abdominal wall position assumed during running speech breathing in the average normal speaker, a position adopted for its mechanical efficiency (Hixon, Mead, & Goldman, 1976). The same speech activities should be used when making comparisons across abdominal wall positions.

Elective Noninvasive Positive Pressure Ventilation

Ventilatory support is dealt with in detail in Chapter 6 (see especially section on noninvasive positive pressure ventilation). Here, the concept of ventilatory support is discussed in relation to a specific application. This application involves the use of noninvasive positive pressure ventilation as an inspiratory supplement for speaking in clients who can breathe on their own.

Noninvasive positive pressure ventilation requires the use of a positive pressure ventilator. A positive pressure ventilator is a device that can be set to deliver a given volume of air every few seconds. This air can be routed through a long tube that has a mouthpiece coupled to its distal end. A client can insert the mouthpiece between his lips and allow air to be pushed into his pulmonary apparatus. Once inspiration ends, the client can release the mouthpiece and speak during expiration in his usual manner. This form of ventilation is called noninvasive because it does not require that the client have a tracheostomy.

A noninvasive positive pressure system allows the client to take deeper inspirations without inspiratory muscular effort. Deeper inspirations often make it possible to produce longer breath groups. And, because the prevailing relaxation pressure is higher at larger lung volumes, speech can be louder (at least at the beginning of breath groups). This use of noninvasive positive pressure ventilation may be especially beneficial for clients who tend to fatigue easily. For such clients, this can mean the difference between being able to speak only a few sentences and being able to speak for a protracted period. This use of noninvasive positive pressure ventilation can also be a powerful tool for relieving dyspnea in certain clients. For example, clients who perceive inspiration as effortful should experience a reduction in effort when using this form of ventilation.

The best candidates for elective noninvasive positive pressure ventilation are clients with muscular weakness of the breathing apparatus due to neuromotor dysfunction. Certain clients with pulmonary disease may also benefit from its use.

Whatever the etiology, it is imperative that the client has good upper airway function to be able to hold the mouthpiece during inspiration. He should also have adequate laryngeal function to produce voice and adequate upper airway function to produce intelligible speech. Also, it is convenient if the client has the use of an upper extremity to hold the mouthpiece, but not necessary. If the client is not able to hold the mouthpiece by hand, it can be mounted on a stand near him so that he can grasp it and release it with his lips.

There is a special case in which the use of elective noninvasive positive pressure ventilation may have additional implications. This is the case of the client with progressive neuromotor disease, such as amyotrophic lateral sclerosis or muscular dystrophy. With this type of diagnosis, a client should realize that there may come a time when he will lose the ability to breathe on his own and that he may be faced with the decision to "go on a ventilator" or die. All too often, this decision comes at a moment of crisis, when the client has suddenly gone into ventilatory failure. And, all too often, the decision to ventilate also involves the decision to be tracheostomized. If such a client were to use noninvasive positive pressure ventilation in the elective manner discussed here, the decision to accept full-time ventilatory support might not seem as psychologically traumatic, and it might not require a tracheostomy. For example, the client might be able to use the same positive pressure ventilator with a nosemask to ventilate himself during sleep.

MUSCLE TRAINING

Muscle training increases strength (ability to produce force) and endurance (ability to sustain force) by modifying the neuromotor system. The most obvious change brought about by muscle training is an increase in muscle girth. Less obvious is that muscle training alters motor commands and changes patterns of activation within and across muscles (Duchateau & Enoka, 2002). These modifications in neuromotor structure and function can enhance the capacity of muscles to do work, which, in turn, can enhance quality of life in clients with various types of impairments.

Muscle training is not the same as general conditioning. General conditioning emphasizes whole-body exercise and can improve overall physical status. By contrast, muscle training targets specific muscles or muscle groups with the goal of increasing their strength and endurance. Muscle training can improve the strength and endurance of breathing muscles, as long as there is residual muscle function available to train. Fortunately, most clients have at least some residual muscle function, even when impairment is profound and widespread.

Muscle training regimens designed to improve strength differ somewhat from those designed to improve endurance (Leith & Bradley, 1976; Pollock, Gaesser, Butcher, Despres, Dishman, Franklin, & Garber, 1998). Strength training is best accomplished through the use of a small number of repetitions with heavy loads and ample recovery time between each set of repetitions. This is sometimes called high-intensity (i.e., high-load) training. By contrast, endurance training is best accomplished by a large number of repetitions with lighter loads. Of course, muscle training regimens can be designed to target both strength and endurance simultaneously by incorporating both high-intensity tasks and a large number of repetitions.

A muscle training regimen for the breathing apparatus should be individually tailored to the specific goals, capabilities, and health of the client. For example, although a high-intensity training regimen is appropriate for many clients, such a regimen may be dangerous for a client who is at risk for cardiovascular dysfunction or orthopedic injury. For this and other reasons, a muscle training regimen for the breathing apparatus is best implemented by a team of healthcare professionals led by a physician, usually a pulmonologist or physiatrist. In most cases, the actual muscle training regimen should be designed by a physical therapist. A speech-language pathologist should provide input to the design by informing the team of the nature of the client's speech breathing disorder and the types of muscular changes that are needed to improve his speech breathing. A respiratory therapist should track changes in the client's breathing function over the course of training, and the speech-language pathologist should provide updates regarding progress in the client's speech breathing function.

Muscle training can benefit speech breathing. For some clients, inspiratory muscle training is the intervention of choice, and for others expiratory muscle training is the intervention of choice. And, for certain clients, a combination of inspiratory and expiratory muscle training may be most appropriate.

Inspiratory Muscle Training

The goal of inspiratory muscle training is to increase the capacity of inspiratory muscles to produce and sustain force. When this goal is met, there can be several positive outcomes for the client. He may be able to generate faster and larger inspirations. He may be able to generate several large inspirations in succession. And he may be able to sustain an inspiratory effort for a longer period. These functional improvements in inspiratory muscle capabilities have important benefits for speech breathing and speech. First, larger inspiratory volumes increase potential expiratory volumes and, therefore, increase the quantity of speech that can be produced during the expiration. Second, larger inspiratory volumes increase the magnitude of the relaxation pressure available so that speech can be louder (at least during the initial portion of expirations). Third, the ability to hold an inspiratory effort longer means that it is possible to brake against relaxation pressure at the beginning of the breath group, if necessary, to maintain a more constant speech loudness. Fourth, the ability to generate faster inspirations can shorten inspiratory time, and, thereby, benefit those clients who have longer-than-desired inspirations. And, fifth, increased strength and endurance can reduce the effort required to inspire during speech breathing.

Most inspiratory muscle training regimens target an inspiratory output variable, for example, pressure. This type of training activates a combination of unspecified inspiratory muscles, rather than targeting specific muscles for activation. Thus, a client may engage the diaphragm, selected rib cage wall muscles, selected neck muscles, or any combination of these, to achieve the inspiratory pressure target.

Inspiratory muscle training often incorporates the use of a hand-held training device through which the client breathes. An example of such a device is one that requires that the client generate a minimum (i.e., threshold) inspiratory pressure. This pressure opens a spring-loaded valve so that air can flow through the device. The client must maintain at least this magnitude of pressure for inspiration to continue. Over the course of training, as the client builds inspiratory strength and endurance, the training regimen can be adjusted so that the client continues to be challenged. For example, the threshold pressure can be increased, the number of repetitions can be increased, the frequency of exercise periods can be increased, or some combination of these.

Inspiratory muscle training regimens can take many forms, depending on the goals of the training (including speech breathing goals) and the client's potential for improvement. A general example of an inspiratory muscle training regimen is described here as an illustration. To begin, the client's maximum inspiratory pressure is obtained as an indicator of his overall inspiratory strength, and repeated maximum inspiratory pressures are obtained as a reflection of his inspiratory endurance (American Thoracic Society/European Respiratory Society, 2002). The largest maximum inspiratory pressure is used to help determine the client's training threshold pressure. For example, if the client's largest maximum inspiratory pressure is 30 cmH_2O, the threshold might be set to 70% of maximum inspiratory pressure, or 21 cmH_2O. Training involves having the client inspire repeatedly through the device for 2 minutes. This is followed by 1 minute of recovery, during which the client sits quietly and breathes normally. This sequence of 2-minute loaded-inspiration periods followed by 1-minute recovery periods is usually repeated multiple times (e.g., 8 times). This training routine is performed daily for several weeks. A new measure of the client's maximum inspiratory pressure is obtained each week, and if it has increased, the threshold pressure is increased accordingly so that it remains at 70% of maximum inspiratory pressure. For example, if the client's maximum inspiratory pressure increased from 30 to 35 cmH_2O, his threshold pressure is adjusted from 21 to 24.5 cmH_2O. At the end of the training period, a maintenance regimen is devised to help the client maintain his new level of inspiratory strength and endurance.

Inspiratory muscle training regimens, such as the one just described, have been used extensively and have been shown to benefit healthy subjects (Leith & Bradley, 1976; Kellerman, Martin, & Davenport, 2000) and subjects with several types of breathing impairments. Such subjects include those with chronic obstructive pulmonary disease (Larson, Kim, Sharp, & Larson, 1988; Larson, Covey, Wirtz, Berry, Alex, Langbein, & Edwards, 1999; Riera, Rubio, Ruiz, Ramos, Otero, Hernandez, & Gomez, 2001; Sturdy, Hillman, Green, Jenkins, Cecins, & Eastwood, 2003), asthma (Weiner, Berar-Yanay, Davidovich, Magadle, & Weiner, 2000; Weiner, Magadle, Massarwa, Beckerman, & Berar-Yanay, 2002) cystic fibrosis (Sawyer & Clanton, 1993), spinal cord injury (Huldtgren, Fugl-Meyer, Jonasson, & Bake, 1980; Rutchik, Weissman, Almenoff, Spungen, Bauman, & Grimm, 1998), muscular dystrophy (Martin, Stern, Yeates, Lepp, & Little, 1986; Wanke, Toifl, Merkle, Formanek, Lahrmann, & Swick, 1994; Koessler, Wanke, Winkler, Nader, Toifl, Kurz, & Zwich, 2001), spinal muscular atrophy (Koessler et al., 2001), and other medically complex conditions (Martin, Davenport, Franceschi, & Harman, 2002). Training regimens that incorporate muscle activity feedback using surface electromyography have also been shown to increase inspiratory muscle strength in subjects with spinal cord injury (Morrison, 1988; Gallego, Perez de la Sota, Vardon, & Jaeger-Denavit, 1993). The benefits of inspiratory muscle training are reflected in increased maximum inspiratory pressure, increased inspiratory capacity and vital capacity, reduced dyspnea, and improved quality of life.

A few studies have looked at the effects of inspiratory muscle training on speaking. These have shown that such training can reduce speaking-related dyspnea in subjects with high inspiratory laryngeal airway resistance resulting from laryngeal papilloma (Sapienza, Brown, Martin, & Davenport, 1999) and bilateral vocal fold paralysis (Baker, Sapienza, & Collins, 2003; Baker, Sapienza, Martin, Davenport, Hoffman-Ruddy, & Woodson, 2003).

The full effects of inspiratory muscle training on speech breathing and speech are not known. However, there is strong reason to believe (and, in some cases, empirical evidence) that such muscle training has the potential to reduce speaking-related dyspnea, increase breath group length, increase loudness (at the beginning of breath groups), improve the ability to counteract loudness bursts at high lung volumes, decrease inspiratory time, or any combination of these. Once a client is engaged in

TURNING UP THE JUICE

Children with cerebral palsy often show weakness in the muscles of breathing. Attempts have been made to assist them by electrically stimulating their muscles. Signals are delivered through electrodes placed on the body surface so that the underlying muscles contract. The method, referred to as "electro-lung therapy," can sometimes result in muscle strengthening. This seems simple. Strengthen the muscles (rib cage wall and abdominal wall) and things should get better. But, they often don't get better, and they may, in fact, actually get worse. A strengthening of both inspiratory and expiratory muscles, but to different degrees, can result in reductions of certain lung volumes and capacities. For example, the expiratory reserve volume has been found to decrease as a result of electro-lung therapy (Jones, Hardy, & Shipton, 1963). Turning up the juice is not always a good thing to do.

an inspiratory muscle training regimen under the guidance of a physical therapist, the speech-language pathologist can capitalize on the improvements in inspiratory muscle function by incorporating them into the speech breathing habilitation or rehabilitation program. Some ideas as to how this might be done are offered here.

If a client reports speaking-related dyspnea, its severity would be expected to decline over the course of inspiratory muscle training. This should be monitored by occasional dyspnea ratings (using "hunger for air," "high effort to breathe," or other appropriate descriptors) immediately following the performance of a standard speech activity. As dyspnea decreases, it may be appropriate for the client to adopt new strategies for his daily speaking behavior. For example, a client who presents with significant speaking-related dyspnea might be counseled to adopt a strategy in which he ceases all other physical activity when speaking. As dyspnea diminishes with muscle training, it may be appropriate to modify this strategy so that speaking can be combined with selected physical activities.

If a client exhibits short breath groups, inspiratory muscle training should improve his potential to produce longer breath groups. This can be incorporated into management by asking that he produce breath groups consisting of an increasingly greater number of syllables. An important component of this exercise is to ensure that the client's natural articulation rate does not change (unless it is judged to be a beneficial change) and that his voice quality does not degrade (by becoming strain-strangled). In certain cases, some form of exteroceptive feedback may help the client learn to incorporate his increasing inspiratory strength into his speech breathing cycle. For example, it may be useful for him to monitor changes in lung volume with a body surface measurement device (such as respiratory magnetometers or respiratory inductance plethysmographs). He could use volume feedback to target a range of inspiratory volumes to be used during speech breathing.

As the client learns to take advantage of his newly acquired inspiratory muscle strength for speech breathing, it may become apparent that he has loudness control problems. For example, he may not capitalize on the higher relaxation pressure available to him at

TURNING DOWN THE JUICE

People with cerebral palsy will often show such severe neuromotor dysfunction that their conditions seem to be intractable. Attempts have been made to help them by enhancing the inhibitory potential of the cerebellum. This is done by electrically stimulating the cerebellum through surgically implanted electrodes. The most important consequence of such stimulation is a lessening of the co-activation of agonist and antagonist muscles. The benefits of stimulation are usually most prominent for gross motor skills. The first of us had the opportunity to listen to tape recordings gathered by Ratusnik, Wolfe, Penn, and Schewitz (1978) on a group of subjects who had chronic cerebellar implants. Using the types of evaluation criteria discussed elsewhere in this book, it was determined that speech breathing was not positively affected by cerebellar stimulation. Thus, turning down the juice was not effective.

the start of the breath group (following a large inspiration) because he opens the larynx and allows air to escape before beginning to speak. In this case, the client should be instructed in how to begin speaking at the onset of expiration. It may even be useful to coach the client to parse his breath groups such that salient words are produced near the beginning of breath groups when speech can be loudest. This strategy requires that the client inspire immediately prior to producing the word of interest. Another type of loudness control problem is exhibited by the client who produces bursts of loudness at the beginning of breath groups. Such bursts might occur if the client is able to inspire to larger lung volumes as a result of his inspiratory muscle training, but then fails to counteract the relaxation pressure when it is greater-than-desired for conversational loudness. In this case, the client should be instructed on how to hold back with inspiratory effort at the start of the breath group.

If a client exhibits abnormally long inspirations during speech breathing, it may be that inspiratory muscle training could allow him to inspire more quickly. This would likely be the outcome if the client continued to inspire his usual volume of air. However, if it is more important that he learn to inspire larger volumes (to increase breath group length and increase loudness, as just discussed), then his inspiratory time may not change. Stated another way, his stronger inspiratory efforts may increase inspiratory flow rather than decrease inspiratory time.

Expiratory Muscle Training

The goal of expiratory muscle training is to increase expiratory muscle strength and endurance. Expiratory muscle training can increase strength for expulsive acts of breathing, such as coughing, and endurance for sustained expiratory efforts, such as speaking.

Expiratory muscle training usually involves the same general principles and procedures as inspiratory muscle training. A hand-held training device can be used, similar to that described above for inspiratory muscle training. In some cases, it is even possible to use the same device for both inspiratory and expiratory muscle training merely by having the client use different ends of the device. An example of a regimen for improving expiratory muscle strength and endurance would resemble that already described for improving inspiratory muscle strength and endurance. In this case, the client's largest maximum expiratory pressure would be used to help determine the threshold pressure for the device and to monitor his progress with training.

Expiratory muscle training, using a pressure-threshold device, has been shown to increase maximum expiratory pressure in healthy subjects (Leith & Bradley, 1976; Suzuki, Sato, & Okubo, 1995; Sapienza, Davenport, & Martin, 2002), in subjects with chronic obstructive pulmonary disease (Weiner, Magadle, Beckerman, Weiner, & Berar-Yanay, 2003), and in those with neuromotor disorders (Smeltzer, Lavietes, & Cook, 1996; Cerny, Panzarella, & Stathopoulos, 1997; Gosselink, Kovacs, Ketelaer,

Carton, & Decramer, 2000). Such training also has been shown to increase vocal sound pressure level in children with hypotonia (Cerny et al., 1997).

There are several benefits of expiratory muscle training for clients with speech breathing disorders. To begin, expiratory muscle training may make it possible for the client to produce louder speech throughout the breath group. This can occur if the client develops enough expiratory strength to be able to supplement the lower expiratory relaxation pressure that prevails at smaller lung volumes and to overcome the inspiratory relaxation pressure that prevails within the expiratory reserve volume. One way to incorporate the client's newly developing expiratory function into his speech breathing performance is to have him target a given oral pressure throughout the breath group (see section above on exteroceptive feedback).

Expiratory muscle training may also allow the client to produce longer expirations and, therefore, longer breath groups. Longer breath groups can be encouraged by progressively increasing the number of syllables the client is to produce on a breath group, being careful that he does not increase his articulation rate or allow his voice quality to degrade. Exteroceptive feedback can be useful in this context as well. For example, the client can monitor lung volume events using body surface measurements and target a specific range of lung volumes within which to terminate his breath groups.

Another benefit of expiratory muscle training is that the effort to speak may diminish as strength and endurance increase. To document this, the client should rate his effort during performance of standard running speech activities. This should be done before training begins, during training, and at the end of training.

Finally, it is relevant to note that a byproduct of expiratory muscle training may be an increase in the client's inspiratory speed. This may occur if the abdominal wall muscles come to be more active during speech breathing as a result of the training. Active abdominal wall muscles can displace the abdominal wall inward, thereby stretching the fibers of the diaphragm and increasing its capacity for generating inspiratory pressure.

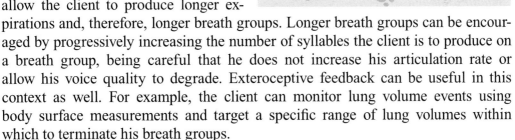

THE PIANO MOVER

During a singing conference, the first of us slipped backstage in advance of an evening session. A young man was there, pushing a piano across the stage. He seemed intent only on pushing it, not on putting it anywhere in particular. Then, the real oddity of it struck. He wasn't pushing with his hands, but with his abdominal wall. When asked about it, he said he was a voice student and his teacher had suggested the activity. He said its purpose was to strengthen his abdominal muscles and increase his "abdominal support" for singing. An informal chat followed. He came to understand that his efforts might play a small role in strengthening his diaphragm, but that they had very little to do with increasing his so-called "abdominal support." He seemed a bit dismayed at these suggestions, but he gradually warmed to them. He expressed thanks and was last seen moving the piano to behind the curtain, pushing it all the while with his hands.

GLOSSOPHARYNGEAL BREATHING

Glossopharyngeal breathing (also known as glossopharyngeal inspiration) is a form of positive pressure breathing that can be used as a compensatory mechanism in clients whose inspiratory muscles are paretic or paralyzed. It is colloquially referred to as "frog breathing" because it bears a strong resemblance to the way a frog inspires. A frog inspires by gulping air into its mouth and then squeezing it (i.e., pressurizing it) through a piston-like stroke of its upper airway. This action pushes air into the pulmonary airways and lungs. The frog inspires this way because it does not have a diaphragm, and, therefore, cannot generate negative pressure to pull air into the lungs in the way that humans and other mammals do.

Humans can mimic the frog's positive pressure inspiration as a strategy to replace or supplement their usual negative pressure generated inspiration. Human-generated glossopharyngeal inspiration proceeds in small volume steps, with each glossopharyngeal stroke increasing lung volume by 50 to 75 cc. Each stroke takes about 0.5 to 0.75 second to effect. Thus, inspiration of a normal-sized tidal breath requires 8 to 10 glossopharyngeal strokes and takes approximately 5 seconds to complete. Although this may seem a tedious way to breathe, it can be a lifesaver as well as an excellent supplement when used for speech breathing purposes.

Glossopharyngeal breathing can be learned spontaneously, by imitating other glossopharyngeal breathers, or as a result of formal instruction (Dail, Affeldt, & Collier, 1955; Dail, Zumwalt, & Adkins, 1955; Kelleher & Parida, 1957; Affeldt, 1964). However it is learned, research has shown (Collier, Dail, & Affeldt, 1956; Lawes & Harries, 1957; Ardran, Kelleher, & Kemp, 1959; Hixon, Putnam, & Sharp, 1983) that glossopharyngeal breathing occurs in four stages, as follows:

(a) with the larynx closed and the mouth open, the cycle is started by taking a mouthful and throatful of air by depressing the tongue, mandible, and larynx and widening the pharynx;

(b) with the larynx still closed, the mouth is closed and the velum is raised to form an airtight cavity consisting of the oral and pharyngeal portions of the upper airway;

(c) the larynx opens, the mandible and tongue are raised, the tongue is moved backward, the pharynx is constricted, and the neck muscles fix the chest wall in position to prevent is footward displacement – actions that collectively compress the air within the upper airway and force it into the trachea, pulmonary airways, and lungs; and

(d) the larynx closes again to trap the air contained within the pulmonary apparatus and complete the cycle – thus, the larynx functions as a one-way inspiratory flow valve.

Glossopharyngeal breathing can only be used during wakefulness because the actions of laryngeal, upper airway, and neck structures require voluntary control. Thus, clients who rely on glossopharyngeal breathing to achieve adequate ventilation while awake need to use some other form of ventilatory support while asleep (see Chapter 6).

Glossopharyngeal breathing can be used alone or in conjunction with inspiratory efforts of the diaphragm, inspiratory rib cage wall muscles, and/or neck muscles. When used alone, glossopharyngeal breathing can make speech production possible. When used in combination with other inspiratory muscle efforts, glossopharyngeal breathing can make speech better by helping to inspire the breathing apparatus to larger lung volumes than might be achieved through the use of inspiratory muscles alone. In either case, a good glossopharyngeal breather should be able to inspire to the total lung capacity by generating a series of glossopharyngeal inspirations (one after another).

There are a number of reasons why speech may improve when using glossopharyngeal breathing to inspire to larger lung volumes. First, when the end-inspiratory lung volume is large, the prevailing relaxation pressure is high. Thus, speech can be produced with a higher alveolar pressure and can, therefore, be louder, at least during the initial portion of the breath group. Second, when the end-inspiratory lung volume is large, the potential expiratory volume for utterance is also large. This means that more speech can be produced per expiration. Third, when glossopharyngeal breaths are inserted into running speech activities, they can maintain the breathing apparatus at a nearly fixed volume (size) if the injected breaths replace the volume expended during the preceding utterance. Thus, a speaker can use glossopharyngeal breaths to "set" his breathing apparatus within a given lung volume range (and within a given relaxation pressure range) and, thereby, maintain a relatively constant speech loudness. The speaker may glossopharyngeal breathe around the lung volume of choice and continue speaking in this way until he either fatigues or his drive-to-breathe requires him to take a

A RIBBITTING EXPERIENCE

The first of us spent a year as a guest researcher in the pulmonary unit of a large Veterans Administration Medical Center. The head of the unit was an advocate of glossopharyngeal breathing and patients on the ward (most with spinal cord injury) touted themselves as the "frog-breathers' brigade." They had taught one another how to frog breathe and how to use it when speaking. During a visit to the ward, a television newscast happened to be featuring a university commencement ceremony and the awarding of a doctoral degree to a paralyzed student. The student was shown in a conversation with the university's president. The camera focused on the student's face and it was clear that he was skillfully frog breathing as he spoke. The ward fell silent and then after a few seconds broke into cheers. The brigade had a new hero. Morale soared up to the ceiling lights. It was undoubtedly the emotional high of the research year.

more substantial breath.

Hixon, Putnam, and Sharp (1983) documented the potential for using glosso-pharyngeal breathing during speech production in a subject with total expiratory muscle paralysis and near-total inspiratory muscle paralysis as sequaelae to acute paralytic poliomyelitis. Physical examination and electrodiagnostic evaluation revealed that the muscles of the subject's rib cage wall, diaphragm, and abdominal wall were paralyzed and markedly atrophied. He was, however, able to spend brief periods of time "free breathing" by using his neck muscles in combination with glossopharyngeal breathing. This subject was taught to use glossopharyngeal breathing for safety reasons and for transition breathing (along with neck breathing) while off his ventilator. However, he came to incorporate his glossopharyngeal breathing into his running speech production and was often unaware that he was doing it.

Below are transcriptions of conversation, counting, reading, and loud reading as performed by the subject studied by Hixon et al. (1983). Each line in these transcriptions represents one "neck breath group" and the small circles above the lines represent individual glossopharyngeal breaths.

- Conversation

  °°Well, I … uh … °like to talk about my fam'lies.
  °I have a wonderful family.
  °I have two children and a wife.
  My boy just got married this summer …
  June third.
  °An … uh … °both him and his wife °moved in this area.
  So he'll be a tremendous help to me.
  Be able to get home on weekends an …
  °Fact, I was invited out
  °To dinner last night °to his house …
  For a spaghetti dinner which I enjoyed very much.
  (Are you froggy breathing at all now?)
  °No, just with my neck muscles.

- Counting

  One, two, three, four
  °Five, six, °seven, °eight, °nine, °ten
  °Eleven, °twelve, °thirteen, °fourteen, fifteen, °sixteen, °seventeen, °eighteen
  Nineteen, °twenty, °twenty-one, °twenty-two, °twenty-three, °twenty-four.

- Reading

  °When
  °The sunlight strikes °°°rain °drops in the air, °they act like a

°Prism and
°Form a rainbow.
°The rainbow is a
°Division
Of white light into many beautiful colors.
°These take the shape
Of a long round,
Arch,
°With it °path high °above
°And it °two ends apparently °beyond the °°horizon?
(I don't know where these glasses are.)
There is,
According to the legend,
°A boiling pot of gold
At the end ... °People look but °°no one ever finds it.
°When a man looks °for °something beyond his reach,
His friends say °be
He is looking
°For a pot of gold at the end of the rainbow.

- Loud Reading (Paragraph read only partially)

When the sunlight strikes raindrops in the air, they act like a pri ...
Prism and form
A rainbow.
The rainbow
Is a division of white light
Into many beautiful colors.

These transcriptions reveal that glossopharyngeal breaths occurred both between words and within words (e.g., "strikes°°°rain°drops"). Note that during conversation the subject was asked "Are you froggy breathing at all now?" and he replied, "°No, just with my neck muscles." Not only had the subject denied using glossopharyngeal breathing, but he even used such a breath during the sentence in which he made his denial. During the counting activity, the subject took individual glossopharyngeal breaths before most numbers. This enabled him to remain at a relatively constant lung volume during the task by quickly "recocking his expiratory spring" to resupply the volume expended during production of the preceding number. Thus, the subject was able to produce a relatively long string of numbers of relatively equal loudness on a single neck breath. Finally, it is interesting to note that the subject did not use glossopharyngeal breaths during loud reading. Rapid depletion of the air supply during loud speech production was probably more than could be easily offset by glossopharyngeal breaths.

Instructional videotapes are available that can help clients learn to glossopharyngeal breathe, including an excellent one by McPherson (1999). This video-tape covers many aspects of glossopharyngeal breathing and features McPherson himself, who has paralysis of the breathing apparatus subsequent to acute paralytic poliomyelitis. This videotape can inform the clinician who is preparing to teach her client how to glossopharyngeal breathe, as well as the client who is interested in learning how to glossopharyngeal breathe on his own. In the videotape, McPherson describes the many benefits and applications of glossopharyngeal breathing, all the while demonstrating superb speech production skills under glossopharyngeal conditions. He describes how glossopharyngeal breathing can be "liberating" to its user, as illustrated by the following two excerpts. Circles above the lines in the transcriptions indicate that glossopharyngeal inspirations were injected both before each breath group and within the flow of each breath group.

- Is it difficult to talk?

    °°°Well, wuh, no, that's one of the things that I probably do best. But, uh, sometimes I run uh out of air when I do it because I have to remember to breathe °°°°when I'm talking cause what happens once in awhile °°is I'll be talking and I won't be ventilating properly. °°And, so after 15 or 20 minutes, I, °°°I start to feel a little light headed maybe or my my nails or my lips start to turn a little bit blue because I'm not °breathing, uh, adequately, so I have to °°°think about it. But when I think about it and I, uh, °°°I actually °°°over ventilate myself sometimes just to get that extra oxygenation when I know I'm going to be giving a speech °°or doing a lot of talking. So, uh, °°°that's a very good question because it does present problems sometimes and I do have to think about it.

- How is your general health improved by "frog" breathing?

    I think definitely, uh, definitely in a number of ways re- because °°°°frog breathing gives me a feeling of independence, well, not only a feeling, it gives me indepen-dence, °uh, for time away from the respirator. °°°It allows me to travel. °It allows me to work. It allows me to go do some playful activities … °°socialization. °°It allows me to exercise. °°Uh, °°°I, I actually do a fair amount of speaking … public speaking. °°°And, so, all these things are very healthy, I think, for an individual. °°And, so, not only it is psychologically liberating, °°°°it is physically very liberating. And, so it's, uh, °°it's been a very useful experience for me and I think its °°not only given me a quality of life which I wouldn't have experienced before, °but it's probably also prolonged my life and the quality of it.

Despite the promise of glossopharyngeal breathing, there are certain clients who are unable to benefit from it. One is the client with significant impairment of the bulbar musculature (i.e., the musculature of the larynx and upper airway). Such a client may not be able to command the strength and coordination for the pumping and valving actions required to generate positive pressure inspiration.

Another is the client with a trachcostomy. Unless the tracheostomy is occluded, the glossopharyngeal inspiration will be lost through the tracheostomy. And another is the client who is simply unable to learn how to glossopharyngeal breathe for one reason or another (e.g., cognitive impairment or motor programming impairment).

Although glossopharyngeal breathing can often improve speech, its use also has some drawbacks. Because multiple glossopharyngeal strokes are often needed to inspire the desired volume of air, speech onset is usually delayed and pauses tend to be abnormally long. Another drawback of glossopharyngeal breathing is that the pumping movements of the face, jaw, and tongue may be distracting, especially to someone who is naïve about this form of breathing. Finally, although this form of breathing is generally considered safe, it may cause undesirable effects for certain clients. For example, because this form of breathing applies positive pressure to the breathing apparatus, it causes an increase in intrathoracic pressure, which, in turn, may decrease the gradient of venous return to the chest and decrease cardiac output. Collier et al. (1956) have suggested that glossopharyngeal breathing may be contraindicated in clients with abnormal vasomotor reflexes. For these reasons, a management program that includes glossopharyngeal breathing should never be initiated without clearance from the client's pulmonologist and other relevant physicians (e.g., cardiologist).

Despite these potential drawbacks, glossopharyngeal breathing can be a powerful mechanism for facilitating speech breathing in many clients with severe or profound chest wall dysfunction. It is relatively straightforward to teach and improves the speech product in several ways. Glossopharyngeal breathing can also save lives.

RELIEVING SPEAKING-RELATED DYSPNEA

Many clients with speech breathing disorders experience dyspnea (i.e., breathing discomfort, as discussed in Chapter 4). Dyspnea can range from mild and intermittent to severe and continuous. Dyspnea usually intensifies when performing physical work, such as walking or lifting, and it may worsen with speaking. Dyspnea often stems from pulmonary, cardiovascular, or neuromotor dysfunction.

For some clients, dyspnea can be a serious and pervasive problem that interferes with activities of daily living. Such clients, especially those who have stable disease of the pulmonary airways and lungs, may be candidates for a pulmonary rehabilitation program administered by a team of healthcare professionals. These programs usually have several components, which may include the following: (a) client education (e.g., information regarding breathing function and disease); (b) general physical exercise (e.g., walking, bicycling); (c) specific muscle training (e.g., inspiratory muscle training); (d) relaxation training (e.g., progressive relaxation); (e) breathing training (e.g., pursed-lip breathing, deep and slow breathing); (f) nutritional counseling; (g) energy conservation; and (h) psychosocial support (i.e., psychological counseling, meditation, stress management, panic control management, support groups). Some clients may also be candidates for pharmacological treatment, ventilatory support, or both.

The focus of this section is on what the speech-language pathologist can do to help clients whose dyspnea is caused or exacerbated by the act of speaking. For some clients, minor modifications of speech breathing behavior may be all that is necessary to relieve speaking-related dyspnea. These modifications may be suggested and directed by the speech-language pathologist, with a priori approval of the pulmonologist. Management strategies discussed here include recognizing the problem, optimizing the communication context, using trade-off strategies, speaking at large lung volumes, making postural and positional adjustments, and engaging in inspiratory muscle training.

Recognizing the Problem

Management often begins by recognizing that speaking-related dyspnea exists. In this sense, the speech breathing evaluation is sometimes the first step in the management process. The evaluation, although designed primarily to provide information and insights to the clinician, may also serve to educate the client about his disorder. For some clients, the speech breathing evaluation may mark the first time he recognizes the association between his dyspnea and his speaking.

Once speaking-related dyspnea is recognized, the clinician and client should attempt to identify the situations in which it occurs and try to determine why it occurs. For example, the client might report that his dyspnea is particularly severe when he speaks to his supervisor in her office. This observation could mean that the dyspnea has an emotional basis and is caused by anxiety related to interacting with his supervisor. Or it could be that there is an environmental irritant in her office that exacerbates his problem. Or it could relate to the fact that the client must walk up a short flight of stairs to get to her office. By analyzing the components of each situation, the clinician can help the client sort out which variables, or combination of variables, need to be addressed to minimize his speaking-related dyspnea.

Optimizing the Communication Context

The next step is to consider how to optimize the communication context so as to reduce the possibility that the client will experience speaking-related dyspnea, or at least minimize its severity. In the example described above, the communication context might be modified in several ways, depending on what variables were contributing to the problem. Potential modifications might include the following: (a) having the client deal directly with emotional issues related to his fear of people in authority by seeking counseling; (b) conducting the meetings in the client's office rather than the supervisor's office; or (c) having the client rest at the top of the stairs for a few moments before entering his supervisor's office.

There are also several general ways to modify the communication context to minimize speaking-related dyspnea. One way is to avoid speaking while performing other physical activities, such as walking or dressing. By speaking while at rest, the client reduces the neuromotor and metabolic demands on the breathing apparatus so that he can allocate the majority of his resources to the act of speech breathing. Other ways to modify the communication context are to reduce background noise in the environment, increase proximity of conversational partners, and ensure that the conversational partners are positioned so that they can see each other. All of these adjustments should reduce the loudness (and, therefore, alveolar pressure) demands on the client. Another suggestion is to have the client explain the nature of his problem to his conversational partner(s). For example, he might say, "I get winded when I talk. Sometimes I have to stop and take a couple extra breaths. Please wait for me to catch my breath, rather than try to finish my thoughts for me." Or, in the case where the source of an environmental irritant is the conversational partner, the client might say, "I would appreciate it if you didn't wear perfume around me. It makes it hard for me to breathe." Such honesty often helps to reduce the stress associated with speaking and improves the quality of the interaction. If the client is more relaxed when speaking, he is likely to feel less dyspneic. Several additional suggestions for improving the environment for clients with speech breathing disorders are discussed in another part of this chapter (see section below on optimizing the environment).

Trade-Off Strategies

Although healthy individuals tend to hyperventilate when they speak, clients with breathing impairments may have to struggle to maintain adequate ventilation while speaking. For some clients, the challenge of balancing the demands of ventilation with those of speech production may be difficult and uncomfortable. One way to ease the stress of this dual task is to incorporate trade-off strategies for speech breathing. Such strategies involve "taking breaks" from simultaneous breathing and speaking to engage in brief periods of breathing only. There are several ways to do this.

One trade-off strategy is to incorporate nonspeech expirations into the speech breathing cycle. A nonspeech expiration is just that, an expiration that is not accompanied by speech. A nonspeech expiration can be produced immediately following a spoken utterance. For example, a client might say, "My name is Jim Smith," followed by a nonspeech expiration and then an inspiration, "I live in Pasadena," followed by a nonspeech expiration and then an inspiration, and so on. Note that only a limited number of syllables is produced per expiration. In the example illustrated, each utterance contains only five to seven syllables. Because each utterance is followed by a quick expiration, the time to the next inspiration is reduced from what it would have been had the client continued to speak throughout the expiratory phase of the cycle. This means that the breathing frequency is increased and, thus, ventilation should be greater than it would have been without the nonspeech expirations. By including nonspeech expirations in the speech breathing cycle, the demands of ventilation can be satisfied. The trade-off is that less speech is uttered per breath.

Another trade-off strategy involves inserting occasional nonspeech breaths between speech breaths. In this context, nonspeech breaths refer to inspiration-expiration cycles that contain no speech. For example, a client might say, "My name is Jim Smith," followed by an inspiration, "I live in Pasadena near the Wrigley Estate," followed by an inspiration-expiration-inspiration, "My house is on Bradford Street near Orange Grove," followed by an inspiration-expiration-inspiration, and so on. In this case, inserting nonspeech breaths between speech breaths enables the client to concentrate on the business of breathing and satisfy his ventilation needs without having to attend to speech goals at the same time. When using this strategy, the client may want to alert others that he needs to pause occasionally to "catch his breath." By doing so, he may be able to avoid being interrupted during the abnormally long pauses associated with nonspeech breaths.

Trade-off strategies can also be executed between conversational partners. This simply means that the client can adopt a conversational style that encourages turn-taking. This allows the client frequent opportunities to breathe quietly while the conversational partner has the floor. This can be accomplished by using a conversational style that involves frequent yielding of the floor to the conversational partner. It may also be handled explicitly by the client at the start of a conversation by stating that he needs prolonged breaks during conversation to "catch up on breathing."

As should be apparent, the idea behind these trade-off strategies is that the client ceases speaking so that he can concentrate solely on breathing. In this way, the client avoids the stress of trying to manage competing demands of meeting speech breathing goals and ventilation needs simultaneously. The concept is a simple one and its implementation will often work wonders for clients who otherwise would choose to avoid speaking.

Speaking at Large Lung Volumes

Speaking at large lung volumes refers to maintaining the breathing apparatus at a larger-than-usual size. For certain clients, this strategy may help to relieve dyspnea. To determine if it does, the client is instructed to take a deep breath before beginning to speak and then to inspire again before expending a great deal of air. That is, the client should terminate breath groups above the resting tidal end-expiratory level. This strategy is easily described to the client by instructing him to "keep yourself big," and may be made more clear by providing him with lung volume feedback (see section above on exteroceptive feedback). Although it is not known why breathing (or speaking) at large lung volumes can relieve dyspnea (Killian, Gandevia, Summers, & Campbell, 1984), it may be due to increased sensory input associated with enlargement of the breathing apparatus.

In some clients, speaking at large lung volumes may not relieve dyspnea, but instead, may make it worse. In such clients, the perception of excessive physical exertion associated with maintaining the breathing apparatus at a large size may exacerbate speaking-related dyspnea. The only way to determine with certainty whether or not speaking at large volumes relieves a client's dyspnea is to have him rate his dyspnea (using the relevant terms identified during the evaluation) under different lung volume conditions.

Postural and Positional Adjustments

Postural and positional adjustments may reduce dyspnea in some clients. For clients with chronic obstructive pulmonary disease, dyspnea is often relieved by leaning forward and bracing the arms on something (Sharp, Drutz, Moisan, Foster, & Machnach, 1980). Such posturing can be achieved in many ways, such as by leaning against a table, the arms of a chair, or even against one's own knees. Interestingly, this postural adjustment appears to do more than just relieve dyspnea. It may actually improve the function of the inspiratory muscles (O'Neil & McCarthy, 1983; Banzett, Topulos, Leith, & Nations, 1988), increase ventilation, and improve gas exchange. A client who benefits from arm bracing may want to consider creative ways to incorporate this posture into daily activities. For example, he might configure his seating arrangement for talking on the telephone so that he can brace his arms. Because this posture is most easily assumed if the client does not have to hold the telephone, he might want to consider using a speaker-phone or a head set.

Adjustments to body position may also be critical to the relief or exacerbation of dyspnea in certain clients. For example, there are several conditions that are associated with orthopnea (i.e., increased dyspnea when moving from an upright body position to a supine body position). Clients who are apt to suffer from orthopnea are those with cardiac dysfunction such as congestive heart failure, obstructive disorders such as chronic obstructive pulmonary disease, or neuromotor disease such as amyotrophic lateral sclerosis. For clients with orthopnea, the supine body position should be avoided for all forms of breathing, not just speech breathing.

The best way to determine the influence of body posture and position on speaking-related dyspnea (and overall speech breathing function) is to experiment (with the permission and oversight of the client's physician). There is no easy "recipe" for knowing which posture and/or position will be most comfortable for the client without testing out the different possibilities. For example, in the client with neuromotor impairment, the degree to which a given posture or position relieves speaking-related dyspnea will depend, at least in part, on the degree to which that posture or position improves spared inspiratory and expiratory muscle function (see section above on body positioning). Because the perceptual consequences of postural/positional adjustments are often not easily predicted, it is imperative to carefully query the client regarding his breathing comfort during both speaking and rest with each adjustment.

Inspiratory Muscle Training

Inspiratory muscle training (discussed in detail in the section above on muscle training) can relieve dyspnea. Inspiratory muscle training has been shown to reduce dyspnea in subjects with neuromotor impairments, such as spinal cord injury (Rutchik, Weissman, Almenoff, Spungen, Bauman, & Grimm, 1998), and obstructive breathing disorders, such as asthma (Weiner, Berar-Yanay, Davidovich, Magadle, & Weiner, 2000) and chronic obstructive pulmonary disease (Riera, Rubio, Ruiz, Ramos, Otero, Hernandez, & Gomez, 2001). Inspiratory muscle training also has been shown to reduce speaking-related dyspnea in subjects with laryngeally based speech production disorders (Baker, Sapienza, & Collins, 2003; Baker, Sapienza, Martin, Davenport, Hoffman-Ruddy, & Woodson, 2003). Although such effects have not been tested in individuals with breathing-based speech impairments, it seems reasonable to predict that inspiratory muscle training could reduce speaking-related dyspnea in certain clients. The decision regarding whether or not a particular client is an appropriate candidate for inspiratory muscle training must be made by the client's physician (e.g., pulmonologist, neurologist, cardiologist).

MONITORING GAS EXCHANGE

Gas exchange may be different during speech breathing than during rest. For example, because healthy individuals tend to hyperventilate when they speak (see section on speaking and ventilation in Chapter 3), the partial pressure of carbon dioxide (PCO_2) in arterial blood is lower after a period of speaking than after a period of rest. Nevertheless, it cannot be assumed that a client with a speech breathing disorder will show the same pattern. In fact, in some clients, the ability to balance speech breathing demands with gas exchange requirements can be a challenge. One way to help such clients achieve the right balance is by monitoring gas exchange during speech breathing.

There are noninvasive indicators of gas exchange that have been described as evaluation tools (see section on instrumental examination in Chapter 4). Two of these are especially appropriate for use in the management of clients with speech breathing disorders. One is oxygen saturation (SpO_2) and the other is end-tidal PCO_2. As is the case for evaluation, the monitoring of gas-exchange variables should be done under the direction of the pulmonologist and alongside a respiratory therapist.

SpO_2 can be monitored with a small and lightweight pulse oximeter. The probe is fixed on the client's finger and the SpO_2 value appears on a digital display. Because a portable pulse oximeter is so easy to operate and carry, the client can usually be instructed in how to use it on his own. Recall that SpO_2 is a critical safety measure. In healthy individuals, SpO_2 is near 100% and reflects the percentage of blood hemoglobin that is saturated with oxygen. Some clients are at risk for desaturating (e.g., SpO_2 falling below 90%, or whatever safe minimum level is set by the pulmonologist). Desaturation can be extremely dangerous because, without hemoglobin being fully (or nearly fully) saturated with oxygen, not enough oxygen will be delivered to the body tissues. Clients in whom SpO_2 should be monitored as part of speech breathing management are those who tend to desaturate when speaking.

End-tidal PCO_2 can be monitored with a portable capnometer, coupled to the client by nasal cannulae. As described in Chapter 4, measures of end-tidal PCO_2 are obtained at end-expiration during resting tidal breathing. Thus, if the clinician wants to measure the client's end-tidal PCO_2 associated with speaking, the best way to do this is by comparing his end-tidal PCO_2 (during resting tidal breathing) immediately before and immediately after speaking. Clients who tend to hypoventilate or substantially hyperventilate when speaking are good candidates for end-tidal PCO_2 monitoring. It is important to note that end-tidal PCO_2 may not be a valid indicator of arterial PCO_2 in certain clients. Even so, it may be a good indicator of change in arterial PCO_2. Whether or not end-tidal PCO_2 is a meaningful measure for any given client should be determined by the pulmonologist.

Two clinical examples are offered here to demonstrate how SpO_2 and end-tidal PCO_2 might be used in the management of speech breathing. The first example pertains to a client with moderate emphysema. Such a client may be able to maintain a high enough level of ventilation to keep his blood gases in a reasonably normal range. However, when he speaks, he may not maintain the same high level of ventilation, and he may desaturate. In his case, a pulse oximeter could be used to monitor his SpO_2 and determine what types of speaking behaviors cause desaturation. This information could be used to identify speech breathing strategies that maintain the client's SpO_2 at an acceptable level (for example, trade-off strategies as described above in the section on relieving speaking-related dyspnea).

The second example is one in which a client is an appropriate candidate for end-tidal PCO_2 monitoring. Consider a client who has amyotrophic lateral sclerosis with moderate-to-severe spinal signs and only mild bulbar signs. Suppose he had just begun to use elective noninvasive positive pressure ventilation to assist his speech breathing (see section above on mechanical aids). Further suppose that he complains of lightheadedness, suggesting that he might be "overdoing" his supplementary ventilation. In such a case, measures of end-tidal PCO_2 might be relatively normal during resting tidal breathing without the ventilator (e.g., 42 mmHg), but drop substantially after speaking with noninvasive positive pressure ventilation (e.g., to 31 mmHg). This would confirm that the client was hyperventilating during ventilator-supported speech breathing. By monitoring end-tidal PCO_2 during management sessions, it should be possible to determine appropriate speech breathing patterns to offset the client's tendency to hyperventilate.

In a sense, the monitoring of gas exchange is a form of exteroceptive feedback. However, it differs in critical ways from the exteroceptive feedback discussed in other parts of this chapter. When exteroceptive feedback is incorporated into a muscle training program, for example, it is done so that the client is provided with information related to the strength of his muscles. The feedback allows the client to determine how well he is achieving his goal of increasing muscle strength. When SpO_2 and end-tidal PCO_2 are monitored during speech breathing management, it is usually done as an ancillary observation. For example, a client may be working to increase his pressure generation and volume excursion with the goals of producing louder speech and longer breath groups. Gas exchange variables are monitored, not to help him achieve these speech goals, but to ensure that he maintains adequate gas exchange in the process of achieving those goals.

MOUTHING AND BUCCAL SPEAKING

Clients with speech breathing disorders often manifest problems generating alveolar pressure that is high enough to oscillate the vocal folds and drive upper airway articulation. Some of the management methods discussed in this chapter are designed to increase alveolar pressure. Nevertheless, sometimes these methods are not fully successful and it may be necessary to come up with ways to compensate for less-than-adequate pressure generating capabilities. Two compensatory strategies that allow a client to continue to "speak," even when alveolar pressure is inadequate, are mouthing and buccal speaking. For these strategies to be successful, the client must have good upper airway control.

Mouthing is defined as speech production movements in the absence of sound. Able-bodied individuals often use mouthing to "speak" silently to a "listener," often with the intention that others nearby will not understand the message. Mouthing is a natural adaptation to not being able to speak aloud and clients often adopt this strategy spontaneously when they are unable to produce voice. One drawback to mouthing is that the receiver of the message must be able to see the speaker's face. Another drawback is that many speech movements, such as those produced in the laryngeal and pharyngeal areas, are not visible to the receiver. Because of this, it is not surprising that many people are poor speech readers (i.e., lip readers), even when the speaker produces perfectly executed movements.

Despite these drawbacks, mouthing can be an effective compensatory strategy for certain clients who cannot produce voice. Mouthing is most successful when used intermittently, rather than continuously. For example, mouthing might be a good option for a client who generates adequate alveolar pressure to produce speech throughout most of the breath group, but loses that ability at small lung volumes (where expiratory relaxation pressure is low or absent). Such a client could extend the breath group by mouthing the last syllable or two. The probability that the listener would understand these syllables is quite good because syntactic and semantic cues provided in the preceding utterance should increase the listener's ability to predict the mouthed words.

Buccal speaking is another compensatory strategy for clients who have difficulty generating adequate alveolar pressure for speech production. This is often called "Donald Duck" speech because it sounds like the speech of the famous cartoon character. The buccal "voice" is produced by pushing air between buccal (cheek) tissue and the maxilla (Weinberg & Westerhouse, 1971). This sets the tissue into motion and creates a sound source that can then be used to produce speech. Another related form of speaking is pharyngeal speaking in which the sound source is created by forcing air between the tongue and the upper alveolus, the palate, or the pharyngeal wall (Weinberg & Westerhouse, 1971). Buccal and pharyngeal speaking have no alveolar pressure requirements because they are generated independently of the breathing apparatus. This is easily demonstrated by producing buccal or pharyngeal speech while breath holding.

As was the case with the mouthing strategy, buccal (or pharyngeal) speaking can be used to add an extra syllable or two to the end of a laryngeally voiced utterance. For example, a client might say, "May I have a glass of orange (juice)?" and produce the last word with buccal (or pharyngeal) speech. This form of speech can also be used to generate full sentences or entire conversations. The presence of a sound source generally renders buccal (or pharyngeal) speaking much more intelligible than mouthing. It also has the advantage that it can be used with the telephone. Some clients adopt this form of speech spontaneously (Hoit & Shea, 1996), whereas others require direct instruction to develop it.

CONVERSATIONAL STRATEGIES

Conversation can be quite difficult for some clients with speech breathing disorders. Typically, the most serious problems are caused by the timing demands that accompany conversational interchange. When two people engage in conversation, there is a turn-taking rhythm that develops as an emergent property of the interaction between their two individual speech breathing rhythms (see section on conversational interchange and speech breathing in Chapter 3). When one of the conversational partners has a speech breathing disorder that disrupts that interactional rhythm, the conversation can become stressful for both.

The primary reason that conversational rhythm becomes disrupted is that the person with a speech breathing disorder exhibits longer-than-expected pauses. Problems arise when the conversational partner begins speaking during the pause because he did not realize that the speaker intended to continue his train of thought. Abnormally long pauses may occur for various reasons. They may be associated with abnormally slow inspirations caused by weak inspiratory muscles, or they may be associated with the need to take an extra breath between speech breaths to relieve dyspnea. One of the most common situations in which abnormally long pauses occur is during ventilator-supported speech breathing (see Chapter 6). When it is not possible to alleviate abnormally long pauses, it is useful to develop strategies that help maintain a natural conversational exchange. The strategies suggested here are linguistic planning, prosodic cueing, and nonverbal signaling.

Linguistic Planning

Linguistic planning can take two forms. One is to plan the breath group so that it terminates at the end of a sentence. Another is to plan the breath group so that it terminates before the sentence is completed. These two planning strategies serve different purposes.

Planning for the breath group to terminate with the end of a sentence is a way to signal that a spoken thought is complete. In the context of conversation, this may serve as a turn-taking cue, indicating that the speaker is yielding the floor. For example, the client might say, "I am ready to go home," leaving the partner to pick up the conversation with a response. Ending the breath group with the end of a sentence is also appropriate for didactic speaking situations, wherein the speaker has control of the floor and there is little risk of being interrupted. Examples of didactic speaking situations include lecturing to an audience or reading aloud to another person. Listeners in these situations generally realize that a pause is not a turn-taking cue and will not attempt to interrupt the speaker. When lecturing to an audience, it may be important to maintain adequate loudness so that everyone is able to hear what is said. In this case, the best strategy may be to terminate the breath group while alveolar pressure is still relatively high, as well as to attempt to break at linguistically acceptable junctures.

The second linguistic planning strategy is to terminate breath groups at what might be considered inappropriate linguistic junctures. This is an effective way to hold the floor during conversation. With this strategy, the breath group is terminated anywhere except at the end of a sentence or at a juncture that could be mistaken for the end of a sentence. Examples of junctures that offer clear signals that the speaker intends to continue speaking after pausing are those that follow conjunctions (e.g., "There were rhinos and elephants, but . . . [pause] . . . no lions at the zoo.") or break noun phrases (e.g., "My bother has a black . . . [pause] . . . cat, and my sister has a yellow . . . [pause] . . . lab."). Such junctures are less likely to elicit interruptions from a conversational partner than those that come before a conjunction (e.g., "There were rhinos and elephants, ... [pause] . . . but no lions at the zoo.") or between noun phrases (e.g., "My bother has a black cat, . . . [pause] . . . and my sister has a yellow lab.").

Prosodic Cueing

There are certain prosodic cues that signal when a speaker wants to hold the floor and others that signal when he wants to yield his conversational turn. One turn-yielding cue is the presence of a pause following the utterance. Another turn-yielding cue is a decrease in loudness near the end of the utterance. Certain clients with speech breathing disorders may exhibit both of these cues routinely. They do so, not intentionally, but because these cues are a direct consequence of a fall in alveolar pressure near the end of the breath group.

One prosodic cue that the client with a speech breathing disorder may still have under behavioral control is the fundamental frequency (pitch) of his voice. Decreasing pitch at the end of an utterance, like decreasing loudness or the presence of a pause, tends to serve as a turn-yielding cue. Thus, if the client wants to hold the floor into the next breathing cycle, he should raise his fundamental frequency slightly on the last syllable or two of the utterance to indicate to his listener that he intends to continue. For clients with a falling pressure profile, this needs to be done consciously because the natural tendency is for fundamental frequency to decrease as pressure decreases.

Nonverbal Signaling

Another way to hold the floor is to use nonverbal signaling as a way to counteract naturally occurring turn-yielding cues (e.g., the presence of a pause and decreasing loudness). Examples of nonverbal signals that can indicate an intention to continue speaking might include maintaining an open mouth posture or holding up a hand or finger (if not paralyzed) in a "wait" configuration throughout the duration of the pause.

Other nonverbal signals can be developed to serve as turn-yielding cues. For example, a client could signal a desire to yield his conversational turn by nodding his head or pointing to the conversational partner. One of the benefits of developing turn-yielding cues is that they can provide a distinct contrast to floor-holding cues.

OPTIMIZING THE ENVIRONMENT

Thus far, this chapter has concentrated primarily on how to manage speech breathing by adjusting the client's behavior and physical status. In this section, the focus turns from management of the client per se to management of his environment. Offered here are several suggestions as to how to enhance communication in general and speech breathing specifically by optimizing auditory cues, visual cues, the physical environment, and the communication competency of others.

Optimizing Auditory Cues

Many clients with speech breathing disorders have difficulty with pressure generation, which means that they have difficulty producing adequately loud speech. In extreme cases, they may not be able to generate enough pressure to produce voice. Others may be able to produce adequately loud speech, but only at a high effort cost. For clients such as these, it is important to minimize the background noise with which their speech must compete. This means that, when the client is speaking, careful attention should be paid to turning off or "muting" the television, turning off the radio, turning down the air conditioner, and otherwise reducing extraneous noise that could mask the client's speech.

Also critical to communication success is the auditory status of the communication partner. If a client's communication partner (e.g., spouse or parent) has a hearing impairment, higher pressure-generating demands will be placed on the client as he attempts to speak louder. Management of the communication partner's hearing impairment (e.g., with hearing aids) should make conversation easier and more successful for both the client and his partner.

Optimizing Visual Cues

Visual cues are not required for communication to be successful under normal circumstances. The ease of telephone communication provides the most obvious example of this. Nevertheless, visual cues can provide an important dimension to communication, especially in the context of a communication disorder.

Visual cues may be essential for successful communication in clients whose speech breathing disorder results in compromised speech intelligibility. With such clients, intelligibility may be enhanced by the addition of visual information associated with speech movements, facial expressions, and gestures. Visual cues may also facilitate conversational interchange in clients whose speech breathing impairment causes long pauses between breath groups.

Certain environmental adjustments can be made to maximize the ability to use visual cues. One is to situate the conversational partner such that he/she can see the client's face and upper body. This will make it possible to see the client's speech movements, facial expressions, and gestures. Sometimes this involves adjustment of the client's posture. For example, if the client tends to drop his head forward, it may be difficult for the conversational partner to access visual cues related to the client's speech movements. Thus, the client's posture should be adjusted so that mutual gaze can be established. Another way to maximize access to visual cues is to ensure that the lighting is appropriate. It should be bright enough to be able to see the client clearly, but not so bright as to be annoying.

Optimizing the Physical Environment

There are often ways to modify the physical environment to make spoken communication easier for the client with a speech breathing disorder. The specific modifications depend on the nature of the client's speech breathing disorder and the nature of his environment.

In some cases, it is important that the physical environment contain a special seating arrangement that allows the client to adjust his posture to maximize his speech breathing function. For example, the seat might need to tilt slightly toward supine. Or the back of the seat might need shoulder straps and a head strap to help hold the client upright.

Conversation is easier if the conversational partners are in close proximity to one another. By being close to each other, the client does not have to speak excessively loudly and the conversational partner can take advantage of visual cues provided by the client. To make it possible for the client to be close to his conversational partners, the client should have access to the areas of the house where communication occurs. Some clients may need an electric wheelchair to move from room to room. Use of a wheelchair (or other ambulation aid) may require that the house be modified for accessibility through doorways and to areas normally accessed by steps. In some cases, it makes sense to alter the way certain rooms are used, so that the client can be "where the action is." For example, a formal dining room located next to the kitchen might be made into a family room so that these two communication-intense areas are in closer proximity.

The air within the home may need to be modified for the client with a speech breathing disorder. For example, the air may need to be humidified. This would mean that there should be a humidifier in the areas where the client is most likely to spend time. As another example, the client may be highly sensitive to smoke and other airborne irritants. It seems obvious that the home of such a client should be smoke-free, and that anyone entering the home should refrain from smoking. Also, it may be important that the people who are around the client refrain from wearing cologne or other fragrant and potentially irritating products.

The unfortunate situation may arise in which a client's home is located at a higher-than-ideal elevation. For certain clients, the additional struggle required to extract oxygen from "thin air" overtaxes an already compromised speech breathing apparatus. In such cases, it may be necessary for the client to move to a lower elevation. This, of course, is an enormous adjustment and one that must be weighed against the disadvantages of having to begin all over again in a new environment.

Optimizing the Communication Competency of Others

The communication competency of the conversational partner can have a major influence on the success of the interaction. The first step toward optimizing the communication competency of those who interact with a client is to educate them about the nature of the client's problem, and the second is usually to offer suggestions as to how to make the interaction easier and more successful. Such education might take different forms for different communication partners. In the case of someone who is actively involved in the client's management (e.g., spouse, close friend), the clinician may have the opportunity to offer direct instruction and demonstration. For example, the clinician might explain that the client has trouble maintaining adequately loud speech for long periods and that communication will be more successful and less stressful if the conversational partner minimizes the background noise, sits close to the client, and waits patiently when the client needs to stop speaking momentarily. In the case of communication partners who are not actively involved in the client's management (e.g., neighbors, casual friends), the client may need to assume the role of educator. For instance, if the client is conversing with someone at a party, he may want to ask his communication partner if they can move away from the crowd so that he can be more easily heard and understood. These issues are discussed further in the section below on counseling.

COUNSELING

Management of a client with a communication disorder should always include some form of counseling. When the client has a speech breathing disorder, counseling may become even more central to the management process. This is because breathing difficulty may threaten survival. Stated simply, breathing is a life-and-death matter and, as such, cuts to the core of the self. A person is seldom more vulnerable than when he is struggling to breathe. Highlighted in this section are those aspects of counseling that are of particular concern to the management of clients with speech breathing disorders, especially those related to emotional support and education.

Both the emotional support and educational aspects of counseling need to be considered in the broad context of the client's social milieu. That is, although the counseling offered by the speech-language pathologist usually focuses primarily on the client, such counseling often includes other significant people in the client's life. In the case of the very young child, parents and sometimes siblings are an integral part of the counseling process. In the case of the school-aged child, teachers and classmates may also be part of the counseling process. With adult clients, spouses, children, grandchildren, and friends often become important partners in counseling interactions. In some cases, it may also be appropriate to include medical caregivers, such as those who attend to the client in an extended care facility or a personal aid who helps the client at home. Significant people, such as those mentioned here, have a strong influence on the client's communication function, including his speech breathing function. It is part of the speech-language pathologist's role to decide which members of the client's social network should be included in counseling, and at what point(s) in the management process they should be included.

The speech-language pathologist should also build her own local network of allied professionals who can offer additional emotional support and/or education for clients with speech breathing disorders. This network might include psychiatrists, psychologists, vocational counselors, pulmonologists, pulmonary nurses, and physical therapists, among others. Professionals included in this local network should be those whom the speech-language pathologist trusts to provide high-quality service. This means that the speech-language pathologist needs to invest time and energy into developing this network and educating these professionals about speech breathing disorders. A strong professional network can enhance the potential for effective and comprehensive management.

Emotional Support

Emotional support is an essential component of counseling. It is part of what the speech-language pathologist brings to the management of the client with a speech breathing disorder (or any other type of communication disorder). Some important forms of emotional support relate to improving the client's attitude, enhancing his independence, and increasing his social well-being. In some cases, the nature of the support required by the client is outside the scope of practice of the speech-language pathologist and calls for the expertise of other professionals.

The client's attitude is critical to what can be accomplished in management. The ideal client is the one who is motivated, happy, and willing to work hard. Nevertheless, the reality is that clients with speech breathing disorders are often depressed and frightened, not just because communication is impaired, but also because breathing difficulties may compromise their quality and quantity of life. As examples, the dyspnea that accompanies some speech breathing disorders can limit participation in certain activities, and the physical deterioration that accompanies progressive conditions can cause premature death. The speech-language pathologist can sometimes help reduce a client's depression and fear merely by acknowledging that these are natural responses to having a discomfort-causing and life-threatening condition. However, in some cases, the client's emotional state is so impaired that help from other professionals must be sought. Sometimes this means that speech breathing management must be delayed until the client is ready to engage in the management process.

The independence of a client with a speech breathing disorder may be restricted. For example, a client with advanced chronic obstructive pulmonary disease may need to be tethered to a supplemental oxygen source. Or a client with a neuromotor-based speech breathing disorder may not be able to drive a car. Loss of independence is

El Toro

He was from the northeast and the slower pace of the southwest was novel to him. His son had a significant neuromotor impairment that was worsening and the family had moved to ease the boy's difficulty in getting around in a wheelchair. The son had significant weakness in his limbs, breathing apparatus, and velopharynx. He was in need of management. At the time, his rural school was not ramped for wheelchair access and the school board refused to provide him with a needed velar-lift prosthesis. Enter the bull. Head down. Easy snorting at first. A light fire in his eyes. Some counseling is heard from a gray-haired man in the grandstand. Get out of the way. Within a month the school is ramped and the school board has convinced a local service agency to buy the needed prosthesis. Occasionally, a well-placed word or two can make all the difference. That's no bull. Help people help themselves.

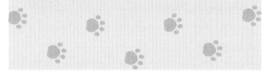

difficult to accept, and requires that the client adapt himself to new circumstances if he is going to be satisfied with his current life. In many cases, the speech-language pathologist can help the client adapt by offering communication strategies to address his limitations. Such strategies cannot free a client from a supplemental oxygen source or enable him to drive a car, but they can help to increase his independence. Speech breathing management strategies, such as those described in this chapter, can increase independence by making it possible for the client to speak for himself instead of relying on others to communicate for him. For some clients, the goal of independence can only be met by gainful employment. Although it may not be reasonable for such a client to return to his old job, it may be possible for him to embark on a new career. Engaging the services of a good vocational counselor can facilitate this process. Often, the combined efforts of the vocational counselor and the speech-language pathologist can maximize a client's potential for success. For example, the vocational counselor might help the client obtain employment that can be conducted from home using the telephone. The speech-language pathologist can then work with the client to identify ways to enhance his speech breathing function in that context. This might involve the use of a telephone with a headset to allow him to posture his breathing apparatus with his arms. It might also involve the construction of a script that is minimally taxing to his speech breathing.

Although some clients have extensive and strong social support systems, others do not. When a client has no support system, or when a client's family and friends do not provide adequate emotional support, other sources of support should be sought. The speech-language pathologist can be instrumental in this process. For example, she can encourage the client to join a support group and assist him in finding the one that best meets his needs (e.g., a support group for individuals with young-onset multiple sclerosis). For a client who is hesitant to join a support group, the speech-language pathologist may be able to arrange to have someone from the group visit him. Even if the client chooses not to join the group, he may derive comfort from his interactions with another person who is facing the same challenges as he is. When appropriate, the speech-language pathologist may also encourage the client's family members to seek out support groups for themselves (e.g., a support group for spouses of people with amyotrophic lateral sclerosis).

Although the speech-language pathologist routinely counsels her clients regarding those aspects of the disorder that relate to speech and communication, sometimes the client's counseling needs extend beyond her scope of practice. For example, a client may evidence a psychogenic hyperventilation syndrome that appears to be linked to early childhood sexual abuse. As another example, a client with a speech breathing disorder secondary to multiple sclerosis may suffer from depression and anxiety that may be best treated pharmacologically. As a final example, a client may have a tremendous fear of "suffocating to death" that appears to be exacerbated by alcohol abuse. In these types of cases, the speech-language pathologist should refer the client to a counselor, psychologist, or psychiatrist. Sometimes it is appropriate to encourage certain clients to seek spiritual counsel as well.

Education

Education is another essential component of counseling. By educating the client about his disorder, the client can become fully engaged in the management process. Speech-language pathologists recognize this and routinely provide education to their clients about speech production, the nature of the speech disorder, and what can be done to improve speech. The same should be done for the client with a speech breathing disorder. For example, the speech-language pathologist might describe how pressure is generated to produce speech, how pressure relates to loudness, and why a client with muscular weakness has difficulty producing loud-enough speech. Or the speech-language pathologist might explain how air moves into and out of the pulmonary apparatus, how ventilation changes when the drive-to-breathe is very high, and why a client with chronic obstructive pulmonary disease may have difficulty ventilating adequately while speaking. The speech-language pathologist educates the client on issues as they relate to speech breathing and communication in general. Nevertheless, when other issues arise that fall outside this realm, it may be necessary to refer the client to other professionals for educational counseling.

There are many other types of referrals that can offer a client appropriate educational counseling. For example, a client might be referred for potential enrollment in a pulmonary rehabilitation program. A pulmonary rehabilitation program usually has several components, including pulmonary education, exercise, breathing training, nutritional counseling, and smoking cessation counseling, among other forms of intervention. Clients who are candidates for pulmonary rehabilitation tend to be those with relatively stable disease of the pulmonary airways and lungs. For clients who have other types of speech breathing disorders (e.g., neuromotor disorders), education regarding breathing status might be provided by a pulmonary nurse, respiratory therapist, or pulmonologist, and education regarding muscle function might be provided by a physical therapist or physiatrist.

Speech breathing disorders can be caused by life-threatening conditions and diseases. Thus, clients with speech breathing disorders may be faced with the possibility of having to make life-and-death decisions regarding their care. Of special relevance to these clients is the need to decide whether or not to accept ventilatory support if self-generated breathing efforts begin to fail. This issue should be faced squarely, in conjunction with family members, and with a full understanding of the consequences of all possible decisions. The speech-language pathologist can offer counsel regarding the speech and communication consequences of various ventilatory support options (see Chapter 6) and can facilitate certain aspects of communication during the decision-making process. Referral for psychological counseling should be made to help the client work through the many other serious emotional and practical issues related to this life-prolonging or life-ending decision. Once the client has come to terms with his decision, he and his family will need legal counsel to formalize the client's wishes. This involves the services of an attorney who will help the client create advance directives (Tippett, 2000a). Advance directives typically include creation of a living will (i.e., establishing limits on the level of palliative care) and designation of a medical power of attorney (i.e., a person who will make specific decisions regarding the client's level of care if he is no longer able to make such decisions).

ASSISTIVE SPEECH DEVICES

A speech breathing disorder can sometimes impair speech to the point that it is no longer functional. In some cases, speech can be made functional with the aid of an assistive speech device. Considered in this section are four types of such devices: speech amplifiers, electrolarynges, buttons and one-way valves, and talking tracheostomy tubes.

Speech Amplifiers

Speech amplifiers (often called voice amplifiers) may benefit clients whose low loudness interferes with their ability to be heard and understood. In some cases, use of an amplifier is adopted only after other interventions have been tried and found to be unsuccessful. In other cases, an amplifier may be used as a supplement to other interventions or for selected applications. For example, a client may not require an amplifier for routine speech breathing activities, but may use it when speaking to a large group or when conversing in a noisy environment.

Speech amplifiers are commercially available and come in several forms. Such amplifiers consist of a microphone and a loudspeaker unit with associated electronics. For most uses, one that is lightweight and "hands free" is preferred. For example, one of the more popular designs is one in which a small microphone is fixed to a plastic band that fits over the head and can be positioned near the speaker's lips (i.e., a head-mounted microphone). Another type of microphone is one that is attached to a flexible cord that hangs around the speaker's neck. And, for clients who have particular difficulty being heard over the telephone, there are telephones available that contain built-in amplifiers that boost the outgoing speech.

Speech amplifiers are most effective for clients with good voice quality and upper airway articulation. They are less effective for clients with breathy or whispered voices. They may be completely ineffective, at least for improving intelligibility, for clients who have poor upper airway articulation. Nevertheless, there may be situations in which a speech amplifier is indicated even for the client who is unintelligible. For example, if a client is able to produce only vowel-like utterances, the amplifier may help him signal caregivers of his need to communicate. He may then use an alternative communication device to convey the actual message.

Electrolarynges

Electrolarynges may be useful for clients who are unable to produce laryngeal voice. In the context of this book, this refers specifically to clients who are not able to generate adequate alveolar pressure to oscillate the vocal folds. Of course, electrolarynx use is associated with conditions other than speech breathing disorders, the most common of which is laryngectomy.

An electrolarynx generates sound that replaces the laryngeally generated voice. Most are electromechanical devices. There are also pneumatic electrolarynges, however, these are not appropriate for clients with speech breathing disorders who have limited pressure and/or volume generation capabilities.

Electrolarynges come in different forms, including neck types and intraoral types. The neck type is held against the neck so as to vibrate the tissue, which, in turn, vibrates the air within the vocal tract. One form of intraoral electrolarynx consists of a tube coupled to a hand-held sound source. The distal end of the tube is inserted into the oral cavity to produce speech. Another form of intraoral electrolarynx consists of a sound generator located within a plastic prosthesis that covers the hard palate and is clipped to the teeth. The sound generator, in this case, is activated and deactivated by a hand-held switch. The switch can also be adapted to be operated by movements of the head, toe, or other parts of the body. This type of electrolarynx may be appropriate for a client who is unable to move his hands and requires a "hands free" voice source.

For an electrolarynx to be useful, the client must have certain attributes. He must have well-controlled upper airway movements so that he is able to create intelligible speech. The client must also have adequate physical strength and dexterity to operate the electrolarynx. In addition, he must have the ability to coordinate the activation of the sound source with his upper airway movements, an ability that often requires skill, training, and ample practice to become a proficient speaker.

Buttons and One-Way Valves

A tracheostomy must be occluded during expiration to produce adequate speech. If it remains open, the majority of the expired air exits through the tracheostomy and little is available to drive the larynx. This is because the resistance of the pathway through the tracheostomy is much lower than the resistance of the laryngeal pathway (during phonation). When the tracheostomy is occluded during expiration, all expired air is routed through the laryngeal airway, as it is during normal speech production. A tracheostomy can be occluded with a finger or thumb, but a more convenient way to occlude a tracheostomy is to use a button or a one-way valve.

There are two general forms of buttons. One is a prosthesis that is inserted directly into the tracheostomy after the tracheostomy tube is removed. This form of button is used for clients who no longer breathe through the tracheostomy, but in whom there may be a future need to do so. A second form of button is a plug that inserts into the distal end of the tracheostomy tube. A client who has a tracheostomy tube, but who does not need to breathe through the tracheostomy at all times, may choose to use such a button. For example, a client with obstructive sleep apnea (whose laryngeal and/or upper airway tissues are sucked inward during sleep) might use a button during the day so that he can breathe and speak normally. At night, the button is removed so that the client can breathe through his tracheostomy while sleeping and bypass the higher resistance of the laryngeal-upper airway pathway. As another example, a client with central hypoventilation syndrome (whose automatic drive to breathe is depressed during sleep) may breathe normally with a button in place during waking hours and remove it at night so that he can connect himself to a ventilator while sleeping. With a button in place, speech breathing can be essentially normal.

One form of a one-way (inspiratory) valve consists of a plastic structure that connects to the distal end of the tracheostomy tube. Inside the structure is a pliable flange that deforms when higher air pressure is applied to one surface (i.e., the surface distal to the client), but remains flat when higher pressure is applied on the other surface (i.e., the surface proximal to the client). During inspiration, the flange deforms and air is free to flow through the tracheostomy into the client's pulmonary apparatus. During expiration, the flange flattens and the air is blocked from exiting through the tracheostomy. There are other types of one-way valves, such as those that are spring-loaded or those that contain a ball that moves into and away from an opening, all of which have the same functional consequence. That is, they allow inspired air to enter the tracheostomy and route expired air through the larynx and upper airway for speech production.

To use a button or a one-way valve, it is imperative that the laryngeal-upper airway pathway be unobstructed. Specifically, the cuff on the tracheostomy tube must be deflated, there must be ample space surrounding the tracheostomy tube for air to flow, and the resistance offered by the larynx and upper airway must not be abnormally high. Sometimes this requires that adjustments be made to the tracheostomy tube itself (e.g., replaced with a smaller tube, replaced with a fenestrated tube). It is also critical that, before the cuff is deflated, the client is able to manage his secretions and/or that appropriate suctioning protocols are performed. Before the button or valve is placed, the client's tracheostomy can be occluded digitally to determine his ability to tolerate the change in airflow and the associated breathing sensations. Further details regarding cuff deflation procedures and the use of buttons and one-way valves are available elsewhere (Tippett, 2000b; Dikeman & Kazandjian, 2002). Note that the present discussion focuses on the use of buttons and one-way valves in clients who can breathe on their own. They are also used with clients who are supported with certain forms of ventilators (e.g., phrenic nerve pacers), but are contraindicated for clients who use ventilatory support that is delivered via a tracheostomy (see section on positive pressure ventilation in Chapter 6).

Talking Tracheostomy Tubes

A talking tracheostomy tube (sometimes called a speaking trachesotomy cannula) is depicted in Figure 5-3. It consists of a tracheostomy tube fitted with a special air-delivery apparatus designed to provide airflow to the larynx when the tracheostomy-tube cuff is inflated. A talking tracheostomy tube supplies this flow by routing air through a narrow catheter located on the top surface of the tube. This catheter is connected at its distal end to a compressed air source (i.e., tank or wall source) and contains an opening (or openings) at or near its proximal end. A port lies between the compressed air source and the opening(s). When the port is occluded, air flows to the larynx and speech can be produced.

Talking tracheostomy tubes are used for clients who must maintain an inflated tracheostomy-tube cuff while receiving ventilatory support (see section on invasive positive pressure ventilation in Chapter 6). Cuff inflation may be indicated to protect against aspiration in cases where the client's swallow is judged to be unsafe. Cuff inflation may also be necessary to maintain ventilation at an appropriate level if the client loses too much of the ventilator-delivered volume through his larynx. To be a candidate for a talking tracheostomy tube, the client must have good laryngeal and upper airway control for speech production.

Speech production with a talking tracheostomy tube is highly successful for some clients and unsuccessful for others (Kluin, Maynard, & Bogdasarian, 1984; Sparker, Robbins, Nevlud, Watkins, & Jahrsdoerfer, 1987; Lohmeier & Hoit, 2003). Several problems have been found to be associated with the use of talking tracheostomy tubes (Tippett & Vogelman, 2000). These include poor voice quality, drying of mucosa in the larynx and upper airway, crimping of the source tube, and clogging of the exit ports with secretions. There is also the drawback that clients with paralyzed upper extremities must rely on someone else to manipulate the flow source, unless a special switch is devised that can be operated by movement of the head or face. Despite these problems, it is worthwhile to test the use of a talking tracheostomy tube with clients who are appropriate candidates. For clients who can use them, the talking tracheostomy tube may mean the difference between having a voice and

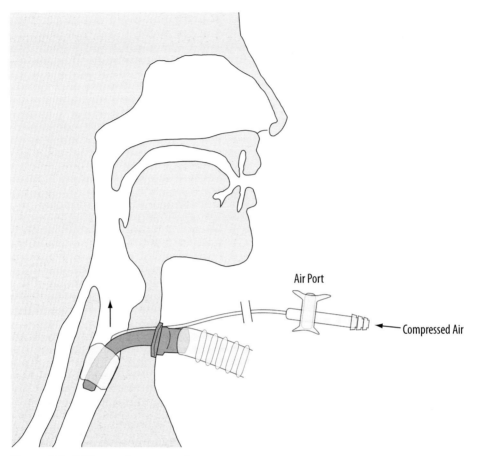

Figure 5-3. Talking tracheostomy tube.

having no voice at all.

The client who is a candidate for a talking tracheostomy tube requires assistance from the speech-language pathologist to maximize his speech production capabilities. To begin, the flow through the talking tracheostomy tube needs to be adjusted to a level that produces the best possible voice quality and is still comfortable for the client (Safar & Grenvik, 1975; Kluin et al., 1984; Leder & Traquina, 1989). If the flow causes discomfort and drying of the surrounding tissues, the air may need to be warmed and humidified. Once the flow is optimized, the client may benefit from behavioral therapy. For example, it may be possible to improve the client's intelligibility by having him slow his articulation rate slightly and increase his articulatory precision (i.e., overarticulate). As another example, it may be possible to improve the naturalness of the client's speech by teaching him to "chunk" his utterances more appropriately. This intervention would target the client who tends to speak continuously (because there is continuous flow to the larynx) and fails to include the natural pauses that listeners expect. Another type of phrasing problem might arise as a consequence of the "mismatch" between the flow to the larynx and the breathing cycle. It has been noted that some clients experience difficulty producing speech during the inspiratory phase of the breathing cycle (Leder & Traquina, 1989), even though the act of speaking is decoupled from the act of breathing when a talking tracheostomy tube is used.

AUGMENTATIVE COMMUNICATION

Although the management approaches described in this chapter are usually successful in improving speech breathing and speech, there are times when such management, no matter how creative or extensive, is not enough. For some clients, speech breathing may not be quite adequate to support intelligible speech, or it may be adequate, but only in certain situations. In such cases, it is often helpful for the client to augment, or supplement, his speech with other modes of communication. By using augmentative communication, a client with poor speech intelligibility may be able to enhance his comprehensibility, that is, the degree to which his message is understood in the context of all available communication cues (Yorkston, Strand, & Kennedy, 1996).

Certain types of augmentative communication require nothing more than the client's body. The client who is able to move his arms and hands can use gesture to aid in communicating his message. Similarly, the client who is able to activate his facial muscles can use facial expression to help communicate the emotional tone of his message. For example, a client with very limited pressure generation capability, and, therefore, very soft speech, can convey an emphatic message (e.g., "No! I don't want to!") by augmenting his speech with a fisted gesture and a frown. Other types of augmentative communication enlist the use of simple devices. One obvious way to augment speech is to use pencil and paper to write the part of the message that cannot be understood with speech alone. Another augmentative communication strategy involves the use of a communication board, a custom-made or commercially produced device that contains words, phrases, and/or pictures that the client can point to as he speaks. A communication board may also con-

---

SCREAMIN' AT THE TOP OF THEIR LUNGS?

There are devices that enable clients who cannot speak to "call out" for assistance. One of their uses is with clients with high-level spinal cord injury who are being weaned from positive pressure ventilation and are not ready to be fitted with assistive speech devices. Such clients may get relief from their feeling of total dependence by being able to signal distress. Burnett and Sutton (1979) developed a device that produces a high-pitched whistle to summon help. It's activated by trapping air in the mouth and then blowing across a sensor, or by touching the tongue to the same sensor. When blowing air, the mouth functions as a pump that's independent of the breathing apparatus. And, when touching the sensor with the tongue, the moisture activates the call and controls how long it'll last. Thus, clients can scream at the top of their lungs even when their lungs are less than half-full.

tain alphabet letters, and the client can point to the first letter of each word as he speaks it. This strategy, called alphabet supplementation (Beukelman & Yorkston, 1977), enhances comprehensibility by offering the communication partner access to visual cues to help with interpretation of the client's speech cues. Fortuitously, alphabet supplementation may also slow the client's speech rate and, thereby, increase his intelligibility. The range of devices that can be used to augment communication is substantial and is limited only by the ingenuity of the speech-language pathologist and the client. Devices used for augmentative communication can also be used for alternative communication (see following section).

ALTERNATIVE COMMUNICATION

There are clients whose speech breathing impairment is so profound that they are not able to produce speech no matter what management approaches are attempted. Such clients usually cannot generate adequate pressure to drive the larynx and upper airway. These are also clients whose laryngeal and/or upper airway valves are so impaired that even the use of assistive speech devices or augmentative communication strategies cannot make them functional communicators. Clients such as these require a form of communication that can replace speech.

This is where the management of speech breathing ends and the introduction of alternative communication begins. The topic of alternative communication is a vast and complex one, and is covered only in very general terms here. Readers who are unfamiliar with alternative communication are encouraged to take advantage of the several good resources available (e.g., Glennen & DeCoste, 1997; Beukelman & Mirenda, 1998).

The decision of whether or not to use alternative communication with a client can be a difficult one. Clearly, if a client is unable to speak, it is critical that some means of communication be established so that he is not cut off from his world. In certain clients who have lost, or have never developed, the ability to speak, alternative communication can be a quality-of-life saver. Nevertheless, there exists the possibility of jumping to the conclusion that a client does not have the capacity to speak, when in fact this may not be true. Such clients may be unwittingly forced to use alternative communication without being given an adequate opportunity to gain or regain speech production skills.

A case report by Workinger and Netsell (1992) is instructive in this regard by documenting the management of a client who had been given alternative communication when it was probably not the best choice. The client was a man in his late 20's who had sustained a traumatic brain injury 12 years earlier. At the time of the evaluation, he was employed in a sheltered workshop and was using a simple letter and word board as his sole means of communication. He was referred to the speech-language pathologist with the request that he be evaluated to determine if he could use a more sophisticated electronic type of communication device. The speech-language evaluation revealed that he had intact language skills, but that all speech production subsystems were impaired. Despite the fact that this client had not spoken for over a decade, the speech-language pathologist decided to attempt to manage his speech production before pursuing additional alternative communication options. Through management that targeted the breathing, laryngeal, and velopharyngeal subsystems, the client was ultimately able to develop functional speech that was 80 to 90% intelligible, and he no longer needed his alphabet board or any other form of alternative communication. The moral of this case report is that the speech-language pathologist should do everything she can to ensure that a client's potential for speech production has been thoroughly defined before surrendering to an alternative mode of communication.

Despite this caution, some clients with speech breathing disorders are ideal candidates for alternative communication. These include clients who have no potential to develop functional speech but who have the cognitive prerequisites, communication drive, and motor skills to use an alternative communication device. Children or adults with severe cerebral palsy or adults with advanced neuromotor disease might fit this category. Clients with profound dyspnea might also benefit from an alternative mode of communication. Other candidates are those who have a temporary need for alternative communication, such as the client whose tracheostomy-tube cuff is inflated and is expected to remain inflated for a few weeks. This might be a client undergoing recovery after sustaining a spinal cord injury or a traumatic brain injury. When a client's speechless state is predicted to be short, an inexpensive communication device or strategy is usually most appropriate.

There are some clients who can speak, but who almost certainly will have a future need for alternative communication. These are generally clients with progressive neuromotor diseases. In such cases, it is preferable to introduce the concept of alternative communication long before the need arises. In this way, the client can become accustomed to the idea gradually. Once the client begins to accept the idea of using another mode of communication, the speech-language pathologist can introduce discussion of the different options. As the client's condition worsens, management can continue to focus on maximizing his speech potential through the use of various behavioral strategies, while, at the same time, introducing the chosen alternative communication approach. By the time the client's speech is no longer functional, the transition to alternative communication should have already been made.

Alternative communication varies widely in its nature and sophistication. A simple alternative communication system might involve the use of a communication board constructed of cardboard or some other inexpensive material that contains words and phrases and/or pictures. It could be just like one used as an augmentative communication aid, except that the client uses it as the sole mode of communication (without speaking). A more sophisticated alternative communication system might be one that is computer-based and provides synthesized speech as its output. With such systems, speech can be generated at the time of the communication interaction, or it can be preprogrammed for later playback. There are a variety of ways to access individual messages on an alternative communication device. For example, the client can point to an item with his finger or with a head pointer, or he can gaze at it with his eyes. Eye-gaze systems often employ a sensor that tracks the position of the client's pupil and allows him to select a target on a visual display merely by maintaining a fixed eye gaze for a brief period.

Alternative communication can be valuable tool for maintaining quality of life when used with the appropriate client. Nevertheless, its use should not prevent attempts to habilitate or rehabilitate speech production skills in clients who have the potential to develop functional speech.

REVIEW

When developing a management plan for a client with a speech breathing disorder, substantial and diverse information must be integrated from the case history interview, the auditory-perceptual examination of the client's speech, reports of the client's perceptions about his speech breathing, the physical examination of the client's breathing apparatus, and the instrumental examination of speech breathing.

The management of speech breathing disorders requires staging that includes consideration of downstream load disorders, consideration of the breathing apparatus proper, and consideration of the collective aspects of a comprehensive management plan.

Management is often begun with direct attempts to adjust the control variables of breathing (pressure, volume, and shape) through practice regimens that are guided by an auditory-perceptual approach and are designed to facilitate the learning or relearning of certain nonspeech and speech breathing behaviors.

Exteroceptive feedback is often useful in the management of speech breathing disorders and can be provided to the client via clinician statements and actions, and through instrumental methods that offer information about control variable outputs, muscle activities, and speech.

Economical valving is a behavioral strategy that can benefit clients with speech breathing disorders, especially those whose lung volume excursions are so limited that they produce only a few syllables per breath group.

Body positioning can effect significant mechanical changes in speech breathing performance that can be used to benefit certain clients with speech breathing disorders, most notably those with neuromotor impairments of the breathing apparatus.

Mechanical aids have a prominent role in the management of clients with speech breathing disorders and include approaches that have to do with general postural support, abdominal wall support, and elective noninvasive positive pressure ventilation.

Muscle training can be used to increase strength and endurance of the inspiratory and expiratory muscles of breathing so as to improve their capacity to do work during speech breathing.

Glossopharyngeal breathing (frog breathing) is a compensatory strategy that uses upper airway adjustments to effect small inspirations that are especially helpful in the speech breathing of clients whose inspiratory muscles are paretic or paralyzed.

Speaking-related dyspnea is breathing discomfort that stems from pulmonary, cardiac, or neuromotor dysfunction and can sometimes be diminished through a pulmonary rehabilitation program, behavioral adjustments, postural and positional adjustments, environmental adjustments, and muscle training.

Noninvasive estimates of blood gas levels can be monitored in clients with speech breathing disorders to ensure that they maintain an appropriate balance between speech breathing demands and gas exchange.

Mouthing and buccal (and pharyngeal) speaking are behavioral strategies for compensating for less-than-adequate pressure generating capabilities that preclude voice production.

Conversational strategies are often important in the management of clients with speech breathing disorders (especially those who exhibit abnormally long pauses) and include linguistic planning, prosodic cueing, and nonverbal signaling.

Management of the client's communication environment is often an essential part of an overall management program and can include optimizing auditory cues, visual cues, the physical environment, and the communication competency of others.

Counseling is an integral part of speech breathing management and includes both emotional support and education for the client and other significant people in the client's life.

Assistive speech devices aid with the production of speech in certain clients with speech breathing disorders and include speech amplifiers, electrolarynges, buttons and one-way valves, and talking tracheostomy tubes.

Augmentative communication may be needed for the client with a speech breathing disorder whose speech breathing may not be quite adequate to support intelligible speech, or may be adequate, but only in certain situations.

Alternative communication may be needed for the client with a speech breathing disorder whose speech breathing impairment is so profound that he is unable to produce speech no matter what management approaches are attempted.

REFERENCES

Affeldt, J. (1964). Neuromotor paralysis. In W. Fenn & H. Rahn (Eds.), *Handbook of physiology. Respiration II, Section 3* (pp. 1509-1518). Washington, DC: American Physiological Society.

American Thoracic Society (1999). Dyspnea mechanisms, assessment, and management: A consensus statement. *American Journal of Respiratory and Critical*

Care Medicine, 159, 321-340.

American Thoracic Society/European Respiratory Society (2002). Statement on respiratory muscle testing. *American Journal of Respiratory and Critical Care Medicine, 166*, 518-624.

Ardran, G., Kelleher, W., & Kemp, F. (1959). Cineradiographic studies of glossopharyngeal breathing. *British Journal of Radiology, 32*, 322-328.

Baker, S., Sapienza, C., & Collins, S. (2003). Inspiratory pressure threshold training in a case of congenital bilateral abductor vocal fold paralysis. *International Journal of Pediatric Otorhinolaryngology, 67*, 413-416.

Baker, S., Sapienza, C., Martin, D., Davenport, P., Hoffman-Ruddy, B., & Woodson, G. (2003). Inspiratory pressure threshold training for upper airway limitation: A case of bilateral abductor vocal fold paralysis. *Journal of Voice, 17*, 384-394.

Banzett, R., Topulos, G., Leith, D., & Nations, C. (1988). Bracing arms increases the capacity for sustained hyperpnea. *American Review of Respiratory Disease, 138*, 106-109.

Beukelman, D., & Mirenda, P. (1998). *Augmentative and alternative communication: Management of severe communication disorders in children and adults* (2nd ed.). Baltimore, MD: Brookes.

Beukelman, D., & Yorkston, K. (1977). A communication system for the severely dysarthric speaker with an intact language system. *Journal of Speech and Hearing Disorders, 42*, 265-270.

Burnett, P., & Sutton, R. (1979). A portable electronic 'calling device' as an aid to 'weaning' ventilator-dependent tetraplegic patients from intermittent positive pressure ventilation. *Paraplegia, 17*, 452-455.

Cerny, F., Panzarella, K., & Stathopoulos, E. (1997). Expiratory muscle conditioning in hypotonic children with low vocal intensity levels. *Journal of Medical Speech-Language Pathology, 5*, 141-152.

Collier, C., Dail, C., & Affeldt, J. (1956). Mechanics of glossopharyngeal breathing. *Journal of Applied Physiology, 8*, 580-585.

Dail, C., Affeldt, J., & Collier, C. (1955). Clinical aspects of glossopharyngeal breathing: Report of use by one hundred postpoliomyelitic patients. *Journal of the American Medical Association, 158*, 445-449.

Dail, C., Zumwalt, M., & Adkins, H. (1955). *A manual of instruction for glossopharyngeal breathing.* New York, NY: The National Foundation of Infantile Paralysis.

Dikeman, K., & Kazandjian, M. (2002). *Communication and swallowing management of tracheostomized and ventilator dependent adults* (2nd ed.). Clifton Park, NY: Thompson-Delmar Learning.

Duchateau, J., & Enoka, R. (2002). Neural adaptations with chronic activity patterns in able-bodied humans. *American Journal of Physical Medicine and Rehabilitation, 81*, 17-27.

Duffy, J. (1995). *Motor speech disorders: Substrates, differential diagnosis, and management.* New York, NY: Mosby.

Fairbanks, G. (1960). *Voice and articulation drillbook* (2nd ed.). New York, NY: Harper and Row.

Farina, D., Merletti, R., & Enoka, R. (2004). The extraction of neural strategies from the surface EMG. *Journal of Applied Physiology, 96,* 1486-1495.

Forner, L., & Hixon, T. (1977). Respiratory kinematics in profoundly hearing-impaired speakers. *Journal of Speech and Hearing Research, 20,* 373-408.

Gallego, J., Perez de la Sota, A., Vardon, G., & Jaeger-Denavit, O. (1993). Learned activation of thoracic inspiratory muscles in tetraplegics. *American Journal of Physical Medicine and Rehabilitation, 72,* 312-317.

Glennen, S., & DeCoste, D. (1997). *Handbook of augmentative and alternative communication.* San Diego, CA: Singular Publishing Group.

Goldman, J., Rose, L., Williams, S., Silver, J., & Denison, D. (1986). Effect of abdominal binders on breathing in tetraplegic patients. *Thorax, 41,* 940-945.

Gosselink, R., Kovacs, L., Ketelaer, P., Carton, H., & Decramer, M. (2000). Respiratory muscle weakness and respiratory muscle training in severely disabled multiple sclerosis patients. *Archives of Physical Medicine and Rehabilitation, 81,* 747-751.

Hixon, T., Mead, J., & Goldman, M. (1976). Dynamics of the chest wall during speech production: Function of the thorax, rib cage, diaphragm, and abdomen. *Journal of Speech and Hearing Research, 19,* 297-356.

Hixon, T., Putnam, A., & Sharp, J. (1983). Speech production with flaccid paralysis of the rib cage, diaphragm, and abdomen. *Journal of Speech and Hearing Disorders, 48,* 315-327.

Hoit, J. (1995). Influence of body position on breathing and its implications for the evaluation and treatment of speech and voice disorders. *Journal of Voice, 9,* 341-347.

Hoit, J., & Shea, S. (1996). Speech production and speech with a phrenic nerve pacer. *American Journal of Speech-Language Pathology, 5,* 53-60.

Huldtgren, A., Fugl-Meyer, A., Jonasson, E., & Bake, B. (1980). Ventilatory dysfunction and respiratory rehabilitation in post-traumatic tetraplegia. *European Journal of Respiratory Disease, 61,* 347-356.

Jones, E., Hardy, J., & Shipton, H. (1963). Development of electrical stimulation in modifying respiratory patterns of children with cerebral palsy. *Journal of Speech and Hearing Disorders, 28,* 230-238.

Kelleher, W., & Parida, R. (1957). Glossopharyngeal breathing: Its value in respiratory muscle paralysis of poliomyelitis. *British Medical Journal, 5047,* 740-743.

Kellerman, B., Martin, D., & Davenport, P. (2000). Inspiratory strengthening effect on resistive load detection and magnitude estimation. *Medicine and Science in Sports and Exercise, 32,* 1859-1867.

Killian, K., Gandevia, S., Summers, E., & Campbell, E. (1984). Effect of increased lung volume on perception of breathlessness, effort, and tension. *Journal of Applied Physiology, 57,* 686-691.

Kluin, K., Maynard, F., & Bogdasarian, R. (1984). The patient requiring mechanical ventilatory support: Use of the cuffed tracheostomy "talk" tube to establish phonation. *Otolaryngology - Head and Neck Surgery, 92,* 625-627.

Koessler, W., Wanke, T., Winkler, G., Nader, A., Toifl, K., Kurz, H., & Zwich, H. (2001). 2 years' experience with inspiratory muscle training in patients with neuromuscular disorders. *Chest, 120,* 765-769.

Larson, J., Kim, M., Sharp, J., & Larson, D. (1988). Inspiratory muscle training with a pressure threshold breathing device in patients with chronic obstructive pulmonary disease. *American Review of Respiratory Disease, 138,* 689-696.

Larson, J., Covey, M., Wirtz, S., Berry, J., Alex, C., Langbein W., & Edwards, L. (1999). Cycle ergometer and inspiratory muscle training in chronic obstructive pulmonary disease. *American Journal of Respiratory and Critical Care Medicine, 160,* 500-507.

Lawes, W., & Harries, J. (1957). Spirographic studies in glossopharyngeal breathing. *British Medical Journal, 5055,* 1205-1206.

Leder, S., & Traquina, D. (1989). Voice intensity of patients using a Communi-Trach I® cuffed speaking tracheostomy tube. *Laryngoscope, 99,* 744-747.

Leith, D., & Bradley, M. (1976). Ventilatory muscle strength and endurance training. *Journal of Applied Physiology, 41,* 508-516.

Lohmeier, H., & Hoit, J. (2003). Ventilator-supported communication: A survey of ventilator users. *Journal of Medical Speech-Language Pathology, 11,* 61-72.

Martin, A., Davenport, P., Franceschi, A., & Harman, E. (2002). Use of inspiratory muscle strength training to facilitate ventilator weaning: A series of 10 consecutive patients. *Chest, 122,* 192-196.

Martin, A. Stern, L., Yeates, J., Lepp, D., & Little, J. (1986). Respiratory muscle training in Duchenne muscular dystrophy. *Developmental Medicine and Child Neurology, 28,* 314-318.

McPherson, G. (1999). *Frog breathing.* Videotape produced by Gary McPherson, Edmonton, Alberta, Canada.

Morrison, S. (1988). Biofeedback to facilitate unassisted ventilation in individuals with high-level quadriplegia: A case report. *Physical Therapy, 68,* 1378-1380.

Murdoch, B., Pitt, G., Theodoros, D., & Ward, E. (1999). Real-time continuous visual biofeedback in the treatment of speech breathing disorders following childhood traumatic brain injury: Report of one case. *Pediatric Rehabilitation, 3,* 5-20.

Netsell, R. (1995). Speech rehabilitation for individuals with unintelligible speech and dysarthria: The respiratory and velopharyngeal systems. *ASHA Special Interest Divisions: Neurophysiology and Neurogenic Speech and Language Disorders, 5,* 6-9.

Netsell, R., & Daniel, B. (1979). A physiologic approach to rehabilitation for adults with dysarthria. *Archives of Physical Medicine and Rehabilitation, 60,* 502-508.

Netsell, R., & Hixon, T. (1978). A noninvasive method for clinically estimating subglottal air pressure. *Journal of Speech and Hearing Disorders, 43,* 326-330.

O'Neil, S., & McCarthy, D. (1983). Postural relief of dyspnea in severe chronic airflow limitation: Relationship to respiratory muscle strength. *Thorax, 38,* 585-600.

Pollock, M., Gaesser, G., Butcher, J., Despres, J., Dishman, R., Franklin, B., & Garber, C. (1998). ACSM position stand: The recommended quantity and quality of exercise for developing and maintaining cardiorespiratory and muscular fitness and flexibility in healthy adults. *Medicine and Science in Sports and Exercise, 30,* 975-991.

Ramig, L., Pawlas, A., & Countryman, S. (1995). *The Lee Silverman Voice Treatment.* Iowa City, IA: National Center for Voice and Speech.

Ratusnik, D., Wolfe, V., Penn, R., & Schewitz, S. (1978). Effects on speech of chronic cerebellar stimulation in cerebral palsy. *Journal of Neurosurgery, 48,* 876-882.

Riera, H., Rubio, T., Ruiz, F., Ramos, P., Otero, D., Hernandez, T., & Gomez, J. (2001). Inspiratory muscle training in patients with COPD: Effect on dyspnea, exercise performance, and quality of life. *Chest, 120,* 748-756.

Rosenbek, J., & LaPointe, L. (1985). The dysarthrias: Description, diagnosis, and treatment. In D. Johns (Ed.), *Clinical management of neurogenic communication disorders* (pp. 97-152). Boston, MA: Little, Brown.

Rubow, R. (1984). Role of feedback, reinforcement, and compliance on training and transfer in biofeedback-based rehabilitation of motor speech disorders. In M. McNeil, J. Rosenbek, & A. Aronson (Eds.), *The dysarthrias: Physiology, acoustics, perception, management* (pp. 207-230). San Diego, CA: College-Hill Press.

Rutchik, A., Weissman, A., Almenoff, P., Spungen, A., Bauman, W., & Grimm, D. (1998). Resistive inspiratory muscle training in subjects with chronic cervical spinal cord injury. *Archives of Physical Medicine and Rehabilitation, 79,* 293-297.

Safer, P. & Grenvik, A. (1975). Speaking cuffed tracheostomy tube. *Critical Care Medicine, 23,* 23-26.

Sapienza, C., Brown, J., Martin, D., & Davenport, P. (1999). Inspiratory pressure threshold training for glottal airway limitation in laryngeal papilloma. *Journal of Voice, 13,* 382-388.

Sapienza, C., Davenport, P., & Martin, D. (2002). Expiratory muscle training increases pressure support in high school band students. *Journal of Voice, 16,* 495-501.

Sataloff, R., Heur, R., & O'Connor, M. (1984). Rehabilitation of a quadriplegic professional singer. *Archives of Otolaryngology, 110,* 682-685.

Sawyer, E., & Clanton, T. (1993). Improved pulmonary function and exercise tolerance with inspiratory muscle conditioning in children with cystic fibrosis. *Chest, 104,* 1490-1497.

Schmidt, R., & Lee, T. (1996). *Motor control and learning: A behavioral emphasis* (3rd ed.). Champaign, IL: Human Kinetics.

Sharp, J., Drutz, W., Moisan, T., Foster, J., & Machnach, W. (1980). Postural relief of dyspnea in severe chronic obstructive pulmonary disease. *American Review of Respiratory Disease, 122,* 201-211.

Smeltzer, A., Lavietes, M., & Cook, S. (1996). Expiratory training in multiple sclerosis. *Archives of Physical Medicine and Rehabilitation, 77,* 909-912.

Sparker, A., Robbins, K., Nevlud, G., Watkins, C., & Jahrsdoerfer, R. (1987). A prospective evaluation of speaking tracheostomy tubes for ventilator dependent patients. *Laryngoscope, 97,* 89-92.

Sturdy, G., Hillman, D., Green, D., Jenkins, S., Cecins, N., & Eastwood, P. (2003). Feasibility of high-intensity, interval-based respiratory muscle training in COPD. *Chest, 123,* 142-150.

Suzuki, S., Sato, M., & Okubo, T. (1995). Expiratory muscle training and sensation of respiratory effort during exercise in normal subjects. *Thorax, 50,* 366-370.

Tippett, D. (2000a). Ethics and ventilator dependency. In D. Tippet (Ed.), *Tracheostomy and ventilator dependency: Management of breathing, speaking, and swallowing* (pp. 267-298). New York, NY: Thieme.

Tippett, D. (2000b). *Tracheostomy and ventilator dependency: Management of breathing, speaking, and swallowing.* New York, NY: Thieme.

Tippett, D., & Vogelman, L. (2000). Communication, tracheostomy and ventilator dependency. In D. Tippett (Ed.), *Tracheostomy and ventilator dependency: Management of breathing, speaking, and swallowing* (pp. 93-142). New York, NY: Thieme.

Wanke, T., Toifl, K., Merkle, M., Formanek, D., Lahrmann, H., & Swick, H. (1994). Inspiratory muscle training in patients with Duchenne muscular dystrophy. *Chest, 105,* 475-482.

Watson, P., & Hixon, T. (2001). Effects of abdominal trussing on breathing and speech in men with cervical spinal cord injury. *Journal of Speech, Language, and Hearing Research, 44,* 751-762.

Weinberg, B., & Westerhouse, J. (1971). A study of buccal speech. *Journal of Speech and Hearing Research, 14,* 652-658.

Weiner, P., Berar-Yanay, N., Davidovich, A., Magadle, R., & Weiner, M. (2000). Specific inspiratory muscle training in patients with mild asthma with high consumption of inhaled β_2-agonists. *Chest, 117,* 722-727.

Weiner, P., Magadle, R., Beckerman, M., Weiner, M., & Berar-Yanay, N. (2003). Specific expiratory muscle training in COPD. *Chest, 124,* 468-473.

Weiner, P., Magadle, R., Massarwa, F., Beckerman, M., & Berar-Yanay, N.

(2002). Influence of gender and inspiratory muscle training on the perception of dyspnea in patients with asthma. *Chest, 122,* 197-201.

Workinger, M., & Netsell, R. (1992). Restoration of intelligible speech 13 years post-head injury. *Brain Injury, 6,* 183-187.

Yates, A. (1980). *Biofeedback and the modification of behavior.* New York, NY: Plenum Press.

Yorkston, K., Beukelman, D., Strand, E., & Bell, K. (1999). *Management of motor speech disorders in children and adults.* Austin, TX: Pro-Ed.

Yorkston, K., Strand, E., & Kennedy, M. (1996). Comprehensibility of dysarthric speech: Implications for assessment and treatment planning. *American Journal of Speech-Language Pathology, 5,* 46-55.

chapter six

Ventilator-Supported Speech Breathing

"When I talk . . . (*4-second pause*) . . . I have to wait . . . (*4-second pause*) . . . for the vent to . . . (*4-second pause*) . . . give me a breath . . . (*4-second pause*) . . . Plus my voice fluctu . . . (*4-second pause*) . . . fluctuates a lot . . . (*4-second pause*) . . . And if I try to talk too (long) . . . (*4-second pause*) . . . my voice fades out . . . (*4-second pause*) . . . like that last 'long.'"

INTRODUCTION

In the present chapter, the focus turns from clients who can breathe on their own to those who use ventilators to supplement or replace their own breathing efforts. Although some of the evaluation and management methods described in previous chapters can be applied to these clients, certain procedures cannot. Other methods require significant modification, and some are unique to clients who use ventilators.

The body of the chapter begins with a discussion of the nature of the task faced by the speech-language pathologist responsible for providing services to clients who use ventilators. The next two sections cover general issues regarding evaluation and management of ventilator-supported speech breathing. Subsequent sections focus on each of five types of ventilators: positive pressure, negative pressure, rocking bed, abdominal pneumobelt, and phrenic nerve pacer. The final section of the chapter provides a summary of these five types of ventilators and their use in supporting speech production.

NATURE OF THE TASK

The task of evaluating and managing speech breathing in clients who use ventilators differs in critical ways from that of evaluating and managing speech breathing in clients who can breathe on their own. The core difference is that the action of the ventilator must be considered a part of the client's speech breath-

A ROSE BY ANY OTHER NAME MAY OR MAY NOT BE THE SAME

As discussed in the main text, a ventilator is a device that supplements or replaces someone's spontaneous breathing. During much of the last century, ventilators were called respirators. Your parents may have visited people in hospitals who were on respirators. Such devices were different from those you're likely to see nowadays in hospitals or on television medical dramas, but they performed similar functions – supplementing or replacing someone's spontaneous breathing. You may have also encountered still another meaning for the term "respirator," a device (usually involving a mask and air filters) that prevents you from breathing in toxic or harmful substances. Maybe you've used one when you spray painted your house. Or, if you're like us, it may be more likely that you've watched your painter use one when he spray painted your house. So, there are respirators that are ventilators and respirators that are not ventilators.

ing behavior, thus adding an entirely new dimension to the clinical task. The nature of this task is discussed under the following headings: ventilators, clients, client-ventilator systems, evaluation and management teams, and communication opportunities.

Ventilators

Ventilatory support is used to sustain life and make breathing more comfortable. Such support also drives (or helps drive) speech production. This means that the act of speaking must be coordinated with the actions of the ventilator, a device that delivers what is usually a very different pattern of aeromechanical drive than that associated with normal speech breathing.

Ventilators come in a variety of forms, ranging from mechanical to neuro-prosthetic. And, even within a given type of ventilator, the operating features can vary widely, depending on the make and model. Because speech-language pathologists provide services to clients who use the full range of ventilator types (Isaki & Hoit, 1997), it is important that they understand the general principles underlying the different types of ventilatory support. Only with such knowledge can they offer the most insightful evaluation and the most effective management possible.

In all considerations regarding the ventilator and its interaction with the client, its function as a "ventilator" must take priority over its role in speech production. Fortunately, it is almost always possible to maintain appropriate ventilation while making mechanical and behavioral modifications that improve speech, reduce the effort to speak, or both.

Clients

Clients who require ventilatory support include adults, children, and infants with a variety of disorders. Some clients need support because they have lost muscle power as a result of acquired neuromotor impairment or because they never developed adequate muscle power as a result of congenital neuromotor impairment. In cases such as these, the ventilator replaces that which is usually accomplished by the muscles of the breathing apparatus. Other clients need a ventilator because they have disease of the pulmonary airways and/or lungs. For example, in a client with chronic obstructive pulmonary disease, a ventilator can improve gas exchange, especially if supplemental oxygen is provided. The ventilator can also help ease the excessive work of breathing that is often imposed by stiff lungs, high airway resistance, and muscles that are placed at mechanical disadvantages because of pulmonary hyperinflation. Ventilatory support may be required by an infant born prematurely and without sufficient surfactant in the lungs (causing him to have to struggle against collapsing alveoli), a child with cystic fibrosis (causing production of excess secretions and poor gas exchange), or an adult with a progressive neuromotor disease (causing muscle paralysis). Sometimes the need for ventilatory support will be temporary. This is usually true for clients with Guillain-Barre syndrome (which causes inflammation of the peripheral nerves and paralysis). By contrast, the need for such support may span years or even decades. This is usually true for clients with traumatic injury to the C1-C2 region of the spinal cord. This chapter, in line with the rest of the book, concentrates on adults with neuromotor disorders. Also, a particular focus in this chapter is on the client who requires long-term support, lasting for a month to a lifetime.

Some clients are not able to breathe on their own at all and need full ventilatory support (i.e., wherein the ventilator does all the work of breathing). Others are able to do some breathing on their own, but their breathing efforts are insufficient to maintain adequate ventilation for more than a short time. Such clients require only partial support from a ventilator (i.e., the client does part of the work while the ventilator does the rest). Some clients require continuous ventilatory support (i.e., all day and all night), whereas others require only intermittent support (i.e., at selected times during the day and/or night). Continuous support is necessary for those clients who are unable to breathe on their own at all or for only a few minutes at a time. Intermittent support is used with clients who can breathe on their own for sustained periods, but who eventually fatigue. Intermittent support can also be in the form of nocturnal ventilation for those who are able to breathe on their own while awake, but who are unable to sustain adequate ventilation while sleeping (e.g., congenital central hypoventilation syndrome).

Client-Ventilator Systems

When evaluating and managing the speech breathing of a client who uses a ventilator, it is important to think of the client and the ventilator as a single functional system. This means that the ventilator is considered to be a part of the breathing apparatus, as much a part as are the muscle, tissue, cartilage, and bone that make up the pulmonary apparatus and the chest wall. In this context, evaluation and management of speech breathing includes the individual components of the system (i.e., the client and the ventilator) and their interactions. Determining how the client interacts physically, physiologically, and behaviorally with the ventilator is an important focus of the clinical process.

Some clients use only one ventilator and require only one speech breathing evaluation and one speech breathing management plan. Some clients use one ventilator, but only part-time. They may require two separate evaluations and two separate management plans, one with and one without the ventilator. Other clients may use two different ventilators and, thus, may require two evaluations and two management plans, one each for each ventilator. The point is that the client alone (i.e., without the ventilator) and each client-ventilator combination must be viewed as a unique system for evaluation and management purposes.

Evaluation and Management Teams

The speech-language pathologist must always collaborate with a pulmonologist and respiratory therapist when evaluating and managing clients who use ventilators. This is because interventions that target speech production often influence ventilation. The speech-language pathologist leads the team regarding issues related to speech and other aspects of communication, but does not proceed with the evaluation procedures or management plan without the express agreement and permission of the pulmonologist. Certain evaluation and management procedures are done alongside the respiratory therapist, especially those related to measuring ventilation and those that include adjusting the ventilator.

There may be situations in which the speech-language pathologist serves as an advocate for a client to help obtain a new or upgraded ventilator. For example, a client who has a ventilator with a limited number of adjustment capabilities may benefit from using a ventilator with a greater range of capabilities. As ventilators become more sophisticated in function, new ways of improving ventilator-supported speech become available. The speech-language pathologist who understands the principles underlying the process of improving ventilator-supported speech will be able to apply those principles to new ventilators and develop original management options for her clients.

The speech-language pathologist may also advocate for the client who would like to switch from one type of ventilator system to another. For example, a client who uses a positive pressure ventilator may be a candidate for phrenic nerve pacers. The speech-language pathologist might offer the argument that the use of phrenic nerve pacers could improve the client's speech. In this way, she can be an influential player in determining those aspects of the client's respiratory care that affect speech.

Communication Opportunities

Historically, ventilators have been selected and adjusted to meet the ventilatory requirements and the comfort demands of the client. Now, given recent understanding of how various ventilator conditions influence speech, it is possible to also include speech-related considerations when selecting and adjusting a ventilator. Two goals of this chapter are to increase awareness and knowledge of how spoken communication can be optimized in clients who use ventilators and to bring this issue to the forefront of the clinical decision-making process.

Today, there is a growing number of communication opportunities that have never before been available. It is now possible for a ventilator user, even if paralyzed, to access the internet, send electronic mail, use a telephone independently, and be relatively mobile with the aid of computer technology and various adaptive devices. Many of these technologies depend entirely on speech or are more easily accessed with speech.

When the speech of a ventilator user is made more fluent and more natural sounding through interventions such as those described in this chapter, significant lifestyle changes may follow. The ventilator user may begin to expand his social circle, seek emotional support from members of listservs, or locate resources for meeting special needs. He may even be able to find gainful employment as a result of his new found speech skill. With greater independence comes better quality of life.

GENERAL PRINCIPLES AND METHODS FOR EVALUATING VENTILATOR-SUPPORTED SPEECH BREATHING

General issues related to the evaluation of ventilator-supported speech breathing are covered in this section. These are included under the following topics: case history supplement, ventilator analysis, auditory-perceptual examination, client perceptions, physical examination, and instrumental examination. This section and the next section on management of ventilator-supported speech breathing lay groundwork for subsequent sections that focus on each of the five types of ventilators.

Case History Supplement

Most of the case history items presented in Chapter 4 (Form 4-1) are appropriate for evaluating a client who uses a ventilator. Nevertheless, it is also important to include items that pertain specifically to ventilator-related issues, such as those found in Form 6-1 at the end of this chapter. These items are discussed below under ventilator history and communication history. Unfamiliar terms in Form 6-1 are defined and discussed later in this chapter.

Ventilator History

A client's ventilator history can be simple (e.g., having used only one ventilator) or complicated (e.g., having used a series of different types of ventilators). The following questions are designed to help the clinician assemble a complete picture of the client's ventilator history.

"What happened that made it necessary for you to start using a ventilator?" and "When did you first start using a ventilator?" These questions are included to elicit information about the relevant injury or disease and how long the client has used ventilatory support.

"Have you used a ventilator ever since then? If not, how many times have you gone on and off a ventilator?" These questions are used to determine if the client has used a ventilator continuously, or if he has a history of going off a ventilator during periods of relative health (e.g., as might occur with myasthenia gravis or post-poliomyelitis syndrome).

"Do you use a ventilator 24 hours a day? If not, what parts of the day and/or night do you use it?" For clients who use a ventilator during part of the day, speech breathing may need to be evaluated and managed both with the ventilator and without it.

"Which of the following ventilators have you used?" Responses to this question can include one or more of the five types of ventilators. The comments section can be used to record the client's experiences with given ventilators, especially experiences related to speech. Although this information may not influence the management plan, there is the possibility that another type of ventilator could be considered if it is known to improve the client's speech.

"What ventilator or ventilators do you use now? (type and brand/model)" and "If you use more than one ventilator, under what circumstances do you use each?" Following these questions, there is space designated for responses regarding two ventilators. If the client uses just one, then only information for Ventilator 1 needs to be filled in. And, if the client uses more than two ventilators, the clinician may add "Ventilator 3" and so on. When more than one ventilator is used, the clinician should gather information regarding the circumstance(s) under which each is used. Such information usually includes time of day (e.g., during the day when out of bed), body position (e.g., upright in wheelchair, supine in bed), social context (e.g., in room with medical staff, at home with family members, in public surrounded by strangers, on the telephone), general environment (e.g., large room, noisy cafeteria, private room), and any other information that may be relevant to communication.

Communication History

The communication history of a client who uses a ventilator may be as varied as his ventilator history. The items presented in Form 6-1 are designed to help elucidate communication problems experienced by the client and any communication strategies that may help to alleviate those problems.

"Did you have any problems with your speech before you started using a ventilator? If so, what were they?" This question is included to help the clinician identify speech problems that may not be directly related to the use of a ventilator. For example, a client may have dysarthria from an earlier cerebral vascular accident.

"Do you have any problems speaking while using your ventilator? If so, what are they?" These are perhaps the most important of all the questions of the case history. The open-ended format allows the client to present perceptions of his speech performance without bias from the clinician. Probes should be used to elicit as much information as possible (e.g., "Can you tell me more about that?").

"How is your speech different now than it was before you started using a ventilator?" This question is most useful for the client who denies that he has problems with his speech. For example, a client who claims that his speech is "fine" in response to the previous question may reply to this question by saying that he has to pause for each breath or that he is not able to finish his sentences.

"How do you coordinate your speech with your ventilator?" This question is included to gain insight into the client's understanding of how speech is produced while using a ventilator and what is involved in the coordination of speaking and breathing. It also is included to help identify client-generated language that could be used later during management.

"Do you ever experience the following speech-related problems?" This question, because it is more direct than the preceding questions in this section, may elicit information not yet volunteered by the client. The list of response items will not be discussed here. Rather, their relevance will become apparent when discussed in relation to each type of ventilator.

"Since you started using a ventilator, have you ever used any of the following to help you communicate? If so, how successful were they?" The response choices are divided into two categories, nonspeech and speech. The nonspeech items represent common communication supplements or alternatives employed by clients who use ventilators. Comments regarding their use can be noted on the form – for example, the circumstances under which they were/are used and the degree to which they were/are successful. Of particular interest in the present context are the client's responses to the speech items. The electrolarynx, one-way speaking valve, and talking tracheostomy tube were described in Chapter 5 and ventilator adjustments are covered in the present chapter. The item "changing speech patterns voluntarily" is intended to elicit information about any behavioral strategies that may have been suggested by a speech-language pathologist or that the client may have developed spontaneously. The last questions in this section ("What strategies do you use to communicate now?" and "How successful are they?") are included to identify the communication strategies, both successful and unsuccessful, currently being used by the client.

Ventilator Analysis

The ventilator analysis is a critical part of the evaluation because the ventilator is an integral component of the client-ventilator system. There are several types of ventilators, and for each type, there are many brands and models that can range substantially in adjustment capabilities. The purpose of the ventilator analysis is for the speech-language pathologist to become familiar with the characteristics of the client's ventilator(s). The best and most efficient way to do this is to consult with the client's respiratory therapist. It is the respiratory therapist who generally has the most knowledge and experience with the operation and care of ventilators.

Form 6-2 can be used during the ventilator analysis to record pertinent information. This record of the client's usual ventilator settings is critical to management procedures that involve changing ventilator settings. If a client has more than one ventilator, a separate ventilator analysis form should be used for each. Not all items listed in the form will be relevant to all ventilators. The adjustment variables and how they apply to speech breathing management are discussed in sections below that pertain to the individual types of ventilators.

Blow Wind – Crack Your Cheeks

The history of mechanical ventilation has been hundreds of years in the making and has included some really interesting events and approaches. Our very favorite has to do with the Amsterdam Society for the Rescue of Drowned Persons, formed in 1767. The Society was concerned with methods of resuscitation that could be used on drowning victims. Rescuers operated in teams and divided their efforts among different activities believed to assist with resuscitation. One volunteer was assigned the task of fumigator. We're not sure if he had first or last choice on this task. Anyway, the fumigator's job was to blow tobacco smoke through a tube inserted into the victim's rectum. That's right. You read it right the first time. Shakespeare's King Lear said, "Blow wind – Crack your cheeks." Do you suppose this was really a part of his encroaching madness, as experts tell us, or was it really resuscitation genius in disguise?

Auditory-Perceptual Examination

The auditory-perceptual examination of speech breathing in a client who is ventilator-supported is different from that for a client who can breathe on his own. It is not based on the three-variable framework of volume, pressure, and shape discussed in previous chapters. Although such a framework offers a powerful approach to the evaluation and management of speech breathing in clients who can breathe on their own, it is not typically well-suited to clients who use ventilators. A better framework for the client who uses a ventilator is one that links pressure, either directly or indirectly, to salient auditory perceptual features of speech (Hoit & Banzett, 1997). This is the framework used in this chapter.

The four speaking activities recommended for the auditory-perceptual examination of clients who use ventilators are the following: (a) sustaining a vowel; (b) reading aloud; (c) extemporaneous speaking; and (d) conversational speaking. For sustaining a vowel, the client is instructed to "Say /ɑ/ for as long and as steadily as you can" (or another vowel may be used). For the three running speech activities, the instructions and materials are the same as those described in Chapter 4 (see section on auditory-perceptual examination). Form 6-3 is provided for recording auditory-perceptual judgments of the client's speech and for recording the client's ratings of dyspnea.

Hallmark Perceptual Features

Abnormalities in utterance duration, pause duration, loudness, and voice quality are hallmarks of ventilator-supported speech and represent frequently targeted areas in speech evaluation and speech management. These are discussed below as they pertain to the use of ventilators in general.

Utterance Duration and Pause Duration

Although utterance duration and pause duration can be varied independently by the client who breathes on his own, these two features tend to covary in the client who uses a ventilator. Thus, they are considered together here. Abnormally short utterance duration and abnormally long (silent) pause duration are common features of ventilator-supported speech and are strongly linked to the prevailing translaryngeal pressure (i.e., pressure difference across the larynx) over the course of the breathing cycle. Recall that a certain minimum translaryngeal pressure is needed to oscillate the vocal folds. As long as translaryngeal pressure is at or above this minimum, it is possible to produce voice. When the pressure falls below this minimum, it is no longer possible to keep the vocal folds oscillating. This minimum pressure can be as low as 2 cmH_2O or it can be higher, depending on the opposing pressure exerted by the larynx.

When voice is produced in the context of a relatively unconstricted upper airway (such as during vowel production), translaryngeal pressure is essentially equal to alveolar pressure. By contrast, translaryngeal pressure is lower than alveolar pressure in the context of certain upper airway constrictions (such as during voiced plosive productions). Nevertheless, for simplicity purposes, the term alveolar pressure (or just pressure) will be used hereinafter.

During ventilator-supported speech production, there can be long periods within the breathing cycle during which pressure is not high enough to produce voice. This is why ventilator-supported speech is characterized by short utterances and long pauses. The ways in which this occurs for each of the different types of ventilators are described in their respective sections.

As the client performs the prescribed speaking activities, the clinician listens to both utterance duration and pause duration. The sustained vowel activity allows examination of how long voicing can be maintained without the additional demands of articulation. Running speech activities (reading aloud, extemporaneous speaking, and conversational speaking) allow examination of utterance duration and pause duration under different linguistic and communication conditions.

Auditory-perceptual ratings and associated comments for each of the four speaking activities are recorded on Form 6-3. The ratings are assigned using the same type of scale as was presented for auditory-perceptual examination of clients who can breathe on their own (see Form 4-2 in Chapter 4). For ratings of utterance duration and pause duration, the scale ranges from normal ("0") to profoundly short ("-4") and profoundly long ("-4"). Abnormally long utterances would be considered rare in ventilator-supported speech. When assigning ratings, the clinician is encouraged to rate the client's average performance. When writing comments, she is encouraged to make reference to variability of performance and to provide information regarding the longest utterance and shortest pause observed during performance of the activity (e.g., "longest utterance was 8 syllables" or "shortest pause was about 1 second").

If the clinician suspects that the client is capable of producing longer utterances than he demonstrates during these prescribed activities, she might also ask him to count aloud. Counting aloud sometimes elicits longer utterances when the instruction is "Count until I tell you to stop. Try to put as many numbers as you can on each breath."

Loudness

Loudness is also linked to alveolar pressure. As pressure increases, loudness generally increases, and as pressure decreases, loudness generally decreases. With ventilators that produce a highly variable pressure waveform, it is common to hear abnormally large variations in speech loudness. Certain ventilators are associated with fading loudness over the course of the utterance. Although these loudness patterns can be attributed to changes in alveolar pressure, it is important to remember that the larynx and upper airway also contribute to loudness adjustments (see section on loudness under auditory-perceptual examination in Chapter 4).

The auditory-perceptual examination includes judgments of average loudness and loudness variability for each of the four speaking activities. If they are normal, a rating of "0" is assigned for each. If average loudness is abnormal, it is rated as abnormally soft (to the left of "0") or abnormally loud (to the right of "0"). If loudness variability is abnormal, then it is rated as abnormally even (to the left of "0") or abnormally variable (to the right of "0"). The "Comments" section should be used to describe any notable patterns in loudness as they relate to the breathing cycle (e.g., "loudness bursts occur at the end of the inspiratory phase of the cycle," "loudness fades toward the end of the expiratory phase of the cycle"). Cycle-related loudness variability is most easily recognized during the sustained vowel activity.

Voice Quality

During normal speech production, the larynx is driven by a relatively steady alveolar pressure. This means that, if activation of the laryngeal muscles remains relatively constant, the pattern of vocal fold oscillation will also remain relatively constant. This is why the quality of the normal voice is perceived to be relatively consistent throughout most of an utterance. By contrast, the pressure driving the larynx during ventilator-supported speech is usually not steady. This means that if laryngeal muscle activation remains fixed, the pattern of vocal fold oscillation will vary. In practice, it appears that clients do not maintain constant activation of laryngeal muscles, but instead alter laryngeal activation to try to manage changes in pressure. For example, a client may increase laryngeal opposing pressure in anticipation of a sharp increase in pressure about to be delivered by the ventilator. The perceptual result might be a pressed voice quality.

Judgments of average voice quality and voice quality variability are made during the client's performance of the four speaking activities. If average voice quality is not rated as normal ("0"), it is rated as either abnormally breathy (to the left of "0") or abnormally pressed (to the right of "0"). The breathy-to-pressed continuum is used for making voice quality judgments because abnormalities along this continuum are common in clients who use ventilators and because these qualities have a strong link to the flow through the larynx and the loss of volume from the pulmonary apparatus. If another voice quality descriptor seems applicable, this should be noted (e.g., "sometimes voice quality sounds strain-strangled and rough"). If voice quality variability is not rated as normal ("0"), it is rated as either abnormally even (to the left of "0") or abnormally variable (to the right of "0"). Abnormally even voice quality would be considered rare in ventilator-supported speech. When voice quality is abnormally variable, the clinician's comments should document how voice quality varies in relation to the breathing cycle (e.g., "voice quality becomes more pressed near the end of expiration").

Associated Perceptual Features

Sometimes auditory-perceptual features other than the hallmark features are detected in the speech of clients who use ventilators. Two of the more common relate to the percepts of pitch and articulatory precision.

Pitch

Pitch is most closely linked to the fundamental frequency of the voice, and most of the control over fundamental frequency is vested in the larynx. Control of fundamental frequency is not necessarily a problem for clients with ventilators, unless there is concomitant cranial nerve X (vagus) impairment or structural impairment of the larynx. Nevertheless, there are clients without such impairments who exhibit an abnormal fundamental frequency. This may reflect a compensatory behavior. For example, a client may raise fundamental frequency when pressure is exceedingly low. Such frequency change is probably accomplished by stretching the vocal folds which, in turn, creates thinner vibrating surfaces (i.e., less mass/length). Thinner surfaces require a lower pressure differential across them to oscillate than do more massive surfaces. By increasing fundamental frequency, the client may be able to prolong voicing slightly as pressure falls. Thus, an abnormal pitch may be a manifestation of the client's attempt to cope with lower-than-desirable pressure.

Perceptual judgments of average pitch and pitch variability are recorded on the auditory-perceptual examination form. Average pitch ratings range from abnormally low (to the left of "0") to abnormally high (to the right of "0"), and pitch variability ratings range from abnormally even (to the left of "0") to abnormally variable (to the right of "0"). Written comments usually concern patterns of pitch variability as they relate to the breathing cycle.

Articulatory Precision

Clients who use ventilators and have normal cranial nerve function and normal muscular and structural integrity of the upper airway do not usually exhibit frank articulatory imprecision. Nevertheless, when the pressure driving the upper airway is inadequately low, high-pressure elements such as plosive, fricative, and affricate consonants may be perceived as imprecise. There may also be occasions when pressure is exceedingly high so that articulatory bursts or excessive spirantization are perceived in the client's speech. In these ways, the prevailing driving pressure may influence the perception of articulatory precision.

There is another, less direct, way that pressure may influence articulatory precision. If pressure is above the voicing threshold for only a short period during the breathing cycle, the client may compensate by speaking rapidly. In general, more rapid articulation is associated with less precise articulation. This reflects a speed-accuracy trade-off, wherein less precise articulation is the price for more speech produced per breathing cycle.

Clients with cranial nerve impairment or upper airway muscular/structural impairment, such as those with amyotrophic lateral sclerosis or certain forms of muscular dystrophy, may exhibit chronic articulatory imprecision. In such clients, articulatory precision may be impaired even when the pressure driving the upper airway is adequate in magnitude and stability. Nevertheless, it is still possible for interventions that improve driving pressure to improve their articulatory precision.

Perceptual judgments of articulatory precision are made during the three running speech activities (not during the sustained vowel activity). Articulatory precision is rated as normal ("0"), abnormally imprecise (to the left of "0"), or abnormally precise (to the right of "0"). An abnormally precise rating is rare and usually indicates compensatory behavior by the client to enhance intelligibility.

Comments on Global Features of Conversational Speaking

Conversational speaking can be considered the most important of all speech breathing activities because it is the context in which most spoken communication occurs. It is also more dynamic than other forms of speech breathing because the behavior of the conversational partner influences the behavior of the client, and vice versa. Unfortunately, the timing problems so common in clients who use ventilators (i.e., short utterance duration, long pause duration, inadequate control over speech initiation) can significantly disrupt conversational interactions.

If possible, the speech-language pathologist should recruit a conversational partner for the client during the evaluation. This makes it easier for her to act as observer instead of having to play the dual role of observer and conversational partner. When observing the client in conversation, the clinician has the opportunity to record more than just ratings of the auditory-perceptual features discussed above. She also has the opportunity to observe global features of the client's conversational communication. The clinician may note whether the client tends to terminate his utterances at linguistically appropriate junctures, or whether he terminates utterances when he is no longer able to speak (whether it be at a linguistically appropriate juncture or not). Also, the clinician should note if the client is interrupted by his conversational partner, and if so, how often and under what conditions. Further, she might observe how well the client seems to be understood by the conversational partner. Does the client have to repeat himself often? Finally, the clinician might note whether or not the client and his partner have a natural conversational rhythm (i.e., alternating pattern of speaking and listening). These and other observations can be recorded in the location indicated on the form.

Notes on Speech Recognition Systems

Speech recognition systems can provide powerful lifelines for certain clients who are supported by ventilators. Often significantly disabled physically and socially, such clients can gain substantial independence and build social networks that would otherwise not be possible. For example, speech recognition systems can be used to operate environmental control units and word processing software. For clients who are users (or potential users) of speech recognition systems, the speech breathing evaluation should include a measure of how well the system recognizes the client's speech. This measure can be used for later comparisons to determine how various management approaches help or hinder speech recognition.

Client Perceptions

Perception of breathing is one of the most critical factors in determining appropriate management strategies for clients who use ventilators. This is because management strategies may involve altering ventilation and this could cause a change in breathing comfort during resting tidal breathing, speech breathing, or both. Therefore, even if a client does not report breathing-related discomfort (i.e., dyspnea) during the case history, it is still important to record his baseline perceptions before initiating management.

Clients who use ventilators, like other clients, may not report dyspnea. Or they may report dyspnea while speaking, but not while breathing at rest. Or they may report dyspnea while speaking and while breathing at rest, but also report that the nature of dyspnea is different under these two conditions (e.g., dyspnea might be described as "hard work to breathe" while speaking and as "shortness of breath" while breathing at rest). The client-selected term or terms determined during the client perception part of the case history (see Chapter 4) are used to obtain ratings of dyspnea during the auditory-perceptual portion of the evaluation. It is important to recognize that a client who is ventilator-supported may use discomfort-related terms that differ from those usually offered by clients who breathe on their own (e.g., "pressure in the chest").

Dyspnea ratings should be obtained from the client during the auditory-perceptual examination immediately after each running speech activity (reading aloud, extemporaneous speaking, and conversational speaking) and during resting tidal breathing. The dyspnea-related term selected by the client during the case history is entered in the space provided, then the client's rating of that term is recorded. Possible ratings are none, mild, moderate, severe, and intolerable. If the client reports experiencing dyspnea, his pulmonologist should be notified immediately.

Physical Examination

If a client uses a ventilator only intermittently and is able to breathe on his own for an extended period, the speech-language pathologist should conduct a full physical examination without the ventilator. This should be done as described in Chapter 4.

If a client uses a ventilator continuously, the usual physical examination cannot be conducted. In some cases, physical observations are limited because the breathing apparatus is encased by the ventilator. Even when the breathing apparatus is visible, it is important to remember that the client's behaviors are not independent of his interactions with the ventilator. Nevertheless, it may be possible to determine if the client assists the ventilator's actions with his own muscular actions (e.g., neck muscle activation) and the degree to which he does so under different conditions (e.g., speaking versus resting tidal breathing).

Instrumental Examination

Instrumental examination can provide valuable insights into the speech breathing of a client who uses a ventilator, and it can help ensure his safety. Instrumental examination is done in collaboration with a respiratory therapist, who, in turn, is overseen by the client's pulmonologist.

Three types of instrumental measurements are recommended when evaluating a client who uses a ventilator. The first type reveals a client's breathing capabilities, and includes measurements of inspiratory capacity, maximum inspiratory pressure, and maximum expiratory pressure. The second type provides explanatory power regarding speech performance and combines estimates of alveolar pressure with the speech signal. And the third type consists of the safety-related measurements of heart rate, blood pressure, oxygen saturation (SpO_2), and end-tidal partial pressure of carbon dioxide (PCO_2). When evaluating clients who use ventilators, it is essential to use safety precautions because, unlike clients who can breathe on their own, they often cannot make voluntarily adjustments to compensate for undesirable changes in ventilation, intrathoracic pressure, or other important physiological variables. The measurements related to speech performance and those related to physiological safety should also be used when testing new management strategies. The instrumentation and procedures associated with all of these measurements have been described in the instrumental examination section of Chapter 4. Nevertheless, a few procedural modifications are recommended when examining clients who use ventilators, as discussed here.

The easiest and most convenient means to determine the inspiratory capacity is with instrumentation that measures lung volume change at the airway opening, such as a spirometer (body surface measurement devices often prove complicated when applied to clients who use ventilators). Inspiratory capacity should be measured from the resting level of the breathing apparatus, when expiration is complete and the next ventilator-generated inspiration has not yet begun. If this period is too short to obtain a measurement, it may be necessary to reduce the breathing rate of the ventilator temporarily. Measures of inspiratory capacity indicate whether or not the client is able to inspire using his own muscular effort. If he can, he may also be able to supplement the ventilator-delivered inspiration during speech breathing.

Measures of maximum inspiratory pressure and maximum expiratory pressure are most easily obtained with an air-gauge manometer. They should be made at the resting level of the breathing apparatus, so as to provide an indication of muscular pressure generation without relaxation pressure contribution. Measures of maximum inspiratory pressure may help determine if the client is able to trigger the ventilator to deliver extra breaths (this requires that the client generate a small sub-atmospheric pressure pulse). Measures of maximum expiratory pressure may help determine if the client can supplement expiratory relaxation pressure with muscular pressure during speech production.

Simultaneous measurements of estimated alveolar pressure and the speech signal can offer valuable insights into ventilator-supported speech performance. If the client has a tracheostomy, alveolar pressure can be estimated continuously from tracheal pressure, and if the client does not have a tracheostomy, alveolar pressure can be estimated intermittently from oral pressure. When sensing the speech signal, it is important to position the microphone so as to maximize the sensing of the client's speech and minimize the sensing of the ventilator-generated noise. Several placements may need to be tested to determine the one with the best signal-to-noise ratio. Recording pressure and speech simultaneously makes it easy to see how changes in pressure influence the client's speech. For example, simultaneous observations can reveal the minimum pressure needed to generate voice in a given client.

GENERAL PRINCIPLES AND METHODS FOR MANAGING VENTILATOR-SUPPORTED SPEECH BREATHING

Clients who use ventilators often report problems with their speech (Lohmeier & Hoit, 2003). Fortunately, ventilator-supported speech can usually be improved. This section covers general principles and methods for managing speech breathing in clients who use ventilators. To begin, special management approaches, not covered in Chapter 5, are described. Next, standard management approaches that were covered in Chapter 5 and that are applicable to clients with ventilators are discussed briefly. Specific applications of all of these approaches are detailed, where appropriate, in the following sections on positive pressure ventilators, negative pressure ventilators, rocking beds, abdominal pneumobelts, and phrenic nerve pacers. A summary of these management approaches is provided in Table 6-1.

Special Management Approaches for Clients Who Use Ventilators

There are two management approaches that are especially designed for clients who use ventilators. They are ventilator adjustments and breath stacking.

Ventilator Adjustments

Ventilator adjustments can improve speech, but they can also change ventilation. For this reason, they must always be carried out in collaboration with a respiratory therapist and with the oversight of a pulmonologist. Typically, it is the speech-language pathologist who suggests the nature of the adjustment to be made, the pulmonologist who determines if the adjustment is safe and if it should be implemented, and the respiratory therapist who actually performs the adjustment. Once an adjustment has been established as safe and comfortable for the client, the pulmonologist may write orders to allow the speech-language pathologist to make that particular adjustment independently. Specific protocols for such procedures differ across institutions.

The ventilator adjustments discussed in this chapter are designed to modify the pressure waveform in ways that address the speech abnormalities common to ventilator-supported speech (i.e., short utterances, long pauses, variable loudness, and variable voice quality). Such adjustments can improve speech immediately, without practice and without training. Nevertheless, practice and training should result in further speech improvement.

When a ventilator adjustment is made to improve speech, the client may decide to use that adjustment during most of his waking hours, whether he is speaking or not. Alternatively, he may decide (or his pulmonologist may advise him) to use the adjustment only when he expects to be speaking. Thus, such adjustments can be thought of as "speech adjustments" to be used on a short-term basis when needed.

When adjusting the ventilator, it is important to remember that the ventilator is only one component of the client-ventilator system. The outcome of a ventilator adjustment depends not just on the adjustment itself, but also on the client's response to the adjustment. Does his larynx respond appropriately to the ventilator adjustment? Does he activate residual inspiratory muscles along with the adjustment? Does he take advantage of increases in potential speaking time offered by the adjustment? These and numerous other behavioral variables influence the relative success of each ventilator adjustment. Presented in this chapter are the potential benefits of selected adjustments for speech and the predicted consequences on ventilation. It will be up to the pulmonologist, respiratory therapist, and speech-language pathologist to determine whether or not a particular adjustment or combination of adjustments is appropriate for a given client. And it will be up to the client to decide

Table 6-1. Summary of management approaches recommended for use with five types of ventilators.

	Invasive Positive Pressure Ventilators	Noninvasive Positive Pressure Ventilators (Volume-Controlled)	Negative Pressure Ventilators	Rocking Beds	Abdominal Pneumobelts	Phrenic Nerve Pacers
Ventilator Adjustments	X	X	X	X	X	
Breath Stacking		X				X
Exteroceptive Feedback	X	X	X		X	X
Economical Valving	X	X	X	X	X	X
Body Positioning		X				X
Mechanical Aids		X				X
Muscle Training	X	X	X	X	X	X
Glossopharyngeal Breathing		X	X	X	X	X
Relieving Speaking-Related Dyspnea	X	X	X		X	X
Monitoring Gas Exchange	X	X	X		X	X
Mouthing and Buccal Speaking	X	X	X	X	X	X
Conversational Strategies	X	X	X	X	X	X
Optimizing the Environment	X	X	X	X	X	X
Counseling	X	X	X	X	X	X
Speech Amplifiers	X	X	X	X	X	X
Buttons and One-Way Valves		X	X	X	X	X
Talking Tracheostomy Tubes	X					
Augmentative and Alternative Communication	X	X	X	X	X	X

whether or not he wants to use it.

To ensure client safety, it is essential that oxygen saturation (SpO_2) be monitored continuously during a ventilator-adjustment session. It is also advisable to check heart rate and blood pressure with each new adjustment. Further, it is informative to monitor end-tidal partial pressure of carbon dioxide (PCO_2) to be able to determine the immediate effect of an adjustment on the client's ventilation. It is not necessarily considered dangerous if ventilation decreases with an adjustment (as indicated by an increase in end-tidal PCO_2), as long as SpO_2 does not fall below the critical value set by the pulmonologist. If an adjustment causes SpO_2 to fall below the critical value or causes the client discomfort, the ventilator should be returned to its usual settings immediately.

The most basic adjustments, and the ones available on essentially all ventilators, are breathing rate (also called breathing frequency) and tidal volume. However, there are many other potential adjustments, depending on the type, brand, and model of the ventilator. Because the same adjustment applied to different types of ventilators may have different speech breathing consequences, specific ventilator adjustments are discussed under the sections below on positive pressure ventilators, negative pressure ventilators, rocking beds, and abdominal pneumobelts. They generally do not apply to phrenic nerve pacers.

Breath Stacking

Breath stacking is the adding of one breath, or part of a breath, to another. If used judiciously, breath stacking can be used to improve speech. When using a ventilator, this means that one ventilator-delivered breath is stacked on top of another. When two breaths are added, the inspired volume is twice as large as usual and the prevailing relaxation pressure is much higher than usual. This increase in lung volume and increase in relaxation pressure can make it possible to produce longer and louder utterances.

A danger of breath stacking is in its potential to generate excessively high intrathoracic pressure. High intrathoracic pressure poses risks of barotrauma (i.e., injury to the lungs caused by overdistention and rupture of alveoli), hypotension, and low cardiac output. Nevertheless, almost all clients can sense pressure change. Even clients with spinal cord injury who have lost afferent input from the chest wall should be able to sense pressure via pulmonary afferents. As long as the client is able to sense pressure and make the appropriate adjustments before the pressure exceeds a safe level, he should be able to use breath stacking without unreasonable risk.

Despite the potential risks, breath stacking also offers health benefits to clients who are not able to breathe on their own. Breath stacking, like deep sighing by an able-bodied person, expands the pulmonary airways and lungs and stretches the muscles and connective tissue of the chest wall in ways that counteract restriction. Even more important is the fact that breath stacking can make it possible for a client to cough and clear airway secretions (Kang & Bach, 2000).

Before a client can be instructed in the use of breath stacking for improving speech, his pulmonologist must approve of its use and the client must demonstrate that he can perceive pressure change. The preferred approach to breath stacking is to determine the appropriate stacking pattern by adding volume gradually. Breath stacking is most applicable to clients who use noninvasive positive pressure ventilation, and may also be useful to those who use phrenic nerve pacers.

Glossopharyngeal breathing (discussed in Chapter 5) is actually a form of breath stacking. The primary difference between glossopharyngeal breathing and breath stacking with a ventilator is that the former is generated actively by the client and incorporates small gulps of air instead of large inspirations. Glossopharyngeal breathing is a safer (but much slower) procedure than breath stacking with a ventilator.

Standard Management Approaches for Clients Who Use Ventilators

Most of the management approaches described in Chapter 5 apply to clients who use ventilators. However, not all approaches are well-suited to all types of ventilators, nor is the effect of a given approach on speech breathing necessarily the same when applied to different types of ventilators. General comments regarding these management approaches are provided here and specific comments are provided under the sections on the individual ventilator types.

Adjusting Breathing Variables

Strategies for adjusting breathing variables behaviorally are generally not useful for clients who use ventilators. In many cases, these clients (especially those with neuromotor disorders) cannot voluntarily change pressure, volume, and shape in the same way that clients who breathe on their own can. Pressure, volume, and shape changes are usually brought about with other management approaches, such as ventilator adjustments, mechanical aids, and breath stacking, among others.

Exteroceptive Feedback

Exteroceptive feedback of the types suggested in Chapter 5 can work well with most clients who use ventilators. A special combination of feedback that includes a continuous tracheal pressure signal and the speech signal is particularly helpful for the subset of clients who interface with the ventilator via a tracheostomy. This is discussed in the section below on invasive positive pressure ventilation.

Economical Valving

Economical valving can be an effective speech breathing strategy for clients who use all types of ventilators. By increasing the resistance to flow through the larynx and upper airway, lung volume can be expended slowly so that more speech can be produced per breath group. The drawback to decreasing flow is that the voice may sound pressed. However, the benefit of being able to produce more speech usually outweighs this drawback.

Body Positioning

Adjustments in body position may improve speech breathing in clients who use positive pressure ventilation delivered via the upper airway and in those who use phrenic nerve pacers. Such adjustments are designed to place selected breathing muscles at favorable mechanical advantages for producing force. Adjustments in body position are not generally helpful for clients who use positive pressure ventilation delivered via a tracheostomy. Changes in body position are not easily implemented (or are impossible to implement) when using negative pressure ventilators, rocking beds, or abdominal pneumobelts.

Mechanical Aids

Certain mechanical aids may help the speech breathing of clients who use positive pressure ventilation delivered via the upper airway and those who use phrenic nerve pacers. These aids, usually in form of binders or trusses, are designed to increase the impedance of the breathing apparatus, place certain muscles at mechanical advantages for producing force, or both.

Muscle Training

Muscle training, specifically inspiratory muscle training, should be a mandatory component of management for clients who use ventilators whenever possible. Many a life has been saved because a client was able to use his residual inspiratory muscles to breathe on his own until help arrived. Ventilators are typically quite reliable, but they can fail. For example, a ventilator can malfunction, the electrical power can go out, the battery can die, or a ventilator can become disconnected from the client. By building residual inspiratory muscle strength and endurance, the client may be able to sustain himself in a crisis. He may also have access to voluntary freedom from the ventilator, even if only for short periods.

Inspiratory muscle training may benefit speech as well. Inspiratory muscle training, if successful, can make it possible for a client to augment ventilator-delivered breaths. By adding a self-generated inspiration to the ventilator-delivered inspiration, the expiratory volume for speech production can be greater and breath groups can be longer. Also, when inspiratory volume is larger, expiratory relaxation pressure is higher. Thus, speech can be louder, at least during the initial part of expiration. Another potential benefit of inspiratory muscle training is that it may allow the client to trigger ventilator-delivered breaths. By triggering a breath, the client has greater control over the timing of his speech. Triggering can be used with either positive pressure ventilators or negative pressure ventilators and is described under those sections.

Expiratory muscle training may also be useful for improving speech in clients who use all types of ventilators. In the present context, the goal of such training is to increase the capacity to generate and control expiratory pressure for speech production.

Glossopharyngeal Breathing

Like inspiratory muscle training, glossopharyngeal breathing should be a high priority component of a management program, at least for certain clients who use ventilators. The most important role that glossopharyngeal breathing can play is that of allowing a client to breathe on his own in the event of ventilator failure. In fact, the ability to inspire with residual inspiratory muscles and the ability to glossopharyngeal breathe may be one of the best skill combinations that a client with a ventilator can develop to help ensure his safety. Many clients should be able to learn to glossopharyngeal breathe. Exceptions are the client with a tracheostomy that is not occluded and the client with laryngeal and/or upper airway control problems.

Glossopharyngeal breathing can improve speech in much the same way that breath stacking with a ventilator can. The client can use glossopharyngeal breathing to supplement the ventilator-delivered inspiration and, thereby, increase the starting volume and starting relaxation pressure of the breath group. This makes it possible for the client to produce longer breath groups and generally louder speech. One drawback is that glossopharyngeal breathing may prolong inspiratory time and, thereby, interrupt the natural flow of speech.

Relieving Speaking-Related Dyspnea

In clients who use ventilators, speaking-related dyspnea may take the form of hunger for air or work/effort. Hunger for air associated with speaking may be found in clients who are ventilated with positive pressure via a tracheostomy. This is because speech is produced, in part, during inspiration. A special strategy is described for reducing air hunger in these clients in the section below on invasive positive pressure ventilation.

Work/effort associated with speaking may occur with all types of ventilators. This form of dyspnea is usually associated with activation of residual inspiratory muscles to supplement the ventilator-delivered volume and to trigger the ventilator to deliver extra breaths. In many cases, the perception of work/effort can be reduced or eliminated with muscle training. The strength and endurance gained from inspiratory muscle training can make the act of speaking less taxing and, therefore, reduce feelings of physical exertion. Sometimes certain ventilator adjustments can also help relieve the work/effort associated with speaking. Another way to treat excessive work/effort is with periods of rest, wherein the client stops speaking temporarily or at least stops activating his muscles to allow the ventilator to take over all the work of breathing.

Monitoring Gas Exchange

Gas exchange should be monitored by the clinician whenever a new management approach is attempted with a client who uses a ventilator. It may also be appropriate to engage the client in the monitoring process as a way to help him understand the influence of various ventilator adjustments or behavioral strategies on gas exchange.

Mouthing and Buccal Speaking

Mouthing and buccal (and pharyngeal) speaking can be used in association with all types of ventilators discussed in this chapter, except when a facemask is used to couple the client to the ventilator. Clients must have relatively intact upper airway function to be good candidates for these two strategies.

Conversational Strategies

One of the most common complaints expressed by clients who use ventilators is that people interrupt them when they speak. Such interruptions are a natural consequence of abnormally long pauses, one of the hallmarks of ventilator-supported speech. Several of the management approaches discussed in this chapter are aimed at reducing pause duration. Nevertheless, it is also useful for clients to develop strategies that will help them hold the floor, especially during conversational interchange. Thus, the strategies of linguistic planning, prosodic cueing, and nonverbal signaling, described in Chapter 5, are especially relevant to clients who use ventilators.

Optimizing the Environment

The same considerations for optimizing the environment that apply to clients who breathe on their own also apply to clients who use ventilators. For example, background noise should be minimized, conversational partners should be positioned so that they can see each others' faces, lighting should be adequate, and the communication abilities of the client's conversational partners should be investigated (e.g., for presence of hearing loss). The issue of background noise can be especially problematic, given that some ventilators can be quite noisy. Although it may not be possible to muffle the ventilator noise, it may be possible to position the conversational partner such that the signal-to-noise ratio is maximized. Other special considerations are described in relation to the use of rocking bed ventilators.

Counseling

Counseling is an essential part of any management program. When counseling clients who use ventilators, it is essential to maintain a strong focus on quality of life (Tippett & Vogelman, 2000). Although many people believe that living with a ventilator is a fate worse than death, this is far from the truth for most clients. In fact, there are numerous studies which document that ventilator users perceive their lives as meaningful and positive, a stark contrast to the perceptions of healthcare professionals who often underestimate the quality of life of their clients who use ventilators (Bach, Campagnolo, & Hoeman, 1991; Bach & Campagnolo, 1992). Thus, it is the responsibility of clinicians involved in the care of these clients to maintain an open mind and not hinder their potential for living productive and happy lives.

A counselor, psychologist, psychiatrist, or minister provides general counseling, and the speech-language pathologist provides counseling related to communication. There are several important communication issues that face clients who need or will need ventilatory support. A client with amyotrophic lateral sclerosis may be told that he will eventually be in need of full support. Will he want a tracheostomy at

WHO'S AFRAID OF THE BIG BAD WOLF?

Until you've looked into the business end of a wolf (not in a zoo), you haven't experienced wilderness. We've been fortunate enough to have done so in a mountain meadow where three of them were in hot pursuit of our beagle. They had designs on her as an hors d'oeuvre. These wolves were magnificent specimens (as is our beagle), but in some respects were less impressive than two drawings of wolves that hang on our wall. Both were drawn with a sketching pen between the teeth of an American Indian man who was paralyzed and used a ventilator. They are meticulously detailed and majestic, capturing the power, cunning, and beauty of their subjects, especially their eyes. None who asks about these drawings can quite believe how they were created. Who could question the quality of the artist's life? He didn't. Each of us contributes in a unique way. By the way, our beagle lived to tell her story.

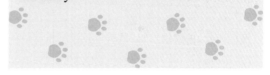

that time? What are the consequences of a tracheostomy on speech and other forms of communication? A client with a spinal cord injury may express the desire to be removed from the ventilator so that he can be allowed to die. Is he able to discuss this desire with his family and his physician? Or is his speech so poor that they cannot understand him? A client with a tracheostomy wants to switch to another form of ventilation that does not require a tracheostomy. What are his options and what are the implications for speech? These are the types of questions that the speech-language pathologist must be able to address, proactively whenever possible.

Another area of concern for clients who must rely heavily on an external system to stay alive is the feeling of dependence. Everything possible should be done to maximize the client's sense of control and independence. This can be addressed in various ways. For example, management might focus on improving speech in ways that facilitate the use of a speech recognition system so that the client can use the internet and operate an environmental control unit. For another example, management might emphasize inspiratory muscle training and glossopharyngeal breathing to improve speech. These management strategies should also enhance the client's independence by giving him the ability to breathe without the ventilator, at least for awhile.

There are many additional reasons that clients who use ventilators may need counseling. The speech-language pathologist is qualified to address those related to speech and communication. For issues that fall outside this realm, appropriate professionals should be sought. Clients who use all the types of ventilators covered in this chapter are candidates for counseling.

Assistive Speech Devices

The assistive speech devices described in Chapter 5 are speech amplifiers, electrolarynges, buttons and one-way valves, and talking tracheostomy tubes. They are discussed briefly below as they relate to clients with ventilators.

Speech amplifiers are appropriate for clients with soft speech and with whom other management options have not been successful. The only difference between managing a client with a ventilator and one without is that placement of the microphone must take into account the noise produced by the ventilator. The microphone should be placed such that it maximizes the speech signal and minimizes ventilator noise. Additional considerations are necessary when using a speech amplifier with a client who uses a rocking bed, as discussed in that section.

Electrolarynges are seldom appropriate for clients who use ventilators. This is because the ventilator almost always provides adequate pressure for speech production during at least part of the breathing cycle. The only time an electrolarynx might be indicated would be in the rare case of the client with ventilatory support, impaired laryngeal function, and excellent articulation.

Many clients who use ventilators are candidates for buttons or one-way valves. Specifically, buttons may be appropriate for clients who use noninvasive positive pressure ventilation, negative pressure ventilation, rocking beds, abdominal pneumobelts, and phrenic nerve pacers. A button allows the tracheostomy to be maintained in the event the client requires suctioning of the pulmonary airways or needs to be connected temporarily to a ventilator via his tracheostomy (e.g., in the event of serious illness). The button occludes the tracheostomy so that expired air is routed through the larynx for speech production (otherwise, most of the expired air would escape through the tracheostomy). A one-way (inspiratory) valve serves the same general function as a button (preventing air leak through the tracheostomy during expiration) and may also be appropriate for certain clients who use the ventilator systems listed above. One-way valves are sometimes used with clients who are ventilated through the tracheostomy. However, this carries serious risks and should be avoided. There are other, safer ways to optimize that form of ventilator-supported speech, as discussed in the section on invasive positive pressure ventilation.

The best candidate for a talking tracheostomy tube is the client with good laryngeal and upper airway function who uses invasive ventilation (i.e., positive pressure ventilation delivered through a tracheostomy), and in whom the ventilator-delivered air is blocked from reaching the larynx. Clients who breathe through the upper airway cannot use a talking tracheostomy tube.

Augmentative and Alternative Communication

Certain clients who use ventilators are candidates for augmentative communication and/or alternative communication. These are usually clients whose upper airway function is severely impaired. If upper airway function is preserved, it is nearly always possible for the client to speak using ventilator-delivered air or a talking tracheostomy tube.

POSITIVE PRESSURE VENTILATORS

This section covers positive pressure ventilators, and includes discussion of positive pressure ventilation in general, invasive positive pressure ventilation, and noninvasive positive pressure ventilation. Of all the types of ventilators discussed in this chapter, the positive pressure ventilator is the one most often encountered in clinical practice.

Positive Pressure Ventilation

Positive pressure ventilation moves air into the pulmonary apparatus by generating pressure near the airway opening that is higher than the pressure within the apparatus. Positive pressure ventilation is analogous to blowing up a balloon, with the balloon representing the pulmonary airways and lungs and the blower representing the positive pressure ventilator. Under normal circumstances, humans do not use positive pressure ventilation. Rather, they ventilate using negative pressure by contracting the diaphragm (and sometimes other inspiratory muscles) to lower pressure within the pulmonary apparatus (relative to atmospheric pressure) and create an inward flow of air.

Positive pressure ventilation can be accomplished in several ways. Positive pressure ventilation can be effected using a mouth-to-mouth approach to revive someone who has stopped breathing. Positive pressure ventilation can also be accomplished through the use of glossopharyngeal breathing, an alternate form of breathing that resembles frog breathing. Or positive pressure ventilation can be driven mechanically by a positive pressure ventilator.

A positive pressure (mechanical) ventilator is a device that pushes air through a tube into the pulmonary airways and lungs. It can be powered pneumatically (with compressed gases), electronically, or both. Air can be driven out of the ventilator in a number of ways. For example, in one type of ventilator, a piston moves through a cylinder to push air out, and in another type of ventilator an air-filled bellows is compressed to move air out of the ventilator. The flow exiting the ventilator can take different forms. It can be relatively constant, it can start high and end low, or it can exhibit other patterns of change. Ventilators include some type of gas-blending mechanism so that oxygen can be added to the air for those clients who require higher-than-usual levels of oxygen. A positive pressure ventilator is depicted in Figure 6-1. This ventilator is large and has many adjustment options. Such a ventilator might be kept next to a client's bed for use while sleeping or while otherwise confined to a room. There are other positive pressure ventilators that are smaller and can be mounted on the back of a wheelchair to allow the client more freedom of movement.

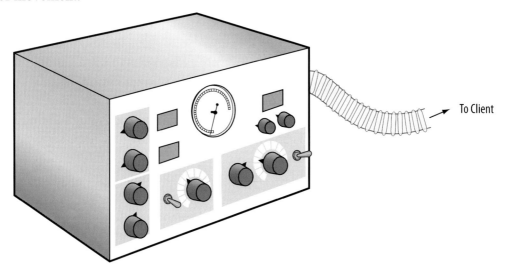

Figure 6-1. Positive pressure ventilator.

Air from the ventilator is routed through a set of tubes, valves, and adapters before reaching the client. This is called a ventilator circuit. The circuit is set up to accommodate humidifiers so that the air can be humidified before reaching the client. Expired air from the client can return to the ventilator through its circuit or it can exit through the client's upper airway, or both.

The function of the client-ventilator system is determined by the manner in which the ventilator is coupled to the client. This coupling can come in three forms. One involves passing a tube, called an endotracheal tube, through the larynx to the trachea. An endotracheal tube is used primarily during surgery, emergency situations that call for immediate life support, or when the need for ventilation is expected to be short-term (usually less than a month). Because this type of tube is routed through the larynx, it is not possible for the client to produce voice. Thus, alternative communication is the most appropriate temporary intervention.

The remaining two forms of client-ventilator coupling are used with clients who are expected to require positive pressure ventilation for an extended period (months or years). The ventilator can be coupled to a tracheostomy tube so that ventilation is delivered through the tracheostomy. Alternatively, the ventilator can be coupled to the upper airway. The former is called invasive positive pressure ventilation, and the latter is called noninvasive positive pressure ventilation. These two client-ventilator systems function quite differently for speech breathing, and are considered separately below.

Invasive Positive Pressure Ventilation

Invasive positive pressure ventilation involves coupling the ventilator circuit to a tracheostomy tube positioned within the client's neck. With this form of ventilation, the ability to produce speech depends heavily on the configuration of the tracheostomy tube.

Some clients who use invasive positive pressure ventilation are not able to speak because the air from the ventilator cannot reach the larynx. This occurs when the tracheostomy tube is unfenestrated (i.e., without openings along the shaft) and the cuff (which encircles the shaft) is inflated to seal against the tracheal wall. This tracheostomy tube configuration is depicted in the upper part of Figure 6-2. The arrows in the figure indicate that, during inspiration, all ventilator-delivered air is routed to the pulmonary apparatus, and that during expiration all air leaving the pulmonary apparatus is routed back to the ventilator. Neither inspiratory flow nor expiratory flow reaches the larynx under this circumstance. With this configuration, the ventilator and pulmonary apparatus function as a closed system.

Fortunately, most clients who are ventilated through a tracheostomy are able to speak using ventilator-delivered air. This is possible because the tracheostomy tube has a fenestration (opening along the shaft), a deflated cuff (or no cuff), or both. A tracheostomy tube with a deflated cuff is shown in the lower part of Figure 6-2. During inspiration, ventilator-delivered air can flow simultaneously through the larynx (if the larynx is open) and to the pulmonary apparatus. During expiration, air can flow both through the larynx (if the larynx is open) and back to the ventilator. With this configuration, the client is able to speak during inspiration and expiration because flow can be routed to the larynx during both phases of the cycle. During inspiration, the driving pressure available for speech production depends primarily on the ventilator-delivered flow, the relaxation pressure of the breathing apparatus, and the impedance offered by the breathing apparatus. During expiration, the driving pressure available for speech production depends primarily on the relaxation pressure of the breathing apparatus and the resistance offered by the ventilator circuit and the larynx. The driving pressure for speech production during both inspiration and expiration can also be influenced by active muscular pressure in clients with the ability to exert such pressure.

Speech breathing during invasive positive pressure ventilation is unlike any other form of ventilator-supported speech breathing. It is the most difficult to understand and the most challenging to evaluate and manage. Included in this section are specific evaluation procedures and management approaches recommended for clients who use this form of ventilation.

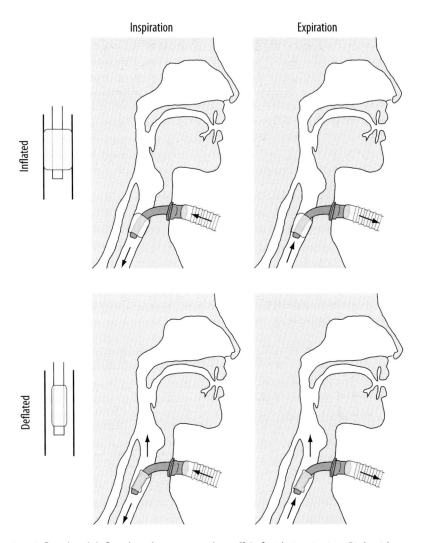

Figure 6-2. Inflated and deflated tracheostomy-tube cuff. Left side inspiration. Right side expiration.

Evaluation of Speech Breathing with Invasive Positive Pressure Ventilation

The groundwork for this section has been laid in this chapter's general discussion of evaluation principles and methods for clients who use ventilators. In the present section, the focus is on specific applications to invasive positive pressure ventilation, including those related to ventilator analysis, auditory-perceptual examination, client perceptions, physical examination, and instrumental examination (case history information is covered in Chapter 4 and in an earlier part of this chapter).

Ventilator Analysis

Positive pressure ventilators range widely in the number of variables that can be adjusted. In general, the more adjustment variables there are, the more options there are for improving speech. Several adjustment variables are described below that may be encountered when examining a positive pressure ventilator. These particular adjustments have been singled out for discussion because they have demonstrated potential for improving speech. They are breathing rate, tidal volume, inspiratory time (or inspiratory flow), end-inspiratory pause, positive end-expiratory pressure, use of a one-way valve (or cork), and pressure-controlled (or pressure-support) ventilation. The ventilator analysis form (Form 6-2) can be used to record adjustment options and the usual ventilator settings for a given client. The type of ventilator (positive pressure) and the method of delivery (via tracheostomy) should be noted on the form. Some of the adjustment variables listed on the form are not discussed in this section because they do not apply to positive pressure ventilators.

Breathing Rate: Breathing rate (or breathing frequency) is defined as the number of ventilator-delivered breaths over a minute. Breathing rate can range from relatively low (e.g., 6 breaths per minute) to relatively high (e.g., 20 breaths per minute). The number of breaths delivered by the ventilator depends on the ventilation mode. If the ventilator is in "control" mode, the ventilator delivers breaths at a set rate and that rate cannot be altered by the actions of the client. For example, if the breathing rate is set at 10 breaths per minute, the ventilator will deliver a breath every 6 seconds. Control mode ventilation is required for clients who are unable to generate adequate inspiratory pressure to trigger the ventilator.

"Assist/control" mode ventilation enables the client to trigger breaths, as long as he can exert inspiratory efforts that exceed a preset trigger threshold. This threshold may be as small as -1 cmH$_2$O. In this mode, the breathing rate indicated on the ventilator is the minimum number of breaths the ventilator will deliver (i.e., the control rate). For example, if the breathing rate is set to 10 breaths per minute and the client does not trigger breaths, the ventilator will deliver a breath every 6 seconds. If the client triggers extra breaths, the ventilator will deliver breaths more often than every 6 seconds and not necessarily periodically.

WANNA BET?

You've probably had arguments in which you were certain you were right and the other person was just as certain he was right. One thing leads to another and soon heels dig in and you're at the stage where bets are being placed. The second of us recalls such an argument when just learning about speech production with invasive positive pressure ventilation. One was convinced that clients spoke only during the inspiratory phase of the ventilator cycle and the other was equally convinced that they spoke only during the expiratory phase of the cycle. Bets were placed and a volunteer was studied. She spoke on both the inspiratory and expiratory phases of the ventilator cycle and the argument was settled. Nobody won or lost the bet. Few bets could have meant more to the second of us. This one launched years of rewarding study into how to improve speech in clients who use invasive positive pressure ventilation.

Tidal Volume: Tidal volume is the amount of air delivered by the ventilator for a given breathing cycle. With some positive pressure ventilators, tidal volume is adjusted directly. With others, it is adjusted indirectly by setting the breathing rate and minute ventilation (defined, in this context, as the volume of air delivered by the ventilator over the course of a minute). To adjust tidal volume, the ventilator must be operating in the volume-controlled mode. This means that the ventilator is set to deliver the designated tidal volume (for a contrast, see section below on pressure-controlled ventilation). Tidal volumes can range from small (e.g., 0.2 L for a child) to large (e.g., 1 L for an adult).

The tidal volume delivered by the ventilator is not always the same as the volume that reaches the client's pulmonary apparatus (i.e., pulmonary tidal volume). The ventilator tidal volume can be larger than the pulmonary tidal volume when some of the air delivered by the ventilator is diverted through the larynx, and it can be smaller than the pulmonary tidal volume when the pulmonary tidal volume is supplemented by the client's own inspiratory effort. The only time ventilator-delivered tidal volume and pulmonary tidal volume are the same is when the client's larynx or upper airway is closed during inspiration or when the client has an inflated cuff and an unfenestrated tracheostomy tube (assuming there is no air leak around the tube). However, neither of these conditions prevails during speech production.

Inspiratory Time or Inspiratory Flow: The rate at which the ventilator tidal volume is delivered can be adjusted in most positive pressure ventilators. The manner of adjustment depends on the ventilator. One way is to change inspiratory time. Inspiratory time can be expressed as an absolute duration (e.g., 2 seconds), as a percentage of the entire breathing cycle (e.g., 25% inspiratory time), or as a ratio of inspiratory to expiratory time (e.g., 1:2 I:E ratio). The shorter the inspiratory time the higher the flow (assuming the ventilator tidal volume does not change). Another way to adjust the rate at which volume is delivered is to adjust inspiratory flow directly. This flow is usually expressed in LPM.

End-Inspiratory Pause: Some ventilators include an adjustment called end-inspiratory pause. This adjustment makes it possible to maintain the expiration valve in the closed position for a given period after inspiration ends. For example, if the pause is set to 10%, the expiration valve will remain closed for a period equal to 10% of the breathing cycle (e.g., 1 second if breathing rate is 6 breaths per minute) before opening. If the pause is set to "0" or if there is no end-inspiratory pause adjustment on the ventilator, the expiratory valve will open as soon as the ventilator's inspiratory flow ceases.

Positive End-Expiratory Pressure: Positive end-expiratory pressure (PEEP) is available as an adjustment option on many positive pressure ventilators. PEEP impedes expiratory flow to the ventilator by adding resistance and a threshold occlusion pressure to the ventilator's expiratory line. When PEEP is set above "0," say at 5 cmH$_2$O, airway pressure remains at 5 cmH$_2$O at end-expiration by closure of the ventilator's expiratory valve (as long as there are no leaks between the ventilator and the client's pulmonary apparatus). For ventilators that do not have PEEP as an adjustment option, PEEP can be applied by attaching a spring-loaded valve to the expiratory port of the ventilator line. External PEEP valves are made to deliver a single level of PEEP (e.g., 5 cmH$_2$O) or an adjustable range of PEEP levels (e.g., 1 to 15 cmH$_2$O).

One-Way Valve (or Cork): This is not a ventilator adjustment as are the previously discussed items. Nevertheless, the presence of a one-way valve (or cork) within the ventilator circuit critically alters the function of the ventilator. A one-way valve is coupled into the ventilator circuit near the distal end of the tracheostomy tube. It opens during inspiration, thereby allowing air to flow freely into the client. The valve closes during expiration so that all flow must exit through the client's larynx and upper airway. A cork placed within the ventilator's expiratory line can have the same functional outcome as the one-way valve (but costs much less).

Pressure-Controlled (or Pressure-Support) Ventilation: Some positive pressure ventilators can deliver pressure-controlled ventilation in which the ventilator targets a predetermined airway pressure. When using pressure-controlled ventilation, tidal volume varies as the prevailing impedance of the breathing apparatus varies. With pressure-controlled ventilation, breaths are delivered at the designated breathing rate and do not depend on client-generated inspiratory efforts.

A variant of pressure-controlled ventilation is pressure-support ventilation, which also targets a pre-set inspiratory pressure. With pressure-support ventilation, the client actively triggers each breath and the duration of his effort determines the duration of the ventilator-delivered inspiration. Pressure-support ventilation is commonly used to wean a client from a ventilator.

Other: Other ventilator-related information can be added to Form 6-2. For example, a client might use a mode of ventilation that has not been associated with specific ventilator-adjustment interventions for speech. One such mode is intermittent mandatory ventilation. Intermittent mandatory ventilation is appropriate for a client who is able to breathe on his own, but still requires additional ventilation. Intermittent mandatory ventilation combines ventilator-delivered breaths with client-generated breaths. A variant of intermittent mandatory ventilation is synchronized intermittent mandatory ventilation in which the ventilator-delivered breaths are activated by the client's inspiratory efforts and are, thereby, synchronized with client-generated breaths. Another example is bilevel positive pressure ventilation, which involves the delivery of two positive pressures, one during inspiration and a lower one during expiration. Another term for bilevel positive pressure ventilation is bilevel positive airway pressure.

Comments: Comments that are not directly related to ventilator adjustments can also be recorded on Form 6-2. For example, the clinician might note that the client uses supplemental oxygen (usually expressed as a fraction of inspired oxygen, F_IO_2, that is higher than 21%). Supplemental oxygen use is most likely to be seen in clients who have impaired gas exchange, such as those with chronic obstructive pulmonary disease. As another example, the clinician might make a note regarding the client's usual tracheostomy-tube cuff inflation (e.g., "client's cuff is partially inflated during the day and is fully inflated at night").

Auditory-Perceptual Examination

Hallmarks of speech supported by an invasive positive pressure ventilator are short utterances, long pauses, variable loudness, and variable voice quality (Hoit, Shea, & Banzett, 1994; Hoit & Banzett, 1997; Hoit, Banzett, Lohmeier, Hixon, & Brown, 2003). Auditory-perceptual signs related to pitch and articulatory precision also may be present. The auditory-perceptual form (Form 6-3) can be used to record these and any other auditory-perceptual signs observed by the clinician while the client performs the prescribed speaking activities (sustained vowel, reading aloud, extemporaneous speaking, and conversational speaking).

As discussed above, these auditory-perceptual features of speech usually can be linked, either directly or indirectly, to pressure. Figure 6-3 shows a schematic illustration of a typical pressure waveform associated with invasive positive pressure ventilation. In this case, the ventilator is delivering a pre-set volume (i.e., volume-controlled mode) at a constant flow (i.e., square-wave flow). During inspiration, the pressure rises rapidly to a peak. Then, during expiration, pressure falls rapidly to zero (atmospheric) and remains there until the next inspiration begins. The dashed line in Figure 6-3 represents the minimum pressure required to oscillate the vocal folds.

The ventilator-delivered pressure waveform is quite different from the waveform for normal speech production. As is illustrated in Figure 6-3, pressure during normal speech production is relatively low, relatively unchanging, and exceeds the minimum voicing pressure throughout most of expiration (the phase of the breathing cycle when normal speech is produced). By contrast, the ventilator-delivered pressure exceeds the minimum voicing pressure for only a short period that spans inspiration and expiration and is below the voicing threshold for much of the cycle. This is why short utterances and long pauses are hallmark auditory-perceptual features of this form of ventilator-supported speech. Also noteworthy is that the "speaking" portion of the pressure waveform (i.e., the portion that exceeds the voicing threshold) changes rapidly and substantially and is highly peaked. This is why abnormal variations in loudness and voice quality are also hallmarks of this form of

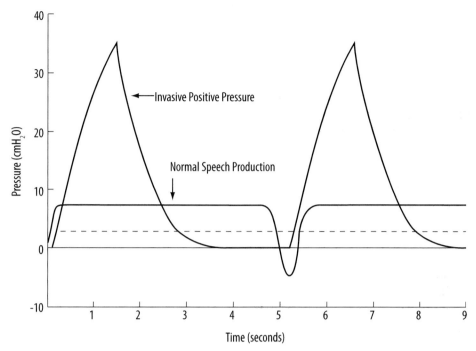

Figure 6-3. Pressure waveforms for volume-controlled positive pressure ventilation and normal speech production. Dashed line shows minimum pressure needed for voicing.

ventilator-supported speech. The ventilator-delivered pressure waveform shown in Figure 6-3 would likely be associated with a burst in loudness near the end of the inspiration (near the pressure peak), and a substantial reduction in loudness during the latter part of the expiration (where pressure approaches zero). Voice quality might vary from clear to breathy to pressed, depending on the laryngeal response to the rapidly changing pressure.

Client Perceptions

Speaking with invasive positive pressure ventilation can reduce ventilation (Shea, Hoit, & Banzett, 1998). This is because the portion of the ventilator-delivered inspiration that is used for speech production does not reach the pulmonary apparatus to participate in gas exchange (i.e., the pulmonary tidal volume is smaller than the ventilator tidal volume). As a result, a client may experience speaking-related dyspnea. Dyspnea is most apt to be associated with a long period of continuous speaking, such as during an extended reading task. Common symptoms, such as feeling "hungry for air," are those related to hypercapnea (too much carbon dioxide in the blood) and hypoxemia (not enough oxygen in the blood). Hypercapnea can also cause symptoms such as fatigue, dizziness, light-headedness, and headache. Some clients might also report symptoms related to work/effort, especially those who trigger the ventilator to deliver extra breaths.

Physical Examination

The physical examination should begin by observing the client during resting tidal breathing. Often the client's only breathing movements are those that are driven directly by the ventilator (unless he is triggering ventilator-delivered breaths or supplementing ventilation with spontaneous breaths). It is instructive to listen to the ventilator and watch the client's breathing movements during inspirations. While doing so, the clinician should pay attention to the rate at which the inspirations are delivered, duration and loudness of the inspirations, and the magnitude and speed with which the client's rib cage wall and/or abdominal wall move. These cues provide information about the inspiratory volume and flow.

While the client continues to rest, all available ventilator data should be recorded from the ventilator's dials and displays (e.g., breathing rate, tidal volume, inspiratory time, etc.). The pressure indicator, which is usually an air-gauge manometer, should be monitored for several breathing cycles to determine the minimum and maximum pressures delivered by the ventilator (note that the maximum pressure is sometimes called the peak pressure). The minimum pressure should occur following expiration, and the maximum pressure should occur at the end of inspiration. If the client does not have a one-way valve (or cork) blocking expiration, minimum and maximum pressures should be recorded with the client's larynx closed or with his upper airway sealed (mouth closed and nares occluded). *If the client uses a one-way valve (or cork), his upper airway must NEVER be occluded because he will not be able to expire.*

The same observations can then be made while the client is speaking. By listening to the ventilator and watching the client's breathing movements, it may be possible to detect differences in the client's chest wall behavior and/or ventilator function as compared to resting tidal breathing. For example, changes in breathing rate may be noted. The client's breathing rate may be higher during speaking than during resting tidal breathing, and the increased rate may be associated with neck, shoulder, and/or other body movements that appear to be time-locked to inspirations. These are clues that the client is triggering extra breaths while speaking. The change in breathing rate can usually be confirmed by checking the ventilator display. As another example, minimum and maximum airway pressures associated with speaking should be noted. Airway pressure values usually vary from cycle to cycle when the client is speaking, but the general pressure range can be estimated. It is especially important to keep track of the client's maximum airway pressure, because this will help ensure that excessive increases in this pressure are not overlooked during management.

Instrumental Examination

When evaluating a client who uses invasive positive pressure ventilation, it is helpful to obtain measures of maximum inspiratory pressure and maximum expiratory pressure, estimated alveolar pressure (combined with the speech signal), heart rate, blood pressure, oxygen saturation, and end-tidal partial pressure of carbon dioxide. Lung volume is generally not measured during speech breathing with this form of ventilation. Accurate lung volume measures are difficult to obtain during speaking because inspired volume can travel either to the pulmonary apparatus or out through the larynx (or both), and expired air can travel back to the ventilator or out through the larynx (or both). Fortunately, lung volume measures are not critical to understanding this type of ventilator-supported speech breathing.

Procedures for obtaining the instrumental measures of interest have been explained elsewhere. Highlighted below are special considerations related to these measures when applied to clients who use invasive positive pressure ventilation.

Maximum Inspiratory Pressure and Maximum Expiratory Pressure: Maximum inspiratory pressure and maximum expiratory pressure measures are good indicators of inspiratory and expiratory muscle strength, respectively. The maximum inspiratory measure is particularly important because it is predictive of whether or not the client can breathe on his own for short periods and if he can generate sufficient inspiratory pressure to trigger a ventilator.

Measures of maximum inspiratory pressure and maximum expiratory pressure are best obtained by coupling a manometer to the client's tracheostomy tube. This requires that the ventilator be disconnected for a brief period. Specifically, the client is told that the respiratory therapist will be disconnecting the ventilator for a breath or two while a pressure-measuring device is attached to his tracheostomy tube. As soon as the device is attached to the client, he is asked to suck as hard as he can (maximum inspiratory pressure measure). Once the measurement is made, the ventilator is reconnected. When the client's breathing feels comfortable again, the procedure is repeated, except that the client is asked to blow as hard as he can (maximum expiratory measure). It is essential to prepare the client with a thorough explanation of this or any procedure that entails disconnecting the ventilator so that he knows exactly what to expect and agrees to it.

The maximum inspiratory pressure and maximum expiratory pressure maneuvers should be performed at the resting level of the breathing apparatus with the larynx closed. The client may spontaneously close his larynx without being instructed to do so. However, if a leak is detected at the upper airway (this can be monitored by the clinician placing her ear or hand near the client's mouth and nose to hear or feel the leak), he should be instructed to close his larynx. If the client is unable to close his larynx voluntarily, he can be asked to close his mouth while the clinician occludes his anterior nares with a noseclip or gloved fingers. If the latter procedure is used, the client should be warned that if he experiences any discomfort in his ears (caused by inflation of the eustachian tubes), he should stop immediately.

Estimated Alveolar Pressure (Combined with the Speech Signal): Tracheal pressure is the best estimate of alveolar pressure in a client who uses invasive positive pressure ventilation. Most of the procedures for measuring tracheal pressure in a client with a tracheostomy and a positive pressure ventilator are the same as those for a client with a tracheostomy, but no ventilator (see Chapter 4). The primary difference is in how the sensing probe is coupled to the client. The pressure-sensing probe (e.g., polyethylene tube) is threaded through a small hole in a swivel adapter made to fit onto the distal end of the tracheostomy tube. The probe should be inserted through the adapter until it is long enough to nearly reach the proximal end of the tracheostomy tube. If it is too long, it will protrude past the end of the tracheostomy tube and may touch the tracheal wall. The pressure probe should fit snugly into the hole so that air does not leak around it. If the fit is not snug, the probe can be wrapped with tape to increase its outer diameter (this also marks the point of entry so that it can be specified if the probe needs to be removed and replaced). The other end of the probe is connected to one side of a mechanical-electrical manometer (i.e., pressure transducer).

Once the probe is positioned in the swivel adapter, it can be coupled into the client's ventilator circuit. The client is told that the respiratory therapist will be disconnecting his ventilator for a breath or two while the adapter is connected. When the connection is complete, the tracheal pressure signal should be visible on the output device (e.g., oscilloscope, computer monitor, or other display device). The tracheal pressure signal should be displayed on one channel of the output device and the speech signal should be displayed on another channel. This makes it possible to see when speech is produced in relation to the pressure cycle (i.e., breathing cycle).

Estimated Arterial Partial Pressure of Carbon Dioxide: Arterial partial pressure of carbon dioxide (PCO_2) provides information about a client's ventilation. In clients who use invasive positive pressure ventilation, this can be estimated from end-tidal PCO_2, but not with nasal cannulae as it is in clients who use other forms of ventilation. This is because at least some of the expired air will exit the tracheostomy and, thereby, be diverted away from the nares. One notable exception is the client whose ventilator circuit contains a one-way valve or a cork that stops air from exiting through the tracheostomy. In this case, nasal cannulae provide the best means for sensing end-tidal PCO_2 by closing the mouth and routing all expired air through the nose. However, if nasal expiration causes the client discomfort, the procedure should be stopped immediately.

In clients who use invasive positive pressure ventilation and do not use a one-way valve or a cork to block expiration, end-tidal PCO_2 is sensed from within the ventilator circuit. The exact set-up depends on the instrumentation being used. One set-up involves placing an adapter within the ventilator circuit to which a probe tube can be attached and routed to a PCO_2 analyzer. Another set-up involves coupling a PCO_2 sensor directly into the ventilator circuit. When obtaining measures of end-tidal PCO_2, it is critical that the client have his larynx or upper airway closed so that all expired air is routed through the ventilator circuit where it will be sensed by the PCO_2 analyzer. The easiest way to do this is to occlude the client's anterior nares with a noseclip and ask him to close his mouth. End-tidal PCO_2 should be monitored for 3 or 4 consecutive resting tidal breaths.

End-tidal PCO_2 cannot be measured accurately while the client is speaking because some of the expired air exits via the upper airway and will not reach the analyzer in the ventilator circuit. Therefore, the best way to determine the effect of speaking on end-tidal PCO_2 (and, therefore, ventilation) is to obtain measures during resting tidal breathing (as just described) immediately before and immediately after the client performs a speaking task. If speaking reduces ventilation (because air is being routed away from the pulmonary apparatus during the inspiratory phase of the breathing cycle), this should be reflected as an increase in end-tidal PCO_2 following speaking.

Management of Speech Breathing with Invasive Positive Pressure Ventilation

When managing a client who uses invasive positive pressure ventilation, the first issue to be considered is whether or not the ventilator's inspiratory flow reaches the larynx. If the client has an unfenestrated tracheostomy tube with an inflated cuff, flow will not reach the larynx and it will not be possible for the client to speak using ventilator-delivered air. When a speech-language pathologist encounters a client with this tracheostomy-tube configuration, she should consult his pulmonologist immediately to determine if the cuff can be deflated. If it can, the client should be able to produce "leak speech" (i.e., by leaking air from the ventilator's flow to the larynx).

Unfortunately, there may be pulmonologists who believe that it is dangerous to deflate the cuff in clients who use invasive positive pressure ventilation, even in clients who are long-term ventilator users and who are medically stable. If a speech-language pathologist meets a pulmonologist with this belief, she might offer one or more of the several published sources indicating that it is usually safe to deflate the cuff. See, for example, Bach & Alba (1990), Tippett & Siebens (1995), and Hoit, Banzett, Lohmeier, Hixon, & Brown (2003), all of which have pulmonologists as authors.

If the cuff can be deflated, then it is important that the client use a balloon-type cuff so that inflation and deflation can be precisely controlled. A foam cuff tends to inflate spontaneously and is not appropriate for clients who use leak speech. Cuff deflation is almost always accompanied by the need to increase tidal volume. This increase in tidal volume is needed to compensate for air lost through the larynx, so that the volume reaching the pulmonary apparatus remains nearly the same as it was before the cuff was deflated.

RIGGED FOR SILENT RUNNING

This isn't about a submarine. It's about clients who use invasive positive pressure ventilators with inflated tracheostomy-tube cuffs. These clients are rigged for silent running. Some of them don't require such rigging, but are doomed to silence anyway. We've met clients who tell stories of having been mute for long periods (sometimes years) under the care of one pulmologist, and who, when transferred to the care of another pulmonologist, had their cuffs deflated immediately. The pulmonologists we work with favor cuff deflation if at all possible. They appreciate that the risks are low for many clients and that the prospects of speech and better mental health outweigh such risks. We aren't here to challenge the wisdom of any pulmonologist. We're here to encourage speech-language pathologists to weigh-in, when appropriate, on the potential speech options for clients with inflated cuffs.

Once the cuff is deflated, it is important to check for air leaks around the tracheostomy tube. Small leaks are common and are not of concern, but a substantial leak can render certain management strategies ineffective. Such air leaks can be challenging to fix, but the respiratory therapist should be able to help in this regard. Two options for occluding leaks include stuffing sterile gauze around the tracheostomy tube, and securing a malleable plastic flange around the tube.

Several management approaches can improve speech and communication in clients who use invasive positive pressure ventilation. As shown in Table 6-1, ventilator adjustments, exteroceptive feedback, economical valving, muscle training, relieving speaking-related dyspnea, monitoring gas exchange, mouthing and buccal speaking, conversational strategies, optimizing the environment, counseling, speech amplifiers, talking tracheostomy tubes, and augmentative and alternative communication may be appropriate for clients who use this form of ventilation. Note also that glossopharyngeal breathing and breath stacking are not recommended for the client who uses invasive positive pressure ventilation. Because the client has a tracheostomy, the only way he can glossopharyngeal breathe or breath stack is if he uses a one-way valve (in the common ventilator line) or a cork (in the expiratory line). However, use of a one-way valve or a cork carries risks, as discussed below.

Most of the approaches listed in Table 6-1 have been described in Chapter 5 and in previous sections of the present chapter. The focus here is on ventilator adjustments, because these usually provide the most powerful means of improving this type of ventilator-supported speech. Remarks are also offered regarding other selected management approaches.

Ventilator Adjustments

Several ventilator adjustments are applicable to improving speech in clients who use invasive positive pressure ventilation. They include increased breathing rate, altered tidal volume, lengthened inspiratory time, end-inspiratory pause, PEEP, pressure-controlled (or pressure-support) ventilation, and selected combinations of these adjustments. It is important to note that these adjustments are best-suited to clients with neuromotor disorders, and that some of them may not be appropriate for clients with significant obstructive airway disease. The use of a one-way valve (or cork) is contraindicated for invasive positive pressure ventilation.

Increased Breathing Rate: Breathing rate can be increased while using control mode ventilation or assist/control mode ventilation. In a client who uses control mode ventilation (i.e., does not trigger breaths actively), breathing rate can be increased by merely adjusting the ventilator directly. Rate should be increased in small steps (by 1 to 2 breaths per minute) to change ventilation as little as possible. When breathing rate is increased, it may be possible to produce more speech over consecutive breathing cycles. Also, pause duration between utterances should be shorter.

If a client is able to generate a small inspiratory pressure, he should be able to trigger ventilator-delivered breaths using an assist/control mode of ventilation. By triggering extra breaths, a client can increase speaking time over consecutive breathing cycles and decrease pause time between utterances. Although the average breathing rate is higher, the breath intervals are not necessarily periodic. The most important advantage of using assist/control mode for speech breathing is that the client can initiate speech breaths more or less at will, rather than having to wait for the next inspiration to be delivered. Another advantage is that, if the client triggers extra breaths only when speaking, his ventilation can remain at the usual level during times of rest.

A client who is not able to generate adequate negative pressure to trigger the ventilator in the standard way may be able to trigger it by using an entirely different approach. This approach involves adding PEEP and setting the trigger level slightly below PEEP. For example, if PEEP is set at 5 cmH$_2$O, the trigger level can be adjusted to 4 cmH$_2$O. With this set-up, the client can trigger breaths by opening the larynx so that pressure drops below the trigger threshold. This approach works only in the case of ventilators that have both internal PEEP and a trigger function.

A potential disadvantage of increasing breathing rate is that the client could hyperventilate. One solution for this is to combine increased breathing rate with decreased tidal volume (as described in the section below on adjustment combinations). However, increased ventilation may be an advantage if the client usually experiences speaking-related hypoventilation.

Altered Tidal Volume: When changing tidal volume, it is important to remember that the ventilator-delivered tidal volume is seldom the same as the tidal volume that reaches the client's pulmonary apparatus. The ventilator-delivered tidal volume may be larger than the pulmonary tidal volume if the client speaks or otherwise opens his larynx during inspiration, and it may be smaller than the pulmonary tidal volume if the client supplements it with spontaneous inspiratory efforts. Thus, even when the ventilator-delivered tidal volume is changed, this does not necessarily mean that the client's pulmonary tidal volume undergoes the same magnitude or even the same direction of change.

A common reason to increase ventilator-delivered tidal volume is to compensate for loss of pulmonary tidal volume. For example, a client who is usually ventilated with an inflated cuff and has his cuff deflated to speak will probably lose tidal volume through the larynx and upper airway. This loss is easily replaced by increasing the ventilator-delivered tidal volume. For another example, if pulmonary tidal volume is lost when inspiratory time is lengthened, ventilator-delivered tidal volume can be increased to return the client's ventilation to its usual level.

In general, tidal volume should not be increased to improve speech without being combined with another adjustment. This is because increasing tidal volume (all else held constant) increases the rate of rise of tracheal pressure during inspiration and increases the maximum pressure. When used alone, an increased tidal volume could improve speech by increasing overall loudness, but it could also make speech worse by causing loudness and voice quality to be more variable.

If tidal volume is decreased (all else held constant), this will reduce the rate of rise of tracheal pressure and also reduce the maximum pressure. This could improve speech by reducing loudness variability and voice quality variability. However, it could also reduce overall loudness. Most clients will not tolerate this adjustment when presented alone because they perceive that they are "not getting enough air." In some cases, it is true that a decrease in tidal volume will cause hypoventilation. In other cases, the client may be chronically hyperventilated so that a reduction in ventilation (via a reduction in tidal volume) is actually beneficial. It is in these latter cases that ventilator adjustments may serve the dual purpose of improving the client's speech and improving the client's blood gas levels. Despite the potential physiological benefit associated with reducing ventilation in a client who is hyperventilated, the client's perception of "not getting enough air" must be respected. Additional adjustments can change this perception and make it possible to decrease tidal volume without causing the client discomfort (see section below on adjustment combinations).

Lengthened Inspiratory Time: Inspiratory time can be lengthened on most ventilators, although the way in which this is done can vary substantially across ventilators (as described above). When inspiratory time is lengthened and tidal volume remains the same, inspiratory flow decreases. When inspiration occupies more than half the total breathing cycle, this is called "inverse ratio ventilation."

When inspiratory time is lengthened (and flow is reduced), the rising (inspiratory) portion of the pressure waveform is longer and has a more gradual slope than usual. This means that there is more time available to speak during inspiration.

Thus, overall speaking time per breathing cycle should increase, and pause time between utterances should decrease (assuming breathing rate either remains unchanged or increases). Often, when inspiratory time is lengthened, the maximum pressure is lower than usual. This is because the client spends more time speaking during inspiration so that more of the ventilator-delivered tidal volume is bled off through the larynx (resulting in a lower pressure maximum). The more gradual (inspiratory) slope and lower pressure maximum should help reduce loudness variability and improve voice quality.

There are clients who are uncomfortable with lengthened inspiratory time because they feel as though they are "not getting enough air." A client may continue to feel this way, even when the larynx is closed and the full pulmonary tidal volume is delivered. Some clients may become accustomed to the lower flow after a few minutes. Others may not, but may feel comfortable with lengthened inspiratory time if it is combined with other adjustments (see section below on adjustment combinations).

When inspiratory time is lengthened, the risk of hypoventilation may increase. This is because the client speaks for a longer period during inspiration so that more of the ventilator-delivered tidal volume is used for speech production and less for gas exchange. Hypoventilation can be countered by increasing tidal volume, reducing the degree to which inspiratory time was lengthened, or instructing the client to close the larynx occasionally during an inspiration.

If inspiratory time is too long, there is a risk that there will not be adequate time for the client to expire the full tidal volume. If this occurs, some of the tidal volume will remain in the pulmonary apparatus and alveolar pressure will be positive at the end of the breathing cycle. This "dynamic hyperinflation" causes what is often called "inadvertent PEEP," "intrinsic PEEP," or "autoPEEP." A client with airway obstruction is most prone to this situation because it often takes him extra time to expire. In such clients, dynamic hyperinflation can be avoided by reducing the degree to which inspiratory time is lengthened. In others, it may not be appropriate to lengthen inspiratory time.

End-Inspiratory Pause: Certain ventilators have an occlusion adjustment, sometimes called an end-inspiratory pause, which makes it possible to delay the opening of the ventilator's expiration valve after inspiration ends. The pressure decreases slowly from its maximum during the period when the expiration valve is closed, then decreases more rapidly once the valve opens. This adjustment can accomplish two speech-related goals. First, it extends the time during which pressure is above the voicing threshold. This can increase speaking time and reduce the pause time between utterances. Second, it can maintain a relatively constant pressure for the period during which the expiratory valve is closed. This can help decrease loudness variability and voice quality variability during that period. Occlusion of the expiratory valve during the initial part of expiration is safer than occlusion throughout expiration, such as occurs with the one-way valve (or cork).

Positive End-Expiratory Pressure: PEEP is one of the most effective interventions available for improving speech with invasive positive pressure ventilation. PEEP is applied by either adjusting the ventilator (in models with this feature) or by coupling an external PEEP valve to the expiratory line. PEEP, when used for speech purposes, usually ranges from about 5 to 15 cmH$_2$O. With PEEP, the pressure decreases more slowly during expiration, and, thereby, remains above the voicing threshold for a longer period. The pressure eventually falls to zero with expiration, because the pressure is bled off during speaking. (Note, however, that if the tracheostomy-tube cuff is inflated or if the larynx is closed, the minimum and maximum pressures should increase by the magnitude of the PEEP). Thus, PEEP makes it possible for a client to speak longer during the expiratory phase of the breathing cycle, thereby increasing speaking time and decreasing pause time between utterances. Interestingly, some clients report that PEEP not only improves speech, but also makes breathing feel more comfortable.

PEEP, like other forms of impeded expiration (e.g., end-inspiratory pause, one-way valve or cork, discussed below), poses safety risks associated with increased intrathoracic pressure. These include barotrauma and reduced cardiac output due to reduced venous return. Thus, extra caution must be used when considering these types of ventilator adjustments in clients with compromised cardiovascular function. As with all other adjustments, the potential risks for any given client are assessed by the client's pulmonologist.

Fortunately, benefits to speech are usually evident at low levels of PEEP (i.e., 5 to 10 cmH$_2$O). As a general rule, it is best to use the lowest level of PEEP that achieves a desirable speech product so as to minimize any safety risks. When using PEEP, it is critical to reduce or eliminate air leaks around the tracheostomy tube. If there is a substantial air leak, PEEP may not be effective.

One-Way Valve (or Cork) is Contraindicated: A one-way (inspiratory) valve opens to allow inspiratory flow from the ventilator to enter the client, and closes to block expiratory flow back to the ventilator. Thus, all expiratory flow is directed through the larynx and upper airway. An equivalent effect can be achieved by simply plugging the expiratory port of the ventilator with a rubber cork.

When considering the pressure waveform generated with a one-way valve (or cork), the inspiratory (i.e., rising) portion of the waveform looks similar to that for the usual invasive positive pressure waveform, but the expiratory portion differs substantially. Without expiratory occlusion (usual condition), the pressure decreases rapidly as the air flows freely through the tracheostomy back toward the ventilator. With the ventilator's expiratory line occluded, the pressure decreases more gradually because resistance is higher. More specifically, the rate of pressure decrease depends on the resistance offered to expiratory flow by the larynx and upper airway. Because pressure changes relatively slowly, speech can last longer and loudness and voice quality are more stable.

Expiratory occlusion carries with it potentially fatal risks. If the upper airway is blocked, or if the tracheostomy-tube cuff is inflated (and there is no fenestration in the tube), the tidal volume delivered by the ventilator cannot be expired. When the next breath is delivered, its volume is added to the already existing volume. And, likewise, the following breath is added to the already large volume. If the ventilator's pressure-limiting device malfunctions, the ventilator will continue to deliver inspirations and severe barotrauma and reduced cardiac output (and reduced venous return) will ensue. If the ventilator's pressure-limiting safety device works properly, the ventilator will stop delivering inspirations and severe hypoventilation will ensue. Either way, the outcome can be deadly.

The serious risks associated with expiratory occlusion make this form of intervention unacceptable to many clinicians (Hoit & Banzett, 2003). A much safer solution is to substitute low PEEP for the one-way valve. If the client is not satisfied with his speech when using low PEEP, then a higher level of PEEP (e.g., 15 cmH$_2$O) can be used. Speech produced with high PEEP has been shown to be indistinguishable from speech produced with a one-way valve (Hoit, Banzett, Lohmeier, Hixon, & Brown, 2003). PEEP is safer than a one-way valve because, if flow through the larynx and upper airway is blocked (e.g., by an inflated tracheostomy-tube cuff), cycles of inspiration and expiration generally can continue, thereby reducing the risk of hypoventilation. PEEP still carries the risk of barotrauma because the overall pressure is higher than usual (by the magnitude of the PEEP applied), but the risk is lower than that posed by a one-way valve.

BELT AND SUSPENDERS

To produce speech during the expiratory phase of positive pressure ventilation, at least some air must pass through the larynx and upper airway. A common way to make this happen is to place a one-way valve between the client and the ventilator. As discussed in adjacent text, another way to do this is to insert a rubber cork into the expiratory line of the ventilator circuit. One of us encountered a client who insisted that both of these be done at the same time. That is, he wore a one-way valve near his tracheostomy and had a rubber cork inserted into the distal end of the expiratory line of his ventilator. When told this was redundant and asked why he wanted both, he simply indicated that he preferred it that way. So, who's to judge? Maybe he just wanted to have a backup system. That's not so strange. How about people who wear a belt and suspenders (at the same time) to hold up their pants? Well, on second thought, maybe it is a little strange.

Pressure-Controlled (or Pressure-Support) Ventilation: To this juncture, discussion has focused on ventilator adjustments as they relate to the use of volume-controlled ventilation (i.e., wherein the ventilator delivers a designated volume of air). With pressure-controlled ventilation, ventilator-delivered breaths target a designated pressure. This mode of ventilation generates pressure waveforms that increase rapidly to the targeted pressure and approximate that pressure for the remainder of the inspiration. When volume is lost through the larynx and upper airway, such as occurs during speech production, the ventilator continues to generate inspiratory flow to maintain the targeted pressure. Once inspiration ends, pressure decreases rapidly. Pressure waveforms associated with pressure-support ventilation are similar to those of pressure-controlled ventilation except that the initiation and duration of inspiration are controlled by the client's efforts. Thus, pressure-supported breaths are not necessarily periodic or of consistent inspiratory duration. An advantage of pressure-controlled (or pressure-support) ventilation is that the pressure can remain relatively constant during inspiration. This stability in the pressure allows for greater stability in loudness and voice quality.

When switching a client's ventilator from volume-controlled to pressure-controlled (or pressure-support) ventilation, the pressure target should not exceed the client's maximum pressure during volume-controlled ventilation (with the laryngeal or upper airway closed), and should be lower than this maximum, if possible. A lower pressure is better for speech production and reduces risks associated with high intrathoracic pressures (e.g., barotrauma, decreased cardiac output). As with all ventilator adjustments, speech-related considerations must be balanced with the primary goal of determining the appropriate level of ventilation for the client as mandated by the pulmonologist.

Adjustment Combinations: There are many combinations of ventilator adjustments that can be used to improve ventilator-supported speech. A few such combinations are described below. With experience, clinical teams will discover other combinations that are effective with their clients and their particular ventilator systems.

Lengthened Inspiratory Time and Positive End-Expiratory Pressure (and Decreased Tidal Volume). Lengthened inspiratory time (by the amount best tolerated by the client) combined with PEEP (5 to 10 cmH$_2$O) is one of the simplest and most successful speech interventions available (Hoit & Banzett, 1997). Lengthened inspiratory time extends potential speaking time during inspiration and PEEP extends potential speaking time during expiration. A client may be more apt to accept this intervention if PEEP is applied before inspiratory time is lengthened. In clients who use assist/control mode to trigger extra breaths, this combination of adjustments sometimes reduces the frequency of triggering and the associated effort to produce speech.

Clients who are chronically hyperventilated may obtain further benefit if tidal volume is decreased along with lengthened inspiratory time and PEEP. Although most clients resist having tidal volume reduced, they may accept less volume if

PEEP is added first. A reduced tidal volume improves speech because it lowers the maximum pressure and, thereby, reduces loudness variability and improves voice quality (Hoit, Banzett, Lohmeier, Hixon, & Brown, 2003).

Increased Breathing Rate and Decreased Tidal Volume. An increase in breathing rate combined with a decrease in tidal volume may improve speech in clients who are not able to trigger extra breaths. The increased rate allows for more speaking time over consecutive breathing cycles. The decreased volume reduces the rate of pressure rise during inspiration and reduces the maximum pressure, and may, thereby, reduce variability of loudness and voice quality. It is important to ensure, however, that the increase in breathing rate does not reduce inspiratory time, or much of the benefit to speech will be lost. The adjustments of breathing rate and tidal volume can be made in a manner that maintains the client's usual minute ventilation. For example, if a client's original rate and volume are 10 breaths per minute and 1 L, respectively, an adjusted rate of 14 breaths per minute and a tidal volume of about 0.71 L will yield approximately the same ventilator-delivered minute ventilation.

Pressure-Controlled (or Pressure-Support) Ventilation and Positive End-Expiratory Pressure (and Lengthened Inspiratory Time). Pressure-controlled (or pressure-support) ventilation improves speech by providing a period during inspiration when the pressure is relatively constant (approximating the type of waveform seen in normal speech production, although the pressure is usually higher). By adding PEEP to this combination, speech can be extended into the expiratory phase of the breathing cycle. In the case of pressure-controlled ventilation, it may also benefit speech to lengthen inspiratory time.

Bilevel positive pressure ventilation, available on certain ventilators, generates a pressure waveform that is quite similar to combined pressure-controlled (or pressure-support) ventilation and PEEP. With bilevel ventilation, the operator sets an inspiratory positive airway pressure and an expiratory positive airway pressure and the ventilator cycles between the two. As long as the expiratory pressure is above the voicing threshold, the client should be able to speak throughout the entire cycle (Prigent, Samuel, Louis, Abinun, Zerah-Lancner, Lejaille, Raphael, & Lofaso, 2003).

Other Adjustment Combinations. Many other adjustment combinations are possible. For instance, increased breathing rate, decreased tidal volume, and PEEP might be combined. Similarly, increased inspiratory time, end-inspiratory pause, PEEP, and decreased tidal volume might be used together. The possibilities are nearly limitless, especially when taking into account the range of values available for each type of adjustment. By being creative, a clinical team has a good chance of finding an adjustment combination that offers appropriate ventilation, increases client comfort, and improves speech.

A FINAL DECISION

He was a vital young man who was always on the move. He worked security at a local club. A bullet severed his spinal cord and left him quadriplegic. The shock to his quality of life was unbearable. The cuff on his ventilator was inflated and he could not speak. He resisted other modes of communication. Depression persisted. He decided that he wanted to be removed from his ventilator on the second anniversary of his injury. He lobbied for this plan. His physician thought that the restoration of his speech might change his perspective. Expert advice was sought. His ventilator was adjusted to enable him to speak. The outcome was judged a success. Although heartened by the change, it was not sufficient to overcome his feelings of hopelessness. The day before the second anniversary of his injury he spoke with television reporters on the evening news about his peace with his decision. By the next evening's news report, he was gone.

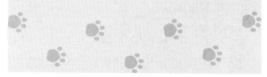

General Comments about Ventilator Adjustments: The adjustments discussed above have been found to improve speech in clients who use invasive positive pressure ventilation when applied individually and in certain combinations. Although ventilator adjustments are generally successful, not all clients benefit from them. Some clients may be too physically fragile to tolerate adjustments to the ventilator. Others may resist the idea of changing a breathing pattern that has become familiar over years of use. And still other clients may show no detectable improvement in their speech no matter what ventilator adjustment or combinations of adjustments are used. Within this last group of clients may be those who have significant laryngeal and/or upper airway problems. Clients with impaired laryngeal function may not be able to take advantage of a more normal pressure waveform. And clients with impaired upper airway function may exhibit improvements in speech timing with new ventilator adjustments (e.g., longer speech duration), but may not have a functional benefit from the intervention if intelligibility is severely compromised. In practice, the only way to determine if a particular client will benefit from adjustments to his ventilator is to test them directly.

When testing ventilator adjustments to improve speech, there are two guiding principles to follow. The first guiding principle is that the client's ventilation, safety, and comfort should never be compromised. To ensure that they are not, ventilator adjustments must be made by a respiratory therapist and overseen by a pulmonologist. Several physiological indicators (heart rate, blood pressure, SpO_2, and end-tidal PCO_2) should be monitored while the adjustments are being tested. And the client must be asked frequently to report on his comfort with each adjustment. The second guiding principle is that the goal of the adjustment(s) is to modify the pressure waveform in a way that has the potential to improve speech. Specifically, the pressure should exceed the voicing threshold for a large portion of the breathing cycle and it should remain as stable as possible. Thus, the goal is to move the abnormal pressure waveform toward normal (for speech production), while adhering to the first guiding principal.

Notes on Other Management Approaches for Speech Breathing with Invasive Positive Pressure Ventilation

Three other management approaches, as applied to clients who use invasive positive pressure ventilation, require comment. These are exteroceptive feedback, relieving speaking-related dyspnea, and use of a talking tracheostomy tube.

Feedback in the form of a continuous tracheal pressure signal combined with the speech signal can be particularly effective for the client who uses invasive positive pressure ventilation. Such feedback is powerful because speech is so strongly linked to pressure in these clients. By watching the on-line display (on an oscilloscope, computer monitor, or other graphic device), the client should be able to see the relation of pressure to speech and gain better control over speech production in ways that take full advantage of the prevailing pressure.

Invasive positive pressure ventilation is the only form of ventilation expected to be associated with speaking-related dyspnea of the "hunger for air" variety. This is because speech is produced, in part, during the inspiratory phase of the breathing cycle so that air is diverted away from the pulmonary apparatus. This competition between speaking and ventilation can cause the client to experience hunger for air and possible hypoventilation. The easiest way to relieve this form of dyspnea is for the client to close his larynx for a few breaths. This strategy works well when engaged in the listening phase of a conversational interchange. However, this strategy does not work well during the speaking phase of the conversational interchange because it interrupts the act of speaking for much too long. A better way to relieve dyspnea while speaking is to close the larynx during inspiration and continue speaking during expiration. This allows the full ventilator-delivered tidal volume to be routed to the pulmonary apparatus for gas exchange. It also allows speaking to continue with the shortest interruption possible. Of course, this means that pressure must be above the voicing threshold for an adequate period during expiration, something that can be accomplished by adding PEEP. It is often helpful to monitor ventilation (via measures of end-tidal PCO_2) while implementing these dyspnea-relieving strategies. In this way, the presence and magnitude of the dyspnea can be related to changes in ventilation. It is always important to monitor SpO_2.

Before a talking tracheostomy tube is considered for a client who uses invasive positive pressure ventilation, the possibility of cuff deflation should first be explored. If the pulmonologist determines that the client's cuff should not be deflated, then the talking tracheostomy tube may be a viable option.

Clinical Summary of Speech Breathing with Invasive Positive Pressure Ventilation

Speech breathing with invasive positive pressure ventilation differs significantly from normal speech breathing. Speech is produced during both inspiration and expiration, the pressure that drives speech production generally is fast-changing and often highly peaked, and speech production competes with ventilation. When evaluating and managing clients who use this form of ventilation, it is extremely important to take safety precautions (i.e., by monitoring the client in ways suggested in the section on general principles of evaluation in this chapter). There are two reasons for this. One is that speaking can cause hypoventilation with this ventilator set-up. The other is that the maximum pressure generated with this form of ventilation can be quite high and it may be undesirable to allow it to be higher.

The most powerful way to manage this form of ventilator-supported speech is through the use of ventilator adjustments. Speech can also benefit from behavioral management, especially with exteroceptive feedback (consisting of the simultaneous display of tracheal pressure and speech), inspiratory muscle training, and conversational strategies. This approach to management is deemed safer than the use of a one-way valve.

Noninvasive Positive Pressure Ventilation

The focus turns here to noninvasive positive pressure ventilation, wherein ventilation is delivered through the upper airway, rather than through a tracheostomy. Positive pressure ventilation can be delivered noninvasively by coupling the client to the ventilator tubing via a mouthpiece, a nosemask (or nasal pillows), or a facemask. Whether invasive or noninvasive positive pressure ventilation is better for the long-term ventilator user is a controversial issue. For a client who is a candidate for either form of ventilation, it is likely that the selection will reflect the philosophical bias of his pulmonologist.

Noninvasive positive pressure ventilation appears to have certain advantages over invasive positive pressure ventilation (Bach, 2002), at least for clients with neuromotor disorders. Its greatest advantage is that the client can avoid the surgery needed to create the tracheostomy and the many potential complications associated with having a chronic tracheostomy (Mehta & Hill, 2001). Noninvasive delivery of positive pressure ventilation may also reduce or alleviate the chronic hyperventilation often associated with invasive delivery of positive pressure ventilation (Bach, Haber, Wang, & Alba, 1995). Importantly, noninvasive positive pressure ventilation may have advantages for speech breathing, especially when volume-controlled ventilation is used.

Speech breathing with noninvasive positive pressure ventilation is quite different from speech breathing with invasive positive pressure ventilation, and, in some ways, easier to understand. During noninvasive positive pressure ventilation, speech is produced during expiration, as it is during normal speech breathing. The driving pressure available for speaking depends on the prevailing relaxation pressure (in clients who have no muscular pressure generating capability) or on the prevailing relaxation pressure plus muscular pressure (in clients with residual inspiratory and/or expiratory muscle function). Discussed below are evaluation and management strategies for clients who are ventilated noninvasively with volume-controlled positive pressure ventilators.

Evaluation of Speech Breathing with Noninvasive Positive Pressure Ventilation

Most of what should be included in the evaluation of a client who uses noninvasive positive pressure ventilation has been covered in the section above on general principles and methods for evaluating ventilator-supported speech breathing. Special issues to be considered with this type of ventilation are highlighted below.

Case History

During the case history interview, information should be gathered about the coupling device or devices that the client uses and under what circumstances he uses them. For example, the client might use a nosemask (strapped in place) at night while sleeping and a mouthpiece (positioned near his mouth) during the day while awake. In this case, speech breathing evaluation and management need only focus on speech produced using the mouthpiece. For another example, the client might use a nosemask when in bed and a mouthpiece when in his wheelchair. If he reports that he speaks in both situations, speech breathing evaluation and management should address both.

Ventilator Analysis

Form 6-2 can be used to perform the ventilator analysis. The type of ventilator (positive pressure) and method of delivery (e.g., via mouthpiece) should be noted at the top of the form. The adjustment variables for positive pressure ventilation are described above under invasive positive pressure ventilation.

Auditory-Perceptual Examination

Auditory-perceptual features of the speech of clients who use noninvasive positive pressure ventilation may include short utterance duration, long pause duration, fading loudness, reduced loudness variability (such as that associated with reduced linguistic stress), and pressed voice quality. The roots of these features can be linked to the alveolar pressure waveform.

When positive pressure ventilation is delivered noninvasively with a volume-controlled ventilator, pressure rises during inspiration (as lung volume increases) and falls during expiration (as lung volume decreases). This is usually followed by a period when pressure remains at zero (atmospheric). The rate at which the pressure falls (and the rate at which lung volume decreases) depends on the relaxation pressure and the resistance offered to expiratory flow by the larynx and upper airway. In clients who are able to activate inspiratory and expiratory muscles, the rate of pressure decrease may also depend on muscular pressure contributions.

The auditory-perceptual features of short utterance duration and long pause duration can be explained by the relatively limited time that the pressure remains above the voicing threshold. The auditory-perceptual feature of fading loudness is linked to the continuous decrease in pressure over the course of the expiration. Restricted loudness variation (for linguistic stress) is associated with a lack of variation in the pressure waveform and is explained by the client's inability to generate muscular pressure pulses. Finally, the auditory-perceptual feature of pressed voice quality is likely a sign that laryngeal airway resistance is high. High laryngeal airway resistance during speaking has the advantage of slowing the rate at which lung volume is expended and extending utterance duration. It is important to note that, although this combination of auditory-perceptual features may be observed in the speech of a client who relies on relaxation pressure alone, it is possible for speech to be essentially normal in a client who retains some active muscle function.

If the client is wearing a nosemask or facemask during the auditory-perceptual examination, it may be difficult to hear certain features of his speech (e.g., nasality, spirantization). Because of this, the best way to perform the auditory-perceptual examination is to have the client use a mouthpiece so that his airway and face are unencumbered during speech production. Of course, the client should also be evaluated with his mask in place to determine the nature and quality of his functional speech and communication.

Physical Examination

A client who uses noninvasive positive pressure ventilation typically does not have a tracheostomy. In fact, the major reason to use noninvasive ventilation is to eliminate the need for one. Nevertheless, in the rare client who uses noninvasive ventilation and still has a tracheostomy, it is important that the clinician check to be sure that it is occluded (e.g., with a button) and that there are no substantial air leaks. To do this, the clinician should listen and feel for air leaks while the client inspires and expires. If a substantial leak is detected, the client's respiratory therapist should be consulted to determine if an adequate seal can be achieved. A substantial air leak may jeopardize attempts to improve speech.

Besides following the usual physical examination procedures described above in this chapter, an additional procedure should be conducted with a client who uses a nosemask or facemask to determine if he can use a mouthpiece. To use a mouthpiece effectively, the client needs to have adequate lip strength and velopharyngeal closure. This can be tested directly by having the client attempt to use a mouthpiece while the clinician watches for lip closure and feels for velopharyngeal closure (via nasal air flow) during inspiration. If lip closure is adequate, but velopharyngeal closure is not, a noseclip may be used (although this may not be a satisfactory long-term solution). If the client is using a mouthpiece for the first time, he might need instruction and practice to be able to make smooth transitions from inspiration to speech production. An infant, a very young child, or an adult with a severe cognitive impairment may not be able to use a mouthpiece. Such clients are better suited for nosemask use.

Instrumental Examination

The instrumental examination is as described under the section on general principles and methods of speech breathing evaluation, with three exceptions. One relates to alveolar pressure estimates and one to estimates of arterial PCO_2. A measure of breath-stacking capacity, also called maximal insufflation capacity (Bach, 2002), can be a useful addition as well.

Usually alveolar pressure during speech production must be estimated from oral pressure, because a client who uses noninvasive positive pressure ventilation typically does not have a tracheostomy. This is done in the manner described in Chapter 4 (i.e., estimated from peak oral pressure during /p/ productions), unless the client's ventilation is delivered via a facemask. To gain access to the oral airway, the mask can be removed for oral pressure measurements during expiration (and speech production). Or the client can be switched to a mouthpiece coupler while measurements are made. Another alternative is to leave the facemask in place and tap oral pressure by providing a connector on the facemask through which a sensing tube can be inserted at the corner of the mouth. If the client happens to have a tracheostomy, measures of tracheal pressure can be obtained and are preferable to estimates of alveolar pressure made from the oral airway.

Arterial PCO_2 can be estimated from end-tidal PCO_2 sensed with nasal cannulae in clients who use a mouthpiece. However, it may be problematic to use nasal cannulae with clients who wear nosemasks or facemasks for noninvasive positive pressure ventilation delivery. In these cases, arterial PCO_2 is more easily estimated from transcutaneous PCO_2, although it has a much longer time-constant than end-tidal PCO_2 (see Chapter 4).

To determine breath-stacking capacity, a respiratory therapist uses a manual resuscitator to deliver consecutive inspiratory strokes to the client. Breath-stacking capacity is measured by having the client expire passively (i.e., without expiratory muscular effort) into a spirometer following a maximum inspiration. This capacity varies according to the client's size, his ability to maintain an adequate lip seal (when using a mouthpiece or nosemask) and velopharyngeal seal (when using a mouthpiece) during inspiration, and his ability to maintain a closed larynx against a high alveolar pressure when breath holding between strokes. Breath-stacking capacity is prognostic of whether or not the client will be able to use breath stacking as a way to improve speech.

Management of Speech Breathing with Noninvasive Positive Pressure Ventilation

The first step in managing the speech breathing of a client who uses noninvasive positive pressure ventilation is to consider the client-ventilator coupler. The best coupler for speech is a mouthpiece. This is because the mouthpiece leaves the face unencumbered during the speaking phase of the breathing cycle. A facemask is the worst option for speech because it restricts upper airway movements and degrades the fidelity of speech. A nosemask is less cumbersome than a facemask, but its presence distorts the acoustic realization of nasal consonants and other speech segments that are influenced by nasalization. Both types of masks also interfere with communication in other ways. A facemask covers parts of the face that can reflect the emotional content of the message (i.e., facial expression), and a nosemask and the ventilator tube to which it is connected can have a distracting appearance. A nosemask can be difficult to use if the nasal pathway is congested. Other problems associated with the use of masks for positive pressure ventilation are air leaks and pressure sores on the face. Masks can cause facial deformations in infants and children. Nasal pillows, which resemble large-bore nasal cannulae, offer an alternative that avoids some of these mask-related problems, but share the drawbacks associated with encumbering the nasal pathway.

The client who is able to use a mouthpiece should be encouraged to do so at times when he is most apt to be speaking. Thus, he could use a mask during sleep and during wakefulness when he is alone, and switch to a mouthpiece when he is going to be in a social situation. If a client uses a lip seal retention device to maintain an adequate lip seal during sleep, he should adopt a tube-like mouthpiece for daytime use, if possible. A client who is just starting to use a mouthpiece may require training and practice to be able to coordinate insertion of the mouthpiece for inspiration and release of the mouthpiece for expiration (including speaking). Also, a client who has just switched from invasive positive pressure ventilation to noninvasive positive pressure ventilation may have difficulty synchronizing the opening of the larynx with the beginning of inspiration. This is because the larynx is usually closed when inspiration is delivered through a tracheostomy (and the client is not speaking).

Nearly all the management approaches listed in Table 6-1 have the potential to improve speech and communication in clients who use noninvasive positive pressure ventilation. These include ventilator adjustments, breath stacking, exteroceptive feedback, economical valving, body positioning, mechanical aids, muscle training, glossopharyngeal breathing, relieving speaking-related dyspnea, monitoring gas exchange, mouthing and buccal speaking, conversational strategies, optimizing the environment, counseling, speech amplifiers, buttons and one-way valves (if the client has a tracheostomy), and augmentative and alternative communication. Description of these management approaches has been provided in Chapter 5 and in other sections above in the present chapter. Additional comments are offered here regarding ventilator adjustments, breath stacking, and other selected management approaches.

Ventilator Adjustments

The positive pressure ventilators used with this form of noninvasive ventilation are the same as those used with invasive ventilation, so they have the same range of ventilator adjustment capabilities. However, the same ventilator adjustment can have different consequences when applied to a noninvasive client-ventilator system compared to an invasive one.

There are fewer adjustment options for improving speech with noninvasive positive pressure ventilation than with invasive positive pressure ventilation. The options available include altered breathing rate, increased tidal volume, and decreased inspiratory time as applied to a volume-controlled positive pressure ventilator.

Altered Breathing Rate: By experimenting, the clinician may find that a particular breathing rate provides a "best fit" for a client's speech breathing behavior. For example, a client who is talkative, prefers to speak in long breath groups, and/or uses low flow during speech production (as a consequence of high laryngeal and upper airway resistance) may do well using a relatively slow breathing rate. This is because such a client is able to sustain the speaking portion of the breathing cycle (expiration) for a relatively long period. This client would also do well with an accompanying increase in tidal volume to improve speech further and to maintain his usual level of ventilation. By contrast, a client who speaks in short breath groups, pauses frequently (e.g., to formulate the upcoming utterance), and/or uses high flow during speech production (as a consequence of low laryngeal and upper airway resistance) may do better with a higher breathing rate. This increase in breathing rate may need to be accompanied by a decrease in tidal volume to avoid hyperventilation. The best way to determine the optimal breathing rate is to test different rates (and possibly different accompanying tidal volumes) while monitoring the client's speech and cardiopulmonary variables.

Another way to improve speech by changing breathing rate is to allow the client to trigger his own breaths using an assist/control mode of ventilation. To use assist/control, the client must be able to generate a small inspiratory pressure. When a client triggers his own breaths, he can have more control over the temporal aspects of his speech production.

Increased Tidal Volume: Increased tidal volume can benefit a client's speech in at least two ways. First, it can supply the client with a larger volume of air with which to produce speech. A larger volume makes it possible to produce more speech per breath, if average expiratory flow remains the same. Alternatively, a larger volume can make it possible to increase the average flow while still producing the same amount of speech. In this way, a client who typically uses a pressed voice quality in association with attempts to conserve volume can reduce laryngeal airway resistance to improve his voice quality.

The second way that increased tidal volume can benefit a client's speech is by the associated increase in relaxation pressure. This is especially beneficial to the client who has little or no expiratory muscle function and who depends heavily on relaxation pressure to drive the larynx and upper airway for speech production. A larger tidal volume results in a higher relaxation pressure at the beginning of expiration, and a higher pressure makes it possible to produce louder speech. However, if the pressure is too high, speech may begin with a louder-than-desirable burst. Thus, the best candidate for increased tidal volume may be the client who has residual inspiratory muscle function and is capable of generating a graded inspiratory pressure that can brake the higher-than-desired relaxation pressure. If the client is able to do this, he can lower the initial pressure to produce the desired loudness. As the utterance continues and available relaxation pressure decreases, inspiratory activity can be reduced. In this way, alveolar pressure can be maintained at a relatively constant level during at least the first part of the breath group.

In the case of the client who uses a mouthpiece, the tidal volume solution is a relatively simple one. The ventilator can be set to deliver a very large tidal volume and the client has the option to use as much of it as he sees fit. For example, while speaking, he can inspire large tidal volumes so that he is able to produce long and loud breath groups. Then, while he is listening to someone else speak, he can inspire much smaller tidal volumes by inspiring only part of the ventilator-delivered tidal volume. One way for the clinician to estimate the relative size of the client's inspired tidal volume is to monitor the pressure gauge on the ventilator. The maximum pressure (at end-inspiration) should correlate with the volume inspired, at least to a first approximation. In the case of the client who uses a nosemask or facemask, an increase in the ventilator-delivered tidal volume may exacerbate leaks around the mask such that there may be no effective increase in the pulmonary tidal volume.

An increase in tidal volume may cause hyperventilation. One way to avoid hyperventilation is to reduce breathing rate. However, this may increase the pause duration between utterances, depending on how the client valves the expiratory volume (see comments above related to altered breathing rate). If the client is able to perceive hyperventilation (e.g., by symptoms such as light headedness or tingling), he may be able to use behavioral strategies to reduce his pulmonary tidal volume, at least temporarily. When using a mouthpiece, this can be done easily. The client merely reduces the pulmonary tidal volume by pulling away from the mouthpiece part way through the inspiration. When using a nosemask, the client can close his larynx part way through the inspiration and open his mouth to allow the remainder of the air to exit. When using a facemask, there is no easy way to reduce pulmonary tidal volume. The only option is to close his mouth and velopharynx and to allow the increasing pressure inside the mask to force a leak at the seal between the face and the mask, but this is not a practical option.

Decreased Inspiratory Time: When inspiratory time is decreased, the pause time between utterances should become shorter. Of course, this means that inspiratory flow will increase (if tidal volume remains the same), and a high inspiratory flow may cause the client discomfort. Thus, the goal is to determine the highest flow (i.e., shortest inspiratory time) that is comfortable for the client.

Breath Stacking

When using noninvasive positive pressure ventilation, it is better to use volume-controlled ventilation (in which a target volume is delivered) than pressure-controlled ventilation (in which a target pressure is delivered), at least for speech purposes. One reason is because volume-controlled ventilation allows the client to breath stack, something that is not possible with pressure-controlled ventilation.

Breath stacking can be an extremely useful strategy for clients who use noninvasive positive pressure ventilation. To stack breaths, the larynx is closed after a tidal breath is delivered. When the next inspiration begins, the larynx is opened to allow additional volume to be inspired, and then it is closed again, and so on. When the client wants to stack a partial breath rather than a full breath, he can do this in the ways discussed above for decreasing tidal volume. That is, if the client is using a mouthpiece, he pulls away from the mouthpiece part way through the inspiration. If the client is using a nosemask, he closes his larynx and opens his mouth part way through the inspiration. If the client is using a facemask, it may not be possible for him to stack a partial breath.

When a client breath stacks, he inspires a larger volume of air. Thus, the advantages to speech are the same as those discussed above for increasing tidal volume (i.e., longer and generally louder breath groups are possible). The major drawback to speech breathing is that speech initiation can be delayed substantially by the time required to inspire an additional breath. However, if the client does not expire fully after breath stacking, he may not need to inspire more than once for each subsequent speech inspiration.

Notes on Other Management Approaches for Speech Breathing with Noninvasive Positive Pressure Ventilation

Most of the management approaches indicated in Table 6-1 need no additional explanation regarding their application to clients who use noninvasive positive pressure ventilation. The exceptions are mechanical aids, mouthing and buccal speaking, and speech amplifiers. These are discussed briefly below.

In the case of noninvasive positive pressure ventilation, the primary reason for using a mechanical aid, such as a binder, is to decrease the compliance (increase the stiffness) of the breathing apparatus. Potential binder configurations for this purpose include an abdominal wall binder, a rib cage wall binder, both an abdominal wall binder and a rib cage wall binder, or a single binder that encompasses both the abdominal wall and the rib cage wall. By decreasing the compliance of the breathing apparatus with a binder, it may be possible to increase the relaxation pressure available for speech production when using volume-controlled ventilation. There are at least two advantages to this management approach. First, because inspiration is driven by the ventilator (and not the client), the decreased compliance of the breathing apparatus does not cost the client muscular effort during inspiration (as it would were the client having to generate inspiration with his own inspiratory muscles). Second, because a higher pressure is achieved without changing tidal volume, it is possible to avoid the hyperventilation that could accompany an increase in tidal volume (which is an alternative way to increase the available relaxation pressure). With greater relaxation pressure available, the client should be able to speak louder. This management approach is most appropriate for the client who uses a mouthpiece and who is able to achieve a strong lip seal around it. This approach may not be as well-suited to the client who uses a nosemask or facemask because the higher pressures associated with the decreased compliance of the breathing apparatus may exacerbate the air leaks around the masks.

There are two management approaches that are substantially affected by the presence of a facemask. One is mouthing and buccal speaking. Although mouthing and buccal speaking are reasonable options for clients who use a mouthpiece or a nosemask, they are not options for clients who use facemasks. The presence of a facemask makes it difficult to see mouth movements or to understand buccally produced speech. Another management approach that is strongly influenced by the presence of a facemask is the use of a speech amplifier. A client who wears a facemask would probably not benefit from an amplifier because, even if speech were amplified, the fidelity would remain poor.

Clinical Summary of Speech Breathing with Noninvasive Positive Pressure Ventilation

Speech breathing during noninvasive positive pressure ventilation differs substantially from speech breathing during invasive positive pressure ventilation and is more like normal speech breathing (when volume-controlled ventilation is used). Evaluation procedures are generally unremarkable, except that it is helpful to obtain a measure of breath-stacking capacity. Nearly all management approaches suggested in this book can be applied to the client who uses noninvasive positive pressure ventilation. Perhaps the most useful approaches are increased tidal volume or breath stacking, inspiratory muscle training, and glossopharyngeal breathing. All of these increase inspiratory volume and allow the client to speak in longer and generally louder breath groups. Binding the chest wall may also augment speech loudness. The best speech is produced when using a mouthpiece interface.

NEGATIVE PRESSURE VENTILATORS

The focus of this section is on negative pressure ventilators. Discussion covers negative pressure ventilation and how speech breathing with negative pressure ventilation is evaluated and managed.

Negative Pressure Ventilation

Humans and other animals with diaphragms use negative pressure ventilation. In contrast to positive pressure ventilation, in which air is pushed into the lungs, negative pressure ventilation pulls (or sucks) air into the lungs. Negative pressure ventilators operate such that their users continue to be negative pressure breathers.

Negative pressure ventilators were at their peak of clinical use during the poliomyelitis epidemic of the 20th century. The most widely recognized negative pressure ventilator is the iron lung (also called a tank respirator). The iron lung consists of a cylindrical tank that encases the body, except for the head. Air pressure inside the tank is lowered by a negative pressure generator (e.g., via a moveable diaphragm located at the foot end of the tank). As air pressure surrounding the body becomes increasingly subatmospheric, the breathing apparatus is sucked outward. As the breathing apparatus expands, the pressure within the pulmonary apparatus (alveolar pressure) lowers and air flows into the lungs (as long as the larynx and upper airway are open). Once alveolar pressure equals atmospheric pressure, inward flow stops. Outward flow begins as the breathing apparatus recoils back to its resting size, causing alveolar pressure to increase. This process mimics normal breathing, except that it occurs without activating breathing muscles.

Negative pressure ventilators come in less cumbersome forms than the iron lung. One is a cuirass (sometimes called a "chest shell") that fits over the anterior rib cage wall. Another is a body suit (sometimes called a "raincoat") made of flexible material that encases the entire upper torso, under which is worn a rigid grid designed to keep the material away from the body wall. Each of these is attached to a negative pressure generator and functions in a manner similar to an iron lung.

Negative pressure ventilation is most often used with clients who require intermittent and/or partial ventilatory support. Examples are clients with chronic obstructive pulmonary disease who need partial support, clients with central hypoventilation syndrome who need full support at night, and clients with neuromotor

---

GOING BACK TO WORK

Going back to work after injury is a big deal, both for the client and his healthcare providers. We've been personally touched by such a situation. He was from another nation and was not a person of means. He had suffered violence and his spinal cord was severely damaged. This meant a ventilator for life. When we met him, his speech was nonfunctional. We spent a lot of time working on ventilator-client adjustments to give him back his power of speech and power of self. He especially wanted to be able to talk on the telephone. It went well. He would brag on the ward about his regained ability and went out of his way to tell others that we had changed his life by reconnecting him to friends through the telephone. Calling one day to follow up on him, we were told by the attending nurse that his "zip code" had changed. He had been busted for dealing drugs. Make up your own moral to this story. We did.

disorders who need partial support periodically during the day to provide relief for fatigued breathing muscles. There are also clients who use negative pressure ventilation full-time and for full support, such as those who are quadriplegic from poliomyelitis.

Negative pressure ventilation is considered to be noninvasive ventilation because it does not require that the client have a tracheostomy. Nevertheless, some clients who use negative pressure ventilation do have a tracheostomy. Often this is to deal with obstructive sleep apnea. Obstructive sleep apnea can occur when breathing is no longer under sufficient central nervous system control, and the cyclical activation of laryngeal and upper airway muscles that usually accompanies breathing disappears. Without such activation, airway tissue becomes floppy and is easily sucked inward by the airway pressure drop associated with inspiratory flow. If the tissue approximates, the airway can obstruct. Clients with cranial nerve impairments (e.g., those with myasthenia gravis or Guillain-Barre syndrome) can experience laryngeal and upper airway obstruction even when awake. If the client has a tracheostomy, the danger of airway obstruction is circumvented.

During negative pressure ventilation, inspiration is driven mechanically by the ventilator. Some clients supplement inspiration using inspiratory muscular pressure. Speech is produced during expiration, as it is during normal speech breathing. Speech production is driven either solely or partially by relaxation pressure, depending on the client's residual muscle function. When expiration is driven by relaxation pressure alone, the magnitude of the prevailing alveolar pressure depends on the prevailing lung volume. The larger the lung volume, the higher the pressure. Also, when driven by relaxation pressure alone, expiration will end at the resting level of the breathing apparatus or at a larger volume. For expiration to end at a lung volume smaller than at the resting level of the breathing apparatus, expiratory muscular pressure is required. When relaxation pressure is supplemented with muscular pressure, alveolar pressure will depend on their sum.

Evaluation of Speech Breathing with Negative Pressure Ventilation

Much of the relevant information about the evaluation of speech breathing in clients who use ventilators has been covered in this chapter's section on general evaluation principles and methods. Selected issues that relate specifically to evaluating clients who use negative pressure ventilation are discussed here under major headings of ventilator analysis, auditory-perceptual examination, client perceptions, and physical examination.

Ventilator Analysis

The Ventilator Analysis form (Form 6-2) is used to note type of ventilator (negative pressure), mode of delivery (e.g., chest shell), and adjustment variables. The adjustments on negative pressure ventilators vary, with newer models generally having a greater range of adjustments than older models. The two adjustments found on essentially all negative pressure ventilators are breathing rate and peak negative (subatmospheric) inspiratory pressure. Additional adjustments are available on some ventilator models and include inspiratory time, expiratory time, and positive expiratory pressure. These adjustments are described here because of their potential value for improving speech.

Breathing Rate

Breathing rate can be adjusted in a negative pressure ventilator, just as it can in a positive pressure ventilator. Rate can be increased or decreased using control mode ventilation. This means that, once set, breathing rate is constant and completely controlled by the ventilator. Typical ranges for negative pressure ventilators are 10 to 30 breaths per minute.

Breathing rate can also be altered through the use of assist/control mode ventilation, which allows the client to trigger his own breaths. With assist/control, breathing rate may fluctuate breath-to-breath, depending on when the client activates the trigger function. To trigger a breath, the client must have adequate inspiratory muscle strength to generate a small pressure pulse. Cannulae are placed at the anterior nares (or tracheostomy, if the client has one) and attached at the other end to the generator. When the generator senses a negative pressure pulse, a breath is triggered.

Peak Negative Inspiratory Pressure

Peak negative inspiratory pressure translates roughly to tidal volume. In general, the greater the peak negative pressure, the larger the tidal volume. Peak negative pressure is determined, in association with breathing rate, to produce the appropriate level of ventilation for a given client. A typical adjustment range for peak negative pressure in a negative pressure ventilator is -5 to -80 cmH_2O.

Inspiratory Time and Expiratory Time

Some negative pressure ventilators, particularly older models, have a fixed inspiratory to expiratory (I:E) ratio. Thus, both inspiratory time and expiratory time are determined by the breathing rate. Typical fixed I:E ratios are 1:1 and 1:2, so that the inspiration occupies one-half or one-third of the breathing cycle. Other negative pressure ventilators allow the operator to adjust inspiratory time or I:E ratio independently of breathing rate, so that the inspiration can occupy variable portions of the cycle.

Positive Expiratory Pressure

Positive expiratory pressure is available on some negative pressure ventilators. When this adjustment is engaged, positive pressure is applied to the breathing apparatus during expiration. A typical range for positive expiratory pressure is 1 to 13 cmH_2O. The purpose of this adjustment is to aid the client with expiration.

Auditory-Perceptual Examination

The auditory-perceptual examination of the speech of clients with negative pressure ventilation is similar to that of clients who use noninvasive positive pressure ventilation. Thus, there is the potential for short utterance duration, long pause duration, low loudness, fading loudness, and pressed voice quality. The similarity in auditory-perceptual features is explained by the similarity in the expiratory (speaking) portion of the alveolar pressure waveforms associated with these two types of ventilation. Specifically, expiration is associated with a continually decreasing pressure, as long as the client relies on relaxation pressure only, without contribution from muscular pressure. As pressure decreases, loudness decreases until pressure drops below the minimum pressure required for vocal fold oscillation and voice ceases. The duration of a given utterance depends on the tidal volume inspired and how rapidly the volume is expired. If volume is expired slowly, the utterance may be long but the voice may sound pressed. The duration of the pause before the next utterance depends on the duration of the previous utterance, the duration of inspiration, the breathing rate set on the ventilator, and whether or not the client is able to trigger the ventilator to deliver breaths.

Client Perceptions

Speaking is not expected to cause hunger for air (or related percepts) in clients who use negative pressure ventilation. This is because speech is produced during expiration, after fresh air has already been delivered to the pulmonary apparatus. It is more likely that such a client would experience dyspnea associated with work/effort, especially if he triggers extra breaths or supplements the ventilator-delivered tidal volume with residual inspiratory muscular efforts.

The client who uses negative pressure ventilation may also experience perceptions of physical discomfort related to the ventilator. For example, if the client wears a cuirass, discomfort associated with pressure points might be exacerbated by certain ventilator adjustments. Or there may be air leaks that are perceptible to the client, and such leaks may increase or decrease with different management approaches.

Physical Examination

A physical examination of the breathing apparatus may be impossible to conduct on a client who uses a negative pressure ventilator, because the breathing apparatus is substantially or completely encased. It may be possible, however, to observe the client's neck to help judge if he is using accessory muscle activity during resting tidal breathing and/or speech breathing.

If the client has a tracheostomy, it should be fitted with a button. If it is open, there will be little pressure drive available for speech production. If a button is in place, it should be checked for leaks during expiration. Such leaks, if large enough, may compromise both the quantity and quality of speech.

Management of Speech Breathing with Negative Pressure Ventilation

There are several management approaches that may be useful for clients who use negative pressure ventilation. They are listed in Table 6-1 and include ventilator adjustments, exteroceptive feedback, economic valving, muscle training, glossopharyngeal breathing, relieving speaking-related dyspnea, monitoring gas exchange, mouthing and buccal speaking, conversational strategies, optimizing the environment, counseling, speech amplifiers, buttons and one-ways valves (if the client has a tracheostomy), and augmentative and alternative communication. These approaches have been covered previously (see Chapter 5 and previous sections of this chapter) and, in most cases, there is little qualification needed when applying them to clients who use negative pressure ventilation. However, ventilator adjustments associated with this form of ventilation warrant additional explanation and are discussed below.

Ventilator Adjustments

There are a few ventilator adjustments that have the potential to improve speech in clients who use negative pressure ventilators. These include increased breathing rate, increased peak negative inspiratory pressure (i.e., increased tidal volume), altered inspiratory time and/or expiratory time, and use of positive expiratory pressure.

Increased Breathing Rate

By increasing the ventilator's breathing rate, the client has more opportunities to speak over consecutive breaths. One way to increase rate is to do so directly using control mode ventilation. Increases should be made in small increments so as to minimize the effect on the client's ventilation. If the resultant increase in ventilation is a concern, the client's tidal volume can be reduced so that his usual minute ventilation is maintained. However, a tidal volume reduction is likely to offset the speech benefits of the increased breathing rate.

Another way to increase rate is to switch to assist/control mode ventilation. Assist/control mode ventilation makes it possible for the client to trigger extra breaths for speaking. Breathing rate usually returns to its control rate when

NO PINK SLIP YET

One of the sidetracks in Chapter 3 talks about Stetson's syllable pulse theory of speech breathing. Experimental phonetician Gordon Peterson offered a challenge to Stetson's theory by reporting on the relatively normal speech of an individual with paralyzed breathing muscles using an iron lung (Peterson, 1958). Some have taken this to be a refutation of Stetson's ideas concerning the syllable pulse and its association with linguistic stress. But it really isn't that easy a dismissal. Normal stressing can be achieved in ways that do not involve raising the alveolar pressure (e.g., raising fundamental frequency and increasing vowel duration). Many on ventilators do sound relatively normal, but investigations have yet to be conducted to examine whether or not the details of their acoustic outputs are comparable to able-bodied counterparts. Stetson doesn't deserve a pink slip yet. But we do see a dilly of a thesis or dissertation topic.

the client is resting. This reduces the risk of hyperventilation and provides the client with greater control over the timing of his speech.

Increased Peak Negative Pressure (i.e., Increased Tidal Volume)

With a negative pressure ventilator, tidal volume is adjusted by manipulating peak negative pressure. In general, tidal volume increases as peak negative pressure increases (i.e., becomes more negative). A larger tidal volume makes it possible for the client to produce longer breath groups. A larger tidal volume also increases the prevailing relaxation pressure at the beginning of expiration so that the client can speak louder, at least during the first part of the utterance. Increased tidal volume can cause hyperventilation and may necessitate a concomitant reduction in breathing rate for certain clients.

Altered Inspiratory Time and/or Expiratory Time

Some negative pressure ventilators have adjustments for inspiratory time and some have adjustments for both inspiratory and expiratory time. Even when there is no designated adjustment for expiratory time, expiratory time can be manipulated indirectly by adjusting inspiratory time and breathing rate to get the desired outcome. For inspiratory time, the goal is to adjust it to be as short as possible (but still comfortable for the client) so that the inspiratory pause between utterances is as short as possible. For expiratory time, the goal is to find the duration that best suits the client's manner of speaking. Primary determinants of this include the client's preferred length of utterance and the average expiratory flow (usually reflected in voice quality). If adjustments in inspiratory time and expiratory time result in a change in breathing rate, it may be necessary to also change tidal volume to maintain the client's usual ventilation.

Positive Expiratory Pressure

A positive expiratory pressure option is available on some negative pressure ventilators. With this option, positive (expiratory) pressure and negative (inspiratory) pressure cycle alternately. This extrinsically exerted positive pressure may benefit speech in those clients without functional expiratory muscles, especially during the latter part of expiration when the prevailing relaxation pressure is very low. An appropriate level of positive expiratory pressure should augment speech loudness, but should not be so high as to cause excessive loudness, particularly at the start of the utterance. Potential speech improvements include increased loudness, increased utterance length, improved voice quality, and, in some cases, more precise articulation and improved intelligibility.

Clinical Summary of Speech Breathing with Negative Pressure Ventilation

Negative pressure ventilation is more like normal breathing than positive pressure ventilation. Evaluation of this form of ventilator-supported speech breathing is generally similar to that of other forms, except that the ability to perform a physical examination of the breathing apparatus is usually quite limited. Several management approaches may improve speech breathing with negative pressure ventilation, including ventilator adjustments, muscle training, and glossopharyngeal breathing.

ROCKING BEDS

Rocking beds comprise a separate type of ventilator because they operate on different principles than positive pressure ventilators and negative pressure ventilators. This section covers rocking bed ventilation and issues pertinent to the evaluation and management of speech breathing in clients who use rocking beds.

Rocking Bed Ventilation

A rocking bed is a simple device consisting of a motor-driven bed that pitches up and down through a range of angles. The ability of the rocking bed to provide ventilation is based on the principle that gravity has a differential effect on the breathing apparatus, depending on the orientation of the body in a gravity field. Rocking bed ventilation is considered a noninvasive form of ventilation because it does not require that the client have a tracheostomy.

To use a rocking bed as a ventilator, the client is positioned on his back. The bed rocks through an arc that can range from a slightly head-down position to a nearly upright standing position. The specific range of angles can be varied and is selected to take into account the client's ventilation needs and comfort. As the client is rocked toward upright, the diaphragm-abdominal unit is pulled toward the foot of the bed. This action decreases alveolar pressure and causes air to flow into the pulmonary airways and lungs. As the client is rocked toward supine (or slightly head-down), the diaphragm-abdominal unit is pushed toward the head of the bed, causing alveolar pressure to increase and air to flow out. Thus, the client inspires and expires as the bed rocks up and down, respectively. Clients who are obese, excessively thin, or have skeletal deformities are not good candidates for rocking bed ventilation.

With rocking bed ventilation, speech is produced during the expiratory phase of the breathing cycle. In the client whose expiratory muscles are paralyzed, pressure for speech production is generated by relaxation pressure alone. The relaxation pressure is greatest at the beginning of expiration and is zero (atmospheric) at the end of expiration (assuming the larynx and upper airway are open). The magnitude of the pressure at any moment depends on lung volume and the position of the body as it rocks (because relaxation volume-pressure relations depend on body position). Speech can be produced as long as pressure is high enough to oscillate the vocal folds.

Evaluation of Speech Breathing with Rocking Bed Ventilation

Part of this chapter above covered the general principles of evaluation for clients with ventilators and Chapter 4 also covered evaluation procedures. Here, discussion focuses on issues related to ventilator analysis, auditory-perceptual examination, client perceptions, and instrumental examination for clients who use rocking bed ventilation.

Ventilator Analysis

Rocking beds have limited adjustment capabilities compared to the other ventilator systems discussed to this point. In fact, there are only two. One adjustment influences the range of angles through which the bed rocks. This is the primary determinant of tidal volume (Hill, 1994). The greatest tidal volume shifts tend to occur between supine and the 40° head-up angle. The second adjustment is rocking frequency, the major determinant of inspiratory and expiratory duration. Rocking frequency is also a secondary determinant of tidal volume. At frequencies above about 16 rocking cycles per minute, tidal volume tends to decrease as frequency increases (rocking angle range held constant). Typical rocking frequencies are from 12 to 16 per minute. Rocking speed is not differentially adjustable for the two directions, meaning that the inspiratory and expiratory duration cannot be adjusted independently. If using the Ventilator Analysis form (Form 6-2), rocking angle range should be noted on the Tidal Volume line and rocking frequency should be noted on the Breathing Rate line.

Auditory-Perceptual Examination

The most disconcerting aspect of evaluating a client with a rocking bed ventilator is that he is almost always moving, and the movements are quite large. This means that certain evaluation procedures need to be modified. During the auditory-perceptual examination, the clinician should be situated so as to be able to see and hear the client clearly. She may want to stand next to the rocking bed and perhaps lean over the client slightly to maintain an observational advantage throughout the rocking cycle. She may also want to perform the auditory-perceptual examination from other, less advantageous positions (e.g., standing behind the head of the rocking bed). This will allow her to determine the influence of listener position on the intelligibility of the client's speech.

Auditory-perceptual features of speech generated with rocking bed ventilation depend, in part, on whether or not the client has functional inspiratory muscles, functional expiratory muscles, or both. Assuming he has neither and that speech is produced using relaxation pressure alone, speech will most likely be characterized by short utterances, long pauses, low loudness, and fading loudness. Voice quality may be pressed if the client uses high laryngeal airway resistance to conserve air during speech production. As with other types of ventilator-supported speech, these auditory-perceptual features can be linked to the prevailing pressure.

Client Perceptions

Client perceptions may not be particularly revealing during the evaluation, because clients who use rocking beds are not expected to experience discomfort with speaking. Nevertheless, their perceptions should be recorded, because it may be that certain management strategies may influence such perceptions. For example, if management includes inspiratory muscle training for supplementing tidal volume, the client may experience a change in work/effort associated with speaking. In addition to the usual perceptual information obtained, the clinician should also question the client regarding his perception of the bed's rock. This baseline perceptual information may become important in the event the client is managed using adjustments to the arc or frequency of the rock.

Instrumental Examination

An instrumental examination is tricky to implement when the client is on a rocking bed. For this reason, the instrumental examination may be omitted, with the exception of continuous monitoring of oxygen saturation. Most other instrumental measures are difficult to obtain or are not expected to offer significant insights with clients who use rocking beds.

If an instrumental examination is conducted, it will require special modifications. Most notably, any leads that couple the client to instruments must be adequately long. This should be carefully ascertained before connecting the client. Also, if high-quality recordings of speech are considered an important feature of the evaluation, they are best made with a head-mounted microphone (or a bed-mounted microphone) so that a constant mouth-to-microphone distance can be maintained throughout the rocking cycle.

Management of Speech Breathing with Rocking Bed Ventilation

Management strategies that could apply to clients who use rocking beds are listed in Table 6-1. They include ventilator adjustments, economical valving, muscle training, glossopharyngeal breathing, mouthing and buccal speaking, conversational strategies, optimizing the environment, counseling, speech amplifiers, buttons and one-ways valves (if the client has a tracheostomy), and augmentative and alternative communication. These have been discussed in Chapter 5 and elsewhere in this chapter (see section on general principles and methods for managing ventilator-supported speech breathing). Some brief comments are offered below regarding ventilator adjustments and other selected management approaches.

Ventilator Adjustments

There are only two possible adjustments on a rocking bed ventilator: range of angles through which the bed swings (tidal volume) and rocking frequency (breathing rate). Adjustment in either or both of these may improve speech (e.g., by increasing utterance length or decreasing the lengths of pauses between utterances). However, only minor adjustments, if any, may be possible, because of ventilation constraints or client discomfort. It is important to keep in mind that adjusting tidal volume and/or breathing rate entail changes in movement of the entire body and may not be tolerated for reasons unrelated to breathing.

Notes on Other Management Approaches for Speech Breathing with Rocking Bed Ventilation

Use of a rocking bed for ventilation presents physical challenges that influence certain aspects of management. Two of these relate to optimizing the environment and to use of a speech amplifier.

The position of the conversational partner is an important consideration when optimizing the communication environment of a client who uses a rocking bed. Because the client is rocking continuously, it may be impossible for a conversational partner to maintain a full-face view throughout the rocking cycle. If the conversational partner sits near the head of the bed, the client's face will be out of view during much of the rocking cycle. The best view of the client can be achieved if the conversational partner is positioned at the side of the bed, slightly toward its foot, and oriented approximately 45° toward the client. The view is further improved if the conversational partner stands upright or sits on a high stool, rather than in a low chair. This makes it easier to make eye contact with the client and for the client to see the face of the conversational partner. If a conversational partner is not able to assume the position suggested (e.g., he/she uses a wheelchair), then it may be necessary to modify certain management approaches. For example, the lack of continuous eye contact may render ineffective strategies such as mouthing, buccal speaking, or nonver-

---

CONTEMPT OF COURT

Conversational interchange is a wonderful thing. The ebb and flow is effortless and those involved in it give the process hardly any thought. Much of the ability to engage in interchange depends on the breathing apparatus. This becomes especially apparent when the apparatus is impaired. Two paralyzed speakers on rocking beds are a good example. Each can speak only during the down rock of the bed. Make the two beds rock 180° out of phase (move in opposite directions up and down) and the two speakers can carry on a conversation quite well, albeit with short phrases. Make the two beds rock in phase (go up and down together) and the two speakers must compete for the same limited "air time." A conversation can proceed, but it begins to sound a bit more like two ill-mannered attorneys trying to talk over one another on a confrontational television talk show.

bal signaling.

Speech amplifiers may be useful for clients who use rocking beds and whose speech intelligibility is impaired by low loudness. However, special consideration must be given to the physical set-up. The microphone must be placed near the mouth and secured so that it does not dislodge with the substantial movements of the client. The loudspeaker component, rather than being fixed to the client or to the bed, is best positioned next to the rocking bed. This helps avoid damage to the loudspeaker and provides a stable sound source for the listener.

Clinical Summary of Speech Breathing with Rocking Bed Ventilation

Evaluation of the speech breathing of a client who uses a rocking bed relies primarily on auditory-perceptual judgments and little on instrumental examination. Management of this form of speech breathing is most likely to be focused on behavioral interventions such as muscle training, glossopharyngeal breathing, economical valving, and conversational strategies.

ABDOMINAL PNEUMOBELTS

Abdominal pneumobelts (also called exsufflation belts) provide yet another form of ventilatory support. This section covers abdominal pneumobelt ventilation and suggests ways to evaluate and manage the speech breathing of clients who use abdominal pneumobelts.

Abdominal Pneumobelt Ventilation

Abdominal pneumobelt ventilation, although not as widely used as positive pressure ventilation or negative pressure ventilation, can be very effective for certain clients. Like the rocking bed, the function of the abdominal pneumobelt depends on the influence of gravity on the breathing apparatus. In fact, rocking beds and abdominal pneumobelts are sometimes classified together as "abdominal displacement ventilators" (Mehta & Hill, 2001). Abdominal pneumobelt ventilation is considered to be a noninvasive form of ventilation because a tracheostomy is not required for its use.

The pneumobelt, depicted in Figure 6-4, consists of an inflatable bladder (resembling a blood-pressure cuff) that overlies the anterior abdomen and is secured by a corset that encircles the entire abdomen. A positive pressure ventilator inflates the bladder. As the bladder inflates, it squeezes air out of the pulmonary apparatus by displacing the abdominal wall inward, pushing the diaphragm headward, and raising alveolar pressure. The bladder is then allowed to deflate and the diaphragm to recoil footward. This decreases alveolar pressure and causes air to flow back into pulmonary apparatus. Thus, expiration is driven by inflation of the bladder and compression of the breathing apparatus, and inspiration is driven by relaxation pressure of the breathing apparatus. For the abdominal pneumobelt to ventilate effectively, the client must be seated upright at an angle no greater than 45° off-vertical. Clients who are obese, overly thin, or have certain structural abnormalities are usually not good candidates for abdominal pneumobelt use.

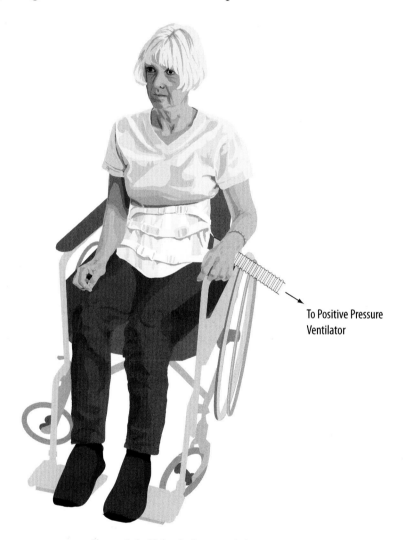

To Positive Pressure Ventilator

Figure 6-4. Abdominal pneumobelt.

Speech is produced during expiration with abdominal pneumobelt ventilation. Clients who have residual muscle function may augment the ventilator-generated tidal volume. In such cases, the client must learn to synchronize his own breathing efforts with the actions of the pneumobelt.

Evaluation of Speech Breathing with Abdominal Pneumobelt Ventilation

Evaluation of speech breathing in clients who use abdominal pneumobelt ventilation follows the general guidelines offered at the beginning of this chapter. Specific comments pertaining to ventilator analysis and auditory-perceptual examination are offered below.

Ventilator Analysis

Abdominal pneumobelts are driven by positive pressure ventilators. Thus, when using the Ventilator Analysis form (Form 6-2), the type of ventilator is positive pressure and the method of delivery is abdominal pneumobelt. Breathing rate is set using control-mode ventilation and can be read directly from the ventilator. By contrast, the tidal volume delivered by the ventilator is not the client's tidal volume. The client's tidal volume is more closely related to the peak bladder inflation pressure. Thus, when noting the client's usual tidal volume on the form, it is useful to note the peak bladder inflation pressure as indicated by the airway pressure gauge on the ventilator.

Auditory-Perceptual Examination

The auditory-perceptual examination of speech produced with abdominal pneumobelt ventilation can reveal speech ranging from essentially normal to impaired. If laryngeal and upper airway functions are intact and if at least some expiratory muscle is spared, speech may sound nearly normal. If the expiratory muscles are paralyzed so that alveolar pressure is dependent on relaxation pressure and the actions of the ventilator, speech may be of low loudness. Shorter-than-normal speech duration and longer-than-normal pause duration are also typical of this form of ventilator-supported speech. These speech signs can be explained by the fact that alveolar pressure may be high enough to produce speech during only part of the breathing cycle. As the bladder inflates, alveolar pressure rises and may remain relatively stable during the expiration (during speaking). When the ventilator's inspiration ceases, the expiration valve on the ventilator opens, the bladder deflates, and alveolar pressure falls rapidly.

Management of Speech Breathing with Abdominal Pneumobelt Ventilation

There are several management approaches that can benefit clients who use abdominal pneumobelt ventilation. As shown in Table 6-1, they are ventilator adjustments, exteroceptive feedback, economical valving, muscle training, glossopharyngeal breathing, relieving speaking-related dyspnea, monitoring gas exchange, mouthing and buccal speaking, conversational strategies, optimizing the environment, counseling, speech amplifiers, buttons and one-way valves (if the client has a tracheostomy), and augmentative and alternative communication. Discussed below are issues related to ventilator adjustments and some notes on other management approaches for speech produced with abdominal pneumobelt ventilation.

Ventilator Adjustments

There are a few ventilator adjustments that may improve speech in a client who uses an abdominal pneumobelt. Ventilator adjustments for positive pressure devices have already been discussed (see section on positive pressure ventilators). However, it is important to recognize that adjusting a positive pressure ventilator to drive an abdominal pneumobelt usually has a substantially different effect on the client than when that same adjustment is applied directly to the airway (either via a tracheostomy or via the upper airway).

Tightened Pneumobelt

It may be possible to increase a client's speech loudness by tightening the abdominal pneumobelt around him. A tightened pneumobelt may increase the client's ability to generate expiratory pressure and, thereby, increase his ability to generate louder speech. However, this strategy has limits. The pneumobelt cannot be too tight or it will not be able to displace an adequately large tidal volume, and it cannot be so tight that it causes the client discomfort.

ARTHUR A. SIEBENS (1921–1996)

Arthur A. Siebens was a driving force behind the management of individuals with spinal cord injury and had a strong interest in the treatment of their communication disorders. He was Chair of the Department of Rehabilitation Medicine at the University of Wisconsin when the first of us was a faculty member there and he later moved east to head up a similar program at Johns Hopkins University. Siebens was an innovative researcher and clinician. He did pioneering work on a device that eliminated the confounding cardiac signal from electromyographic recordings of the diaphragm and worked on problems of mechanical degrees of freedom of the paralyzed chest wall. He is fondly remembered for his motorcycle travels around Madison, Wisconsin, during which he always wore a flowing red scarf and seemed to embody Snoopy's characterization of the Red Baron. Art was a friend to all who were physically impaired. He had an important life.

Increased Breathing Rate

Breathing rate can be increased by adjusting the ventilator (using control-mode ventilation). If breathing rate is increased (and tidal volume remains unchanged), it may be possible for the client to produce more speech over consecutive breathing cycles. When attempting this adjustment, small increases should be used (e.g., 1 breath per minute). The degree to which breathing rate can be increased may depend, in part, on ventilator expiratory time (which is client inspiratory time), because the client must have time to fully inspire.

Increased Tidal Volume

Tidal volume can be adjusted directly on some ventilators and indirectly on others (by adjusting minute ventilation along with breathing rate). When adjusting tidal volume for a client with an abdominal pneumobelt, the target variable is airway pressure (this is the inflation pressure of the bladder). In general (and within a range), the higher the airway pressure, the larger the tidal volume of the client. The potential advantage of increased tidal volume is that speaking time per breath may be longer. However, it may not be possible to increase tidal volume because of client discomfort. This is because, when the tidal volume is greater, the pressure exerted on the abdominal wall and the abdominal content is greater.

Lengthened Ventilator Inspiratory Time (Lengthened Client Expiratory Time)

A typical inspiratory-to-expiratory (I:E) ratio for an abdominal pneumobelt ventilator is 1.5:1 (or a client I:E ratio of 1:1.5). In some cases, it may benefit speech to lengthen the ventilator inspiratory time so as to increase client expiratory time. The potential benefit is longer speaking time per breath. Nevertheless, it is important to realize that if this adjustment is made without altering tidal volume, flow will be lower and, therefore, bladder inflation speed will be slower. Reduced bladder inflation speed may result in a reduction in speech loudness.

Increased Ventilator Inspiratory Flow (Increased Client Expiratory Flow)

Most positive pressure ventilators allow adjustment of the ventilator-delivered inspiratory flow. In clients with soft speech, increased ventilator inspiratory flow (i.e., increased client expiratory flow) may help augment loudness. Of course, without an associated increase in tidal volume, this adjustment could also have the disadvantage of reducing potential speaking (expiratory) time.

Notes on Other Management Approaches for Speech Breathing with Abdominal Pneumobelt Ventilation

Issues regarding certain management approaches for speech breathing with an abdominal pneumobelt require additional comment. These relate to the behavior of the larynx during speech breathing and the effect of active inspiratory muscular efforts on speech breathing. The behavior of the larynx has a substantial influence on alveolar pressure during expiration. If the larynx remains open while the pneumobelt's bladder inflates, volume is expired rapidly and alveolar pressure is positive, but low. If the larynx is closed at or before the moment the bladder begins to inflate, no volume is expired and alveolar pressure builds rapidly. Thus, by closing the larynx before bladder inflation begins, the client is able to initiate speech production early in the expiration and with a substantial positive alveolar pressure. This should allow loudness to build early in the utterance, as well as help increase speech duration and decrease pause duration.

One of the most important management approaches for all types of ventilator-supported speech breathing involves the development of strategies to supplement the ventilator-delivered inspiration (and to be able to breathe independently in case the ventilator fails). This is also true for speech supported by abdominal pneumobelt ventilation. However, the effect on alveolar pressure is somewhat different than it is for the other forms of ventilation. When the bladder deflates, the breathing apparatus inspires to its resting volume. The client can further inspire the breathing apparatus by using inspiratory muscular effort, glossopharyngeal breathing, or a combination of the two. At the termination of the active inspiration, the client can close the larynx to create a positive alveolar pressure (because relaxation pressure is positive at this lung volume). Then, as the ventilator-driven expiration begins, the bladder pressure adds to this already existing pressure. In this way, it may be possible to increase the pressure for speech production and, thereby, increase speech loudness.

Clinical Summary of Speech Breathing with Abdominal Pneumobelt Ventilation

Some clients who use abdominal pneumobelt ventilation have good speech, whereas others may have speech that is inadequately loud and broken by long pauses. Evaluation follows the same general procedures as those described for other forms of ventilator-supported speech breathing. Management may include a combination of ventilator adjustments and behavioral strategies. Ventilator adjustments are not as powerful for improving speech as they are when positive pressure ventilation is delivered at an airway opening, but they may be helpful in certain cases. Behavioral strategies that facilitate inspiratory supplementation (i.e., inspiratory muscle training and glossopharyngeal breathing) are important components of management for clients who use abdominal pneumobelt ventilation. When low loudness cannot be remediated using these management approaches, a speech amplifier may be the best solution.

PHRENIC NERVE PACERS

Phrenic nerve pacers (sometimes called diaphragmatic pacers) are not mechanical ventilators like the others discussed so far. Rather, they are neural prostheses that activate the phrenic nerves. This section covers issues related to phrenic nerve pacer ventilation and how speech breathing is evaluated and managed in clients who use this form of ventilation.

Phrenic Nerve Pacer Ventilation

Phrenic nerve pacer ventilation has been used clinically for long-term ventilatory support for several decades (Judson & Glenn, 1968). As shown in Figure 6-5, the phrenic nerve pacer consists of an electrode placed behind a phrenic nerve and a radiofrequency receiver implanted beneath the skin. The receiver is coupled

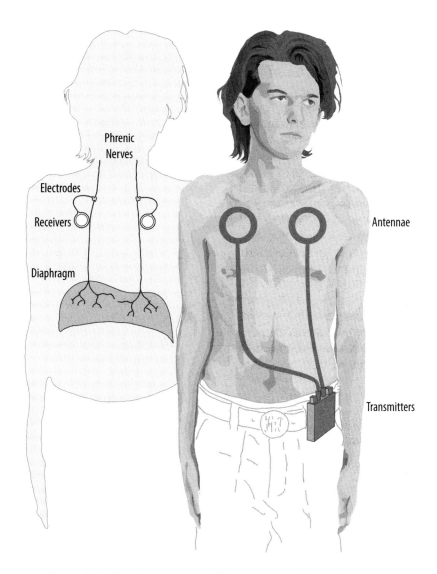

Figure 6-5. Phrenic nerve pacers. (After www.averylabs.com)

inductively to a radiofrequency transmitter located outside the body. Pacers can be implanted to stimulate both phrenic nerves. When the phrenic nerves are stimulated, the diaphragm contracts and alveolar pressure lowers. Air flows into the pulmonary apparatus in essentially the same way it does during normal inspiration, although the flow pattern is somewhat different. Once stimulation ceases, the breathing apparatus recoils back to its resting size, thereby driving air back out of the pulmonary apparatus. Stimulation variables for phrenic nerve pacers include pulse frequency, pulse train duration, and pulse train repetition rate. These are set to meet the client's ventilation requirements. Such variables are usually set to maximize tidal volume.

Most people who use phrenic nerve pacers have high cervical spinal cord injury

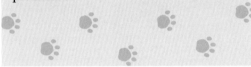

or central hypoventilation syndrome. Those with spinal cord injury generally use the pacers around-the-clock, whereas those with central hypoventilation syndrome generally use them only while sleeping. A tracheostomy is not needed with phrenic nerve pacers, however, most who use pacers have one. A tracheostomy makes it easier for caregivers to perform pulmonary hygiene tasks (e.g., suctioning) and for the user to switch to positive pressure ventilation when necessary (e.g., when having the pacers serviced or when a severe pulmonary infection requires more ventilation than that provided by the pacers).

During phrenic nerve pacing, speech is produced during the expiratory phase of the breathing cycle. In many clients, the tracheostomy is occluded so that inspiratory flow and expiratory flow are routed through the upper airway. In clients who have a one-way (inspiratory) valve in the tracheostomy, inspiratory flow is routed primarily through the tracheostomy and expiratory flow is routed through the upper airway. It is critical that the tracheostomy be occluded during expiration for adequate speech to be produced.

Evaluation of Speech Breathing with Phrenic Nerve Pacer Ventilation

The essential points concerning the evaluation of clients with phrenic nerve pacers have been covered in the general section on evaluation of clients with ventilators. Nevertheless, a few additional comments regarding ventilator analysis and auditory-perceptual examination are offered here.

Ventilator Analysis

Pacer parameters, once set, are generally not changed. Thus, no ventilator analysis is necessary because ventilator adjustments are not used to improve speech in clients with phrenic nerve pacers. Nevertheless, it may be a good idea to make a note of the values for the pacer stimulation variables (pulse frequency, pulse train duration, pulse train repetition rate) and whether the pacer(s) is/are unilateral or bilateral (simultaneous or alternating), in the event the pacers are changed later.

Auditory-Perceptual Examination

As with all other types of ventilators, the auditory-perceptual features of the speech of a client who uses phrenic nerve pacers can be linked to the pressure waveform. In the client who relies on relaxation pressure alone (without active muscular contribution), pressure decreases continuously during expiration. Utterance can continue until pressure drops below the voicing threshold. In a client without expiratory muscle function, utterance duration is determined by the tidal volume and the resistance offered to airflow by downstream structures during speech production.

Common auditory-perceptual features of speech in clients who use phrenic nerve pacers are low loudness, fading loudness, and long inspirations (Hoit & Shea, 1996). Other features can include short utterance duration or pressed voice quality. If the client has spared expiratory muscle function, speech can be essentially normal (with the exception of longer-than-usual inspirations).

Management of Speech Breathing with Phrenic Nerve Pacer Ventilation

Most of the management approaches described in Chapter 5 and in the present chapter can benefit clients who use phrenic nerve pacers. These include breath stacking, exteroceptive feedback, economic valving, body positioning, mechanical aids, muscle training, glossopharyngeal breathing, relieving speaking-related dyspnea, monitoring gas exchange, mouthing and buccal speaking, conversational strategies, optimizing the environment, counseling, speech amplifiers, buttons and one-way valves (if the client has a tracheostomy), and augmentative and alternative communication. Below are some brief comments on breath stacking and other selected management approaches.

Breath Stacking

Some clients with phrenic nerve pacers may be able to breath stack (as long as there is no tracheostomy or the tracheostomy is occluded during expiration). To breath stack, the client closes his larynx at the end of inspiration and keeps it closed until the beginning of the next inspiration. When the next inspiration begins, the client opens his larynx and allows some air to flow in. It may not be possible to stack a full breath (because the prevailing expiratory relaxation pressure may overcome the inspiratory pressure). Another way to breath stack is to produce glossopharyngeal breaths immediately after the phrenically stimulated inspiration ends. Either method of breath stacking will increase the available volume and pressure for speech production (and, therefore, increase breath group length and loudness).

Notes on Other Management Approaches for Speech Breathing with Phrenic Nerve Pacer Ventilation

There are some additional comments to be made regarding body positioning and mechanical aids in clients with phrenic nerve pacers. These are offered below.

Clients with phrenic nerve pacers who do not have functional expiratory muscle may produce better speech when in the supine body position. This is because the abdomen drives the diaphragm headward and stretches its fibers. Given the same stimulator input, a stretched diaphragm creates a greater negative pressure change and a larger tidal volume. The larger the tidal volume, the longer and louder the speech can be. This does not mean that a client should be advised to remain in a supine body position, but it does mean that moving him toward supine might benefit speech. For example, a semi-recumbent (off-vertical toward supine) seated position might be preferable to an erect upright seated position.

Mechanical aids that can improve the speech of clients who use phrenic nerve pacers are those that displace the abdominal wall inward. Inward abdominal wall displacement stretches the fibers of the diaphragm so that a greater negative pressure change is produced for a given stimulus, and a greater pressure change can generate a larger tidal volume. With a larger tidal volume, utterance can be longer. Also, expiratory relaxation pressure is greater so that speech can be louder, at least at the beginning of the expiration. Abdominal support not only can make speech longer and louder, it can also reduce the effort to speak in cases where the increased tidal volume relieves the client of the need to engage his own inspiratory efforts during speech breathing (Hoit, Banzett, & Brown, 2002).

Clinical Summary of Speech Breathing with Phrenic Nerve Pacer Ventilation

Of all the forms of ventilation discussed in this chapter, phrenic nerve pacing most closely resembles normal speech breathing, at least for the inspiratory phase of the speech breathing cycle. This is because the diaphragm drives inspiration, like it does under normal circumstances. However, without additional internal (muscular) or external (mechanical) pressure contributions, speech will not be normal. Evaluation of speech breathing is conducted as described in Chapter 4 and other parts of this chapter, except that there is no need for a formal ventilator analysis. Potential management approaches are numerous, although ventilator adjustments are not among them. Perhaps one of the best means of improving speech breathing in clients who use phrenic nerve pacers is to combine inspiratory muscle training, glossopharyngeal breathing, and the use of abdominal support. This combination provides an effective way to augment inspired volume so that breath groups can be longer and louder, often with a reduction in work/effort.

SUMMARY OF VENTILATOR-SUPPORTED SPEECH BREATHING

The focus of this chapter has been on how to evaluate and manage speech breathing in clients who use ventilators. As background to its focus, this chapter has provided general coverage of the topic of ventilatory support for each of the five types of ventilators discussed. Nevertheless, clinicians responsible for providing services to clients who use ventilators are strongly advised to seek additional knowledge of ventilatory support, the nature of such support for various diseases and conditions, and the specific characteristics of currently available ventilators. For speech-language pathologists, much can be learned through interactions with pulmonologists and respiratory therapists, and by further reading about the principles and practices associated with ventilatory support (Kirby, Banner, & Downs, 1990; Tobin, 1994), the role of the speech-language pathologist in the care of clients who use ventilatory support (Tippett, 2000; Dikeman & Kazandjian, 2002), and the personal experiences of people who have lived with ventilatory support (Sternburg & Sternburg, 1986; Reeve, 1998; Hankins, 2003).

The five types of ventilators discussed in this chapter – positive pressure ventilators (using invasive and noninvasive client-ventilator coupling), negative pressure ventilators, rocking beds, abdominal pneumobelts, and phrenic nerve pacers – have different mechanisms of action for breathing and speech production. These are summarized in Table 6-2. For inspiration, air can be pushed (positive pressure ventilators) or sucked (negative pressure ventilators, rocking beds, abdominal pneumobelts, and phrenic nerve pacers) into the pulmonary apparatus. For expiration, air can be driven out of the pulmonary apparatus by positive relaxation pressure (positive pressure ventilators, negative pressure ventilators, and phrenic nerve pacers), by gravitational drive to the diaphragm-abdomen unit (rocking beds), or by externally applied pressure to the abdominal wall (abdominal pneumobelts). Speech is produced during expiration in all cases, except with invasive positive pressure ventilation, wherein speech is produced during both inspiration and expiration. The alveolar pressure associated with speech production (assuming no muscular pressure contribution) can rise and fall sharply to zero (positive pressure ventilators using invasive client-ventilator coupling), continuously decrease to zero (positive pressure ventilators using noninvasive client-ventilator coupling, negative pressure ventilators, rocking beds, and phrenic nerve pacers), or change gradually (abdominal pneumobelts). The auditory-perceptual features of ventilator-supported speech can be explained, in large part, by the nature of the alveolar pressure waveform. Several of the management approaches suggested in this chapter are designed to modify this pressure waveform in ways that can improve speech.

The ability to speak has a profound impact on quality of life. Perhaps this is especially true of clients who use ventilators. Because the physical impairments of these clients can be so limiting, it is often the ability to speak which can open doors that would otherwise be closed to them. There are many ways to improve speech in clients who use ventilators, as described in this chapter. Many of these management approaches influence ventilation and other aspects of breathing function, and, therefore, must be carried out with extreme care and with the direct oversight of a pulmonologist. Fortunately, it is often the case that a client's ventilation concerns and his speech concerns can be addressed simultaneously. For this reason, the clini-

Table 6-2. Speech breathing for each of the five types of ventilators.

	Positive Pressure Ventilators with Invasive Coupling	Positive Pressure Ventilators with Noninvasive Coupling	Negative Pressure Ventilators	Rocking Beds	Abdominal Pneumobelts	Phrenic Nerve Pacers
Inspiration	Air is pushed in through the tracheostomy	Air is pushed in through the upper airway	Chest wall is sucked outward and air is sucked in	Gravity pulls the diaphragm-abdomen footward while rocking toward upright and air is sucked in	Bladder deflates and air is sucked in by negative relaxation pressure	Phrenic nerves are stimulated to contract the diaphragm and air is sucked in
Expiration	Relaxation pressure pushes air out	Relaxation pressure pushes air out	Relaxation pressure pushes air out	Gravity pulls the diaphragm-abdomen headward while rocking toward supine and air is pushed out	Bladder inflates and pushes air out	Relaxation pressure pushes air out
Speech Production	Inspiration and expiration	Expiration	Expiration	Expiration	Expiration	Expiration
Alveolar Pressure Waveform for Speech Production (without muscular pressure)	Rising to peak, then falling to zero (volume-controlled)	Continuously decreasing to zero (volume-controlled)	Continuously decreasing to zero	Continuously decreasing to zero	Gradually changing	Continuously decreasing to zero

cal decision-making process of selecting and configuring a client's ventilation system can benefit substantially from the input of the speech-language pathologist.

REVIEW

A ventilator is a device that supplements or replaces spontaneous breathing and which can be used to support speech breathing in clients who cannot breathe on their own.

Ventilators come in a variety of forms that range from mechanical to neuroprosthetic and they can be used with adults, children, and infants.

Ventilators, and the clients who use them, constitute a system that must be evaluated and managed as a unit through a team effort involving the pulmonologist, the respiratory therapist, the speech-language pathologist, and others.

General principles and methods apply to the evaluation and management of ventilator-supported speech breathing, but different types of ventilators have unique features that must be taken into account.

Positive pressure ventilators push air into the pulmonary apparatus, either through a tracheostomy (invasive) or through the upper airway (noninvasive).

Negative pressure ventilators pull air into the pulmonary apparatus by lowering pressure around the breathing apparatus and sucking it outward.

Rocking bed ventilators take advantage of the pull of gravity on the abdominal content and move air into and out of the pulmonary apparatus.

Abdominal pneumobelt ventilators encircle the abdominal wall and squeeze air out of the breathing apparatus (expiration) during their activation.

Phrenic nerve pacer ventilators are implanted electrical devices that stimulate the nerve(s) that control the diaphragm, causing it to contract and inspire the breathing apparatus.

For all of the ventilators discussed, the potential impact of their use on speech breathing has much to do with the pressure waveform and how it can be altered to enhance speech and maintain adequate ventilation.

Because the physical impairments of clients on ventilators can be so limiting, improvements made in their speech can often have a profound impact on their quality of life.

The speech-language pathologist has a central role in the evaluation and management of ventilator-supported speech breathing and is the primary team resource on matters pertaining to communication.

REFERENCES

Bach, J. (2002). *Noninvasive mechanical ventilation.* Philadelphia, PA: Hanley and

Belfus, Inc.

Bach, J., & Alba, A. (1990). Tracheostomy ventilation: A study of efficacy with deflated cuffs and cuffless tubes. *Chest, 97*, 679-683.

Bach, J., & Campagnolo, D. (1992). Psychosocial adjustment of post-poliomyelitis ventilator assisted individuals. *Archives of Physical Medicine and Rehabilitation, 73*, 934-939.

Bach, J., Campagnolo, D., & Hoeman, S. (1991). Life satisfaction of individuals with Duchene muscular dystrophy using long-term mechanical ventilatory support. *American Journal of Physical Medicine and Rehabilitation, 70*, 129-135.

Bach, J., Haber, I., Wang, T., & Alba, A. (1995). Alveolar ventilation as a function of ventilatory support method. *European Journal of Physical Medicine and Rehabilitation, 5*, 80-84.

Dikeman, K., & Kazandjian, M. (2002). *Communication and swallowing management of tracheostomized and ventilator-dependent adults.* (2nd ed.), Clifton Park, NY: Thompson-Delmar Learning.

DiMarco, A., Onders, R., Kowalski, K., Miller, M., Ferek, S., & Mortimer, J. (2002). Phrenic nerve pacing in a tetraplegic patient via intramuscular diaphragm electrodes. *American Journal of Respiratory Critical Care Medicine, 166*, 1604-1606.

Hankins, G. (2003). *Rolling on: The story of the amazing Gary McPherson.* Edmonton, Alberta: The University of Alberta Press.

Hill, N. (1994). Use of the rocking bed, pneumobelt, and other noninvasive aids to ventilation. In M. Tobin (Ed.), *Principles and practice of mechanical ventilation* (pp. 413-425). New York, NY: McGraw-Hill.

Hoit, J., & Banzett, R. (1997). Simple adjustments can improve ventilator-supported speech. *American Journal of Speech-Language Pathology, 6*, 87-96.

Hoit, J., & Banzett, R. (2003). Je peux parler! *American Journal of Respiratory and Critical Care Medicine, 167*, 101-102.

Hoit, J., Banzett, R., & Brown, R. (2002). Binding the abdomen can improve speech in men with phrenic nerve pacers. *American Journal of Speech-Language Pathology, 11*, 71-76.

Hoit, J., Banzett, R., Lohmeier, H., Hixon, T., & Brown, R. (2003). Clinical ventilator adjustments that improve speech. *Chest, 124*, 1512-1521.

Hoit, J., & Shea, S. (1996). Speech production and speech with a phrenic nerve pacer. *American Journal of Speech-Language Pathology, 5*, 53-60.

Hoit, J., Shea, S., & Banzett, R. (1994). Speech production during mechanical ventilation in tracheostomized individuals. *Journal of Speech and Hearing Research, 37*, 53-63.

Isaki, E., & Hoit, J. (1997). Ventilator-supported communication: A survey of speech-language pathologists. *Journal of Medical Speech-Language Pathology, 5*, 263-272.

Judson, J., & Glenn, W. (1968). Radiofrequency electrophrenic respiration: Long-term application to a patient with primary hypoventilation. *Journal of the American Medical Association, 203*, 1033-1037.

Kang, S., & Bach, J. (2000). Maximum insufflation capacity: The relationships with vital capacity and cough flows for patients with neuromuscular disease. *American Journal of Physical Medicine and Rehabilitation, 79*, 222-227.

Kirby, R., Banner, M., & Downs, J. (Eds.) (1990). *Clinical applications of ventilatory support.* New York, NY: Churchill Livingstone.

Lohmeier, H., & Hoit, J. (2003). Ventilator-supported communication: A survey of ventilator users. *Journal of Medical Speech-Language Pathology, 11*, 61-72.

Mehta, S., & Hill, N. (2001). Noninvasive ventilation. *American Journal of Respiratory and Critical Care Medicine, 163*, 540-577.

Peterson, G. (1958). Some observations on speech. *Quarterly Journal of Speech, 44*, 402-412.

Prigent, H., Samuel, C., Louis, B., Abinun, M., Zerah-Lancner, F., Lejaille, M., Raphael, J., & Lofaso, F. (2003). Comparative effects of two ventilatory modes on speech in tracheostomized patients with neuromuscular disease. *American Journal of Respiratory and Critical Care Medicine, 167*, 114-119.

Reeve, C. (1998). *Still me.* New York, NY: Random House.

Shea, S., Hoit, J., & Banzett, R. (1998). Competition between gas exchange and speech production in ventilated subjects. *Biological Psychology, 49*, 9-27.

Sternburg, L., & Sternburg, D. (1986). *View from the seesaw.* New York, NY: Dodd, Mead.

Tippett, D. (Ed.) (2000). *Tracheostomy and ventilator dependency: Management of breathing, speaking, and swallowing.* New York, NY: Thieme.

Tippett, D., & Siebens, A. (1995). Preserving oral communication in individuals with tracheostomy and ventilator dependency. *American Journal of Speech-Language Pathology, 4*, 55-61.

Tippett, D., & Vogelman, L. (2000). Communication, tracheostomy, and ventilator dependency. In D. Tippett (Ed.), *Tracheostomy and ventilator dependency: Management of breathing, speaking, and swallowing* (pp. 93-142). New York, NY: Thieme.

Tobin, M. (Ed.) (1994). *Principles and practice of mechanical ventilation.* New York, NY: McGraw-Hill.

FORM 6-1
CASE HISTORY SUPPLEMENT FOR CLIENTS WHO USE VENTILATORS

Client: _____   Date: _____

Date of Birth: _____   Examiner: _____

Sex: _____

VENTILATOR HISTORY

What happened that made it necessary for you to start using a ventilator?

When did you first start using a ventilator?

Have you used a ventilator ever since then?
     If not, how many times have you gone on and off a ventilator?

Do you use a ventilator 24 hours a day?
     If not, what parts of the day and/or night do you use it?

Which of the following ventilators have you used?

_____ positive pressure ventilator
     _____ invasive (with tracheostomy)
     _____ noninvasive (mouthpiece, nosemask, nasal pillows, facemask)

_____ negative pressure ventilator
     _____ iron lung
     _____ cuirass ("chest shell")
     _____ body suit ("raincoat")

_____ rocking bed

_____ abdominal pneumobelt

_____ phrenic nerve pacer(s)

Comments:

What ventilator or ventilators do you use now (type and brand/model)?

Ventilator 1:

Ventilator 2:

If you use more than one ventilator, under what circumstances do you use each?

Ventilator 1:

Ventilator 2:

COMMUNICATION HISTORY

Did you have any problems with your speech before you started using a ventilator?
If so, what were they?

Do you have any problems speaking while using your ventilator?
If so, what are they?

How is your speech different now than it was before you started using a ventilator?

How do you coordinate your speech with your ventilator?

Do you ever experience the following speech-related problems?

_____ short phrases
_____ not being able to finish a sentence
_____ the need to talk fast to finish a sentence
_____ getting interrupted
_____ long pauses
_____ frequent pauses
_____ overly loud speech
_____ overly soft speech
_____ fading of loudness at the ends of phrases
_____ changes in loudness during a breath
_____ too high a pitch
_____ too low a pitch
_____ changes in pitch during a breath
_____ changes in voice quality during a breath
_____ muffled speech
_____ not being understood by other people
_____ not being understood by a speech recognition system
_____ feeling out of breath when speaking
_____ the need to stop and take extra breaths when speaking for a long time
_____ the need to put a lot of effort into speaking
_____ difficulty coordinating speaking with breathing

Anything else?

Since you started using a ventilator, have you ever used any of the following to help you communicate? If so, how successful were they?

Nonspeech:

_____ pencil and paper writing
_____ picture or word board
_____ electronic or computer system
_____ sign language/gestures
_____ mouthing
_____ other (specify)

Comments:

Speech:

_____ electrolarynx
_____ one-way speaking valve
_____ talking tracheostomy tube
_____ ventilator adjustments
_____ changing speech patterns voluntarily
_____ other (specify)

Comments:

What strategies do you use to communicate now? How successful are they?

FORM 6-2
VENTILATOR ANALYSIS

Client: _____   Date: _____

Date of Birth: _____   Examiner: _____

Sex: _____

Type of Ventilator: _____

Make/Model: _____

Method of Delivery: _____

Adjustment Variables	Usual Settings
Breathing Rate (control mode)	
Trigger Sensitivity (assist mode)	
Tidal Volume	
Minute Ventilation	
Inspiratory Time	
Inspiratory Flow	
End-Inspiratory Pause	
Positive End-Expiratory Pressure (PEEP)	
One-Way Valve (or Cork)	
Pressure-Controlled Ventilation	
Pressure-Support Ventilation	
Peak Negative Inspiratory Pressure	
Positive Expiratory Pressure	
Other (specify)	

Comments:

FORM 6-3
AUDITORY-PERCEPTUAL EXAMINATION
FOR CLIENTS WHO USE VENTILATORS

Client: _____   Date: _____

Date of Birth: _____   Examiner: _____

Sex: _____

Auditory-Perceptual Key: 0 = normal; -1 = mildly abnormal; -2 = moderately abnormal;
 -3 = severely abnormal; -4 = profoundly abnormal.

Dyspnea Key: N = none; m = mild; M = moderate; S = severe; I = intolerable.

SUSTAINED VOWEL

	Abnormally Short					Abnormally Long			
	-4	-3	-2	-1	0	-1	-2	-3	-4
Utterance Duration									

Comments:

	Abnormally Short					Abnormally Long			
	-4	-3	-2	-1	0	-1	-2	-3	-4
Pause Duration									

Comments:

	Abnormally Soft					Abnormally Loud			
	-4	-3	-2	-1	0	-1	-2	-3	-4
Average Loudness									

Comments:

	Abnormally Even					Abnormally Variable			
	-4	-3	-2	-1	0	-1	-2	-3	-4
Loudness Variability									

Comments:

	Abnormally Breathy							Abnormally Pressed	
	-4	-3	-2	-1	0	-1	-2	-3	-4
Average Voice Quality									

Comments:

	Abnormally Even							Abnormally Variable	
	-4	-3	-2	-1	0	-1	-2	-3	-4
Voice Quality Variability									

Comments:

	Abnormally Low							Abnormally High	
	-4	-3	-2	-1	0	-1	-2	-3	-4
Average Pitch									

Comments:

	Abnormally Even							Abnormally Variable	
	-4	-3	-2	-1	0	-1	-2	-3	-4
Pitch Variability									

Comments:

READING ALOUD

	Abnormally Short							Abnormally Long	
	-4	-3	-2	-1	0	-1	-2	-3	-4
Utterance Duration									

Comments:

	Abnormally Short							Abnormally Long	
	-4	-3	-2	-1	0	-1	-2	-3	-4
Pause Duration									

Comments:

	Abnormally Soft						Abnormally Loud		
	-4	-3	-2	-1	0	-1	-2	-3	-4
Average Loudness									

Comments:

	Abnormally Even						Abnormally Variable		
	-4	-3	-2	-1	0	-1	-2	-3	-4
Loudness Variability									

Comments:

	Abnormally Breathy						Abnormally Pressed		
	-4	-3	-2	-1	0	-1	-2	-3	-4
Average Voice Quality									

Comments:

	Abnormally Even						Abnormally Variable		
	-4	-3	-2	-1	0	-1	-2	-3	-4
Voice Quality Variability									

Comments:

	Abnormally Low						Abnormally High		
	-4	-3	-2	-1	0	-1	-2	-3	-4
Average Pitch									

Comments:

	Abnormally Even						Abnormally Variable		
	-4	-3	-2	-1	0	-1	-2	-3	-4
Pitch Variability									

Comments:

	Abnormally Imprecise					Abnormally Precise			
	-4	-3	-2	-1	0	-1	-2	-3	-4
Articulatory Precision									

Comments:

Dyspnea Rating

Term:		N	m	M	S	I
Rating						

EXTEMPORANEOUS SPEAKING

	Abnormally Short					Abnormally Long			
	-4	-3	-2	-1	0	-1	-2	-3	-4
Utterance Duration									

Comments:

	Abnormally Short					Abnormally Long			
	-4	-3	-2	-1	0	-1	-2	-3	-4
Pause Duration									

Comments:

	Abnormally Soft					Abnormally Loud			
	-4	-3	-2	-1	0	-1	-2	-3	-4
Average Loudness									

Comments:

	Abnormally Even					Abnormally Variable			
	-4	-3	-2	-1	0	-1	-2	-3	-4
Loudness Variability									

Comments:

Clinical Applications

INTRODUCTION

Applications of the evaluation and management principles and methods discussed in this book are available in published case studies. These include studies of clients with profound hearing loss, motor neuron disease, Friedreich's ataxia, acute paralytic poliomyelitis, functional misuse of the breathing apparatus, spinal cord injury, and spasmodic dysphonia (Hixon, 1982; Hixon & Putnam, 1983; Hixon, Putnam, & Sharp, 1983; Sataloff, Heur, & O'Connor, 1984; Hoit & Shea, 1996). The reader is encouraged to consult these case studies as a supplement to the clinical applications considered here.

This chapter provides the reader with opportunities to think about and apply the principles and methods discussed in this book. It does so through the presentation of eight clinical scenarios, each of which reflects composite features of evaluation and management of more than a single client. Client initials are fictional and case histories and client performances have been modified to ensure anonymity. These scenarios are designed to illustrate how clients with speech breathing disorders behave and how principles and methods of evaluation and management can be used to quantify and change their behavior. No claims are made that the approaches discussed in these scenarios are the only reasonable ones. They are, however, well-tested from many years of clinical experience.

Having said all this, it is important to point out that the reader's engagement is as much a focus of this chapter as the clinical scenarios themselves. The scenarios are meant to serve as vehicles to enhance learning and challenge the reader. Questions are posed and comments are made throughout the scenarios. Answers to the questions will be obvious from the text that follows them. Or, in some cases, a review of earlier chapters in the book will provide the answers.

DOWN AND OUT

RT was a 30-year-old male classical singer. He was an accomplished baritone with a demanding practice and performance schedule. He self-referred and reported that he was in good general health. His complaints were that he "tired" when singing and "lacked stamina" when performing strenuous operatic roles. He further reported that he felt a "need for air" when singing and that he thought there might be something wrong with his breathing.

He had consulted a physician 4 months before coming to the clinic and reportedly had been advised that his problem related mainly to being overweight. He was placed on a weight-loss diet and told to do aerobic exercise three times a week. His physician also suggested that he might be experiencing "performance anxiety."

The case history was unremarkable, except that RT had changed singing teachers a year earlier because his former teacher had moved. RT was following the ad-

HI HO SILVER

Singing teachers often describe voice production as a process in which "the tone rides on the breath" or "the breath carries the tone." Neither description is accurate. When you sing, air moves through you in only one direction. It leaves your lungs, traverses your larynx, and goes out your mouth and/or nose. By contrast, tone moves through you in two directions. It leaves your larynx and goes out your mouth and/or nose. At the same time, it travels down your trachea and vibrates your chest. This is not like the slow mass flow of the breath. Rather, the tone is an extremely rapid, to-and-fro bumping of air molecules, in which each stays near home and passes energy on to its neighbors. Thus, the so-called breath and the so-called tone involve two entirely different energy flows.

vice of his physician, but his symptoms persisted and were continuing to bother him. He offered that they "might, in fact, be getting worse." Seasonal pollen allergies were reported, but were discounted as a possible contributor because of the time of year. He had no signs or symptoms of upper airway infection and reported having none during the previous 5 months. His life was stressful, but not overly so, and he showed no indication of any psychogenic bases for his complaints.

The physical examination was generally negative, although RT was substantially overweight and had major fat deposits throughout his chest wall. The evaluation of general breathing function was negative. Measured values for vital capacity, inspiratory capacity, and expiratory reserve volume were within normal limits for his age, height, and weight.

Speech and voice were normal when he read aloud, spoke extemporaneously, and engaged in conversational speaking. He had no signs of a speech breathing disorder, denied any speaking-related dyspnea, and reported no other symptoms related to everyday speech and voice use.

Given the information provided thus far, which of the following do you think might be causing the client's problems?

> *(a) excess body weight*
> *(b) progressive neural disease*
> *(c) conversion disorder*
> *(d) functional misuse disorder*

RT was observed while he sang two arias that he considered to be taxing of his performance skills. Tape-recorded piano accompaniment was used. Respiratory magnetometers were fixed to his rib cage wall and abdominal wall and signals from the two were displayed against one another on a storage oscilloscope. The display was in the form of a relative diameter diagram (rib cage diameter increasing upward and abdominal diameter increasing rightward) and was calibrated to enable lung volume to be read directly (i.e., converted to a relative volume diagram).

RT was found to breathe through only a limited portion of his vital capacity during performance. His pattern was to start his singing phrases from midrange lung volumes and to run out of air prematurely. Specifically, he initiated most of his breath groups from near 70 %VC and, for some of these, he was observed to expire modestly before engaging in voice production. Thus, singing phrases often terminated at inopportune times and he was forced to take catch breaths to keep pace with the musical score. For certain passages, his performance gave the appearance of being poorly planned and unrehearsed, even though the arias were memorized and highly practiced. For much of his singing, he used smaller rib cage wall volumes and larger abdominal wall volumes than are characteristic of highly trained classical singers. As well, the excursions of his abdominal wall were restricted in comparison to the excursions typically used by highly trained classical singers. His abdominal wall often moved paradoxically outward as he sang, especially at lower lung volumes. RT appeared to have a breathing strategy that sought to maintain his abdominal wall in a relatively outward position during both the inspiratory and expiratory phases of the breathing cycle for singing.

Data on the breathing adjustments of highly trained male and female classical singers can be found in Watson and Hixon (1985) and Watson, Hixon, Stathopoulos, and Sullivan (1990), respectively. Information on breathing behavior during the performance of a novel aria by a highly trained classical singer can be found in Watson and Hixon (1996) and may have relevance to the management of singers with breathing-related disorders of singing.

The mechanical events associated with RT's singing were clearly disadvantageous to his performance. Both his starting lung volumes and his lung volume excursions were smaller than they should have been. His rib cage wall was less elevated than it should have been to function optimally. Also, his abdominal wall was positioned farther outward than it should have been and it moved paradoxically so as to be counterproductive to lung volume change. A corollary to the problem with his abdominal wall position was that his diaphragm was flatter than it should have been for optimal performance during inspirations. Were one to consciously design a strategy for breathing that would have caused RT to tire quickly, to lack stamina, and to feel a need for air, this would be the strategy. But why would this constellation of problems emerge in a highly trained classical singer who had previously not had difficulties?

Hixon and Hoffman (1979) have discussed the relative merits of "down and out" and "up and in" breathing strategies for classical singing. Mechanical considerations clearly favor the "up and in" strategy. In fact, despite what singers are taught or believe, almost all accomplished classical singers eventually come to use the "up and in" strategy. There is a certain wisdom of the body in using this strategy and those who try other strate-gies often encounter problems with their singing over the long term.

The answer came from RT himself. Questioning revealed that he had received conflicting advice from his former teacher and current teacher with regard to "prop-er breathing technique" for classical singing. His current teacher was a so-called "down and out" advocate who focused on an outwardly positioned abdominal wall, whereas his former teacher was a so-called "up and in" advocate who focused on an inwardly positioned abdominal wall. RT indicated that he was focusing much of his performance attention, especially during practice, on the new "down and out" strategy that he had been working on since changing teachers. He offered that his former teacher and current teacher "had very different ways of doing things" and that his current teacher was a "stickler for technique" and thought that there was "only one right way to breathe for singing." Adoption of his new teacher's "down and out" strat-egy apparently contributed to his current problems. A change needed to be made.

Given what you know to this juncture, which of the following would be the cornerstone of your recommendation for the client?

    (a) referral to a psychiatrist
    (b) referral to a neurologist
    (c) exteroceptive feedback and behavioral management
    (d) counseling for stress reduction

The mechanical disadvantages of "down and out" breathing were explained to RT and he was encouraged to return to the clinic to participate in a management program that would focus on visual feedback of lung volume and chest wall shape, and behavioral adjustments. A relative volume diagram, displayed on an oscillo-scope, was used to help him understand the nature of his breathing behavior and then modify it. Management was planned for four 1-hour treatment sessions. Be-cause RT lived a considerable distance from the clinic in a different city, he decided it would be best to participate in two sessions a day (morning and afternoon) on two different days separated by a week. He chose not to talk with his current teacher about his new knowledge and his plan to seek outside advice, at least not just yet.

Now that you know the client's signs and symptoms, which of the follow-ing would be your first point of attack in his management?

    (a) chest wall shape
    (b) starting lung volume
    (c) rib cage wall position
    (d) abdominal wall paradoxing

The first management session focused on starting lung volume. A 90 %VC iso-volume line (same lung volume at all shapes) was drawn with a grease pencil on the face of the storage oscilloscope. This line traced diagonally downward from left to right on the relative volume diagram. RT was instructed to use this line as a target for the depth of his inspirations during singing. He was told that he should breathe in far enough that his singing phrases started above this line on the relative volume diagram. He responded very quickly to visual feedback and increased his starting lung volumes with ease. He caught on quickly to the "feel" of larger starting lung volumes in relation to their display on the relative volume diagram. It took him longer to stop initiating his breath groups with nonphonated expirations. He had trouble "feeling" this expiration and, in fact, denied it until it was shown to him on the oscilloscope several times. After 35 minutes of practice, he had a clear grasp of the importance of larger starting lung volumes and of not wasting (with a brief expiration) the air he had inspired. He proceeded during the remainder of the hour to extend his breath groups. He also reduced the number of inspirations, including catch breaths, compared to the number he had taken during the evaluation. The first session ended with the assignment that he take his "new feel" for lung volume and work at making these large starting lung volumes and longer phrasing adjustments more routine in his practice of the two arias he considered taxing. He was encouraged to practice as much as he wanted before his afternoon session (5 hours later).

The first part of the second management session was spent refining his starting lung volume and phrasing strategy, and then its focus turned to dealing with his chest wall shape. He had no difficulty carrying forward his morning's work on starting lung volume, but he did require further visual feedback of what continued to be brief expirations following some of his inspirations. Efforts at changing his chest wall shape began with instructing him to initiate his breath groups within a circumscribed range of chest wall shapes that had been represented on the relative volume diagram. This area encompassed relatively large rib cage wall volumes and moderate abdominal wall volumes. The range of shapes chosen was consistent with the range typically used by highly trained classical singers.

RT's task was to learn to position his rib cage wall and abdominal wall in such a way as to start singing breath groups within the target area. Much of this was trial and error until he became adept at understanding what the positions on the diagram meant in relation to his own movements. His chest wall shape habits were not as easily broken as were his starting lung volume habits. His main difficulty was with the position of his abdominal wall. He could feel when his abdominal wall was in different positions, but he could not effectively dissociate its position from the position of his rib cage wall. He persisted in wanting to keep his abdominal wall relatively outward. To counteract this tendency, his abdominal wall was held in an inward position manually by the clinician while RT watched his chest wall shape on the oscilloscope. He was then taught to hold his abdominal wall in an inward position with his own hands. By the end of the second session, he could voluntarily position his abdominal wall and rib cage wall within the target area on the oscilloscope, but not without watching the display. He was given the homework assignment of using his hands to position his abdominal wall inward and to practice singing while using this inward displacement cue until the next session. He was also asked to bring in tape-recorded piano accompaniment for two new arias.

The following week RT returned for his third and fourth management sessions. He arrived eager to begin and said that he had practiced diligently using his "feeling" of large starting lung volumes and using his hands to position his abdominal wall inward. The third management session focused mostly on chest wall shape at the start of his singing phrases in the arias he had used the previous week. After about 30 minutes, RT was able to start at consistently large lung volumes, at large rib cage wall volumes, and without having the abdominal wall significantly distended. He had acquired the "feel" of abdominal wall position and no longer required the use of his hands or the use of visual feedback.

Attention was then turned to the extended performance of his singing breath groups. Two items were targeted. One was increasing his abdominal wall excursions and the other was eliminating his abdominal wall paradoxing. The rib cage wall input to the relative volume diagram was grounded and RT was instructed to attend to the abdominal wall signal alone. Using this paradigm, he was told to perform his singing breath groups (expirations) with a large range of displacements of his abdominal wall and not to allow the abdominal wall signal to move rightward (paradox) on the display (rightward movement was expected to occur during inspiration). RT learned relatively quickly to increase his abdominal wall movement, but it took him longer to break his habit of abdominal wall paradoxing. He was eventually able to transfer from visualization of his abdominal wall movements in the relative volume diagram to being able to monitor such movements by looking down at the front of his abdominal wall.

The fourth management session continued to refine his control of chest wall shape by attempting to strengthen the link between visual feedback from the oscilloscope and his sensations about the positions of his abdominal wall and rib cage wall. By this final session, he could voluntarily control his starting lung volumes, starting chest wall shapes, and singing chest wall shapes with considerable skill. It took conscious effort to put all of his new skills together for singing, but he was able to do so. As a test of his ability to generalize, he was asked to perform the two new arias he had been asked to bring to see how different musical scores and demands would influence his new technique. He was successful at such generalization, with only occasional problems. Rapid passages gave him more difficulty, but he had at his command all the monitoring tools to know when he had deviated from course and all of the corrective tools to adjust for it.

By this point in management, the client had mastered several new perfor-mance skills and a helpful contrast for him might have included which of the following?

> *(a) louder singing*
> *(b) a distraction technique*
> *(c) other styles of singing*
> *(d) negative practice*

By the end of the fourth management session, RT had a firm understanding of the differences between an "up and in" strategy and a "down and out" strategy and could execute either easily (a form of negative practice for the latter). He was able to do this without the benefit of the relative volume diagram as a feedback guide. He reported the "up and in" strategy to be less effortful and less tiring than the "down and out" strategy and said that he was going to adopt the "up and in" strat-egy for his practice and performance.

A month after his last management session, RT returned to the clinic for a follow-up session. He had maintained his ability to execute the new strategies at will and reported that he was routinely using the "up and in" strategy for all of his singing. He reported that his symptoms had subsided substantially and attributed this to his new understanding of breathing technique and his improving physical condition. He confided that he had talked with his current singing teacher about the drawbacks of "down and out" singing and how he had sought help with his problems. A change in teacher was discussed between RT and his new teacher, but not pursued. The teacher allowed that he taught the way he himself had been taught, but that he was open to other ideas that would make his student successful.

RT telephoned the clinic several months after his follow-up session. He reported that he was without symptoms and asked if he could bring his teacher by when the two were in town for a regional singing competition. RT wanted to show his teacher how respiratory magnetometers worked.

SUPPORT YOUR LOCAL FIREFIGHTER

AE was a 23-year-old female who had worked summers as a smokejumper. She fell during a let-down rappel from a tall tree and suffered a C6 spinal cord injury. She was quadriplegic, save some minimal function in her arms and hands. Her first visit to the clinic was 15 months after her injury. She was referred by her physiatrist for concerns about her voice.

The case history revealed a well-educated young woman with an undergraduate degree in psychology. She was about to enter law school at the time of her injury and wanted to continue to pursue that goal. She was living with her parents and had obtained a service dog to aid her with some of her physical challenges. Her demeanor was remarkably upbeat and she reveled in a continuing relationship with a young man she referred to as her "main squeeze." She complained that her voice "lacked power." This generally bothered her, but was particularly problematic when attempting to maintain voice control of her service dog at a distance. Fatigue was also a problem for AE when she spoke continually for any protracted period. She was apprehensive about what her speech problems might mean for her chances at a law career and was eager to get on with the rest of her life. She reported mild-to-moderate dyspnea in association with extended speaking and indicated that the best description of her speaking-related discomfort was simply "it takes a lot of work to breathe."

The auditory-perceptual examination revealed difficulties with reading, extemporaneous speaking, and conversational speaking. Her speech was low in loudness and she spoke in short breath groups (usually about 6 to 8 syllables each) that were interspersed with relatively slow inspirations. Her phrasing was often abnormal and her voice routinely trailed off at the ends of breath groups. The use of prescribed utterance activities indicated that she had difficulty adjusting loudness and stress and that she could only minimally increase the lengths of her breath groups.

The physical examination revealed paralysis of the abdominal wall and severe paresis of the rib cage wall for both inspiration and expiration. During forced inspiratory activities, rib cage wall paradoxing was observed and the intercostal spaces were sucked inward. Neck muscle function was found to be intact and diaphragm function was spared. When in an upright position, her abdominal wall distended slightly and her rib cage wall was in a lower-than-normal position. Upright sitting required that her trunk be supported. Her cough was moderately weak.

The evaluation of general breathing function showed AE to have an inspiratory capacity and an expiratory reserve volume that were significantly smaller than normal. Specifically, her inspiratory capacity was 40% of its predicted value and her expiratory reserve volume was 4% of its predicted value. The maximum inspiratory pressure she could generate at the resting tidal end-expiratory level was -23 cmH$_2$O, and the maximum expiratory pressure she could generate at the same level was 2 cmH$_2$O. She was considered to have moderate-to-severe impairment of inspiratory function and severe-to-profound impairment of expiratory function.

Given what you know about the client thus far, which of the following do you think might be the most appropriate intervention?

    (a) phrenic nerve pacers
    (b) abdominal wall support
    (c) myoelectric feedback
    (d) body position adjustment

Manual bracing of the abdominal wall was effected by the clinician as a preliminary test of an abdominal wall support intervention. Results were positive. The client was able to inspire deeper than usual, and her inspirations seemed to be more vigorous. She was able to produce noticeably longer breath groups during manual bracing and her voice sounded louder.

Given the findings to this juncture, which of the following do you think would be the best course to follow?

    (a) bind the abdominal wall
    (b) start a program to strengthen the inspiratory muscles
    (c) institute electro-lung therapy
    (d) consult with her pulmonologist

The pulmonologist was consulted to determine the advisability of binding the abdominal wall as a strategy for improving the client's speech breathing. Binding was approved for 4 hours a day during waking hours and while in the upright body position. The prescription authorized the respiratory therapist to make adjustments to the binder. Later, the prescription was changed to authorize the speech-language pathologist to also make adjustments.

An elastic wrap-around binder was used. It was positioned so as to encroach only modestly upon the lower rib cage wall. The binder held the abdominal wall inward and provided some trunk support to the client. The client wore the binder while seated (usually about 20° off-vertical toward supine in a wheelchair).

The positioning of an elastic wrap-around binder is not as simple as it might seem. It is important to ensure that lower rib cage wall movement is not overly restricted. Otherwise, peripheral portions of the lungs may not be well ventilated. One consequence of binding inappropriately is that it can lead to pneumonia. It should never be done without a prescription from a physician, preferably a pulmonologist. There is an art to applying an abdominal wall binder, and it should only be done by a skilled practitioner. Watson and Hixon (2001) abdominally trussed subjects with spinal cord injury using a custom-made mechanical device that could precisely control the position of the abdominal wall. Their work shows the care required when using any device to fix the abdominal wall in position. It is worth a read to see the challenge faced when binding or trussing the abdominal wall in individuals with abdominal wall paresis or paralysis.

Following a week of accommodation, AE was re-evaluated for general breathing function and for running speech activities with the binder in place. Favorable changes were noted in her inspiratory capacity (from 40% of predicted to 55%

of predicted). Her expiratory reserve volume remained essentially the same as before binding. Maximum inspiratory pressure also changed favorably (from -23 to -28 cmH_2O), whereas maximum expiratory pressure showed essentially no change. Clearly, abdominal wall binding had moderately improved the client's inspiratory function.

Following binding, the client reported less severe speaking-related dyspnea during running speech activities. She tended to speak in somewhat longer breath groups (usually 2 to 3 more syllables per breath group than without binding) and at higher loudness levels. Her inspirations for running speech activities were notably quicker with the binder in place and approached the speeds observed in normal speakers.

At this juncture, what, if anything, should be done with the client?

    (a) discharge her from speech management
    (b) turn her management over to the respiratory therapist
    (c) expand her management into other areas
    (d) refer her for psychological testing

Two additional components of management were instituted after further consultation with AE's pulmonologist. The first was inspiratory muscle training to try to increase the strength of her inspiratory muscles. This training was conducted with her abdominal wall binder in place. The training did not isolate individual muscles, but focused on her overall capability to deliver inspiratory force to the breathing apparatus. The speech production goal of this training was to increase her starting lung volumes for speech production so that her breath groups might be longer and her utterances initially louder (because of the higher expiratory relaxation pressure available at larger lung volumes).

Inspiratory muscle training can be conducted in a number of ways. It can focus on individual muscles, groups of muscles, or all muscles that may contribute to the development of inspiratory force. Which focus to choose depends on the client, the availability of certain special instrumentation, and where the training is to be conducted. In the case being discussed here, much of the training was to be conducted at home. Thus, a simple protocol was desirable and one that the client could execute with a minimum of assistance. Had this client been managed daily in a clinical setting, it might have been profitable to also attempt some neck muscle training with her that employed myoelectric feedback.

AE's inspiratory muscle training program was designed through collaborative efforts of a physical therapist and the speech-language pathologist. The program included a simple device that AE could take home and use on her own. The device contained a spring-loaded valve that was set so that she had to generate a given (negative) pressure to be able to breathe in through it. Her task was to breathe through the device for 20 minutes a day, 5 days a week, for 8 weeks. During her daily 20-minute training sessions, she was to inspire repeatedly through the device for about 2 minutes and then rest for about 1 minute. She was then to inspire through the device for about 2 minutes more and then rest for about 1 minute more, and so on. The pressure threshold was set to 75% of her maximum inspiratory pressure with her abdominal wall binder in place. AE returned to the clinic at the end of each training week so that a new maximum inspiratory pressure measure could be obtained and her device adjusted.

Re-testing for general breathing function was conducted at the end of the 8-week training period and revealed that inspiratory function had changed favorably. AE's inspiratory capacity had increased by 65% from its pre-training value. As expected, her expiratory reserve volume was unchanged. Maximum inspiratory pressure had increased from -28 to -54 cmH$_2$O, whereas maximum expiratory pressure remained at its pre-training value of 2 cmH$_2$O. A maintenance regimen was then established so that AE could retain her newly gained strength and endurance.

The behavioral training component of AE's management began after inspiratory muscle training was completed. This phase of management concentrated on optimizing her speech performance against the background of her gains from abdominal wall binding and improvements in inspiratory muscle function. There were three parts to this phase of her management.

The first part sought to take advantage of the residual function she had in her arms and hands. She was taught to use this residual function to compress her abdominal wall when speaking. Thus, her arms and hands served as surrogate abdominal muscles, albeit weak ones. She could perform best if her arms were extended. Toward this end, a thick, lightweight, foam block was cut to fit the contour of her abdominal wall. This block was covered with a pillowcase and positioned on her lap so that she could gain leverage and pull it toward her body. Through this maneuver, AE was able to supplement the expiratory drive provided by expiratory relaxation pressure and her weak expiratory muscles. Use of this strategy enabled her to raise her maximum expiratory pressure from its usual 2 cmH$_2$O to 8 cmH$_2$O.

The second part of AE's behavioral training concentrated on her speech breathing during conversational interactions. AE had complained that conversations were difficult for her because sometimes her speech was not loud enough and it took many breaths for her to get her points across. These problems were less severe since AE had started using an abdominal wall binder, but they were still not solved. The speech-language pathologist noted that, when AE was engaged in conversation, she exhibited nonspeech expirations at the beginnings of her breath groups. These nonspeech expirations not only reduced the amount of speech she could produce, but they also reduced the pressure available at the beginning of utterance. Thus, her breath groups were not as long or as loud as they could have been. She was surprised that she had this "bad habit." Several strategies for changing her behavior were tried. The most successful strategy proved to be one in which she "held herself up" at the beginnings of breath groups with her newly strengthened inspiratory muscles. This was particularly effective when she had to pause after an inspiration (either for cognitive processing reasons or because she was being interrupted by her conversational partner). She practiced using this new strategy while conversing and did quite well. Her task was to be aware of her nonspeech expirations and to remember to use this new speech breathing strategy during conversations outside the clinic.

There was another reason that AE's conversational interactions were more difficult than they needed to be. After questioning her about the nature of her daily conversations, it became clear that her conversational environment could be improved. She was counseled about the effects of background noise, physical orientation of conversational partners, and issues related to the status of the conversational partner. A determination was made that her conversational environment could potentially be enhanced by the following: (a) decreasing background noise (e.g., muting the television, turning off the radio); (b) sitting closer to her conversational partner and ensuring that they could make eye contact; and (c) suggesting to her father (one of her frequent conversational partners) that he have his hearing tested.

By the end of the second part of AE's behavioral training, she was capable of generating longer breath groups (18-syllable potential), speaking with considerable loudness, and had acquired performance strategies that enabled her to better hold the floor in conversations. She had made application to a regional law school and was planning to move out of her parents' home. She had maintained her relationship with her "main squeeze" and was discussing marriage with him. But one thing remained to be done in her behavioral management program.

A final part of AE's behavioral training included work with her service dog. One of her original concerns was her inability to consistently control her dog with voice commands, especially at a distance. Given her new skills, this proved a relatively simple challenge. AE was instructed to inspire near maximally before issuing commands and to deliver such commands while pulling in on her abdominal wall. Each command was to be short, crisp, and emphatic and she was to be consistent in their repeated forms. She also was taught to routinely give initial alerting commands to the dog to ensure his attention before delivering action commands. All went extremely well with this part of AE's management program. Her final question before being released from management was whether or not some of these command strategies might work on her "main squeeze."

Trained service dogs are an important part of the lives of many individuals with neuromotor impairments. They function as assistants (not to mention companions) in a wide variety of habilitation and rehabilita-

tion capacities. Given their value and status, would you say the following statement is true or false?

Food, shelter, and veterinary care for a trained service dog are tax deductible.

AN APPLE FOR THE TEACHER

JB was a 63-year-old psychology instructor at a branch campus of a major university. Six months before coming to the clinic, she had been diagnosed as having chronic obstructive pulmonary disease. She had been a heavy smoker for most of her adult life. She complained of breathing difficulty during classroom teaching and reported that her difficulty was progressively worsening. Her physician had suggested that she consider an early retirement from teaching. She did not want to entertain this option. She enjoyed teaching and expressed that she was "not ready to walk away from it." She indicated that much of her reluctance was financially based. She was the sole support of her elderly mother and herself. Her husband had died from lung cancer 4 years earlier.

JB was teaching introductory and intermediate undergraduate courses that had relatively large enrollments. Her teaching load was three courses a semester. She was typically a very energetic person, but was recently finding herself physically and emotionally exhausted at the end of each teaching day. She had 2 years of service to complete before she would have full retirement benefits and full social security benefits. These, she thought, would meet her financial needs.

JB's physician had made the referral to the speech-language clinic. He requested that testing be done to determine whether or not there might be speaking strategies that would relieve her dyspnea. JB, herself, was clear about what she wanted: "Teaching is getting harder. Breathing and talking is the problem. I just want to make it through 2 more years. I can't afford to quit. I need help with this."

JB's medical records indicated that her chronic obstructive pulmonary disease was primarily characterized by emphysema. Recent pulmonary function testing revealed a vital capacity that was 80% of predicted, a forced expiratory volume in 1-second that was 65% of predicted and, when expressed as a percentage of her forced vital capacity, was 60% of predicted. All testing signs were consistent with obstructive pulmonary disease.

*Given an accurate medical diagnosis and valid pulmonary function data, which of the following would **not** be a probable sign or symptom for the client?*

(a) chacexia
(b) chest tightness
(c) normal oxygen saturation
(d) normal blood gases

Auditory-perceptual examination revealed that JB's speech was characterized by normal loudness and loudness variation, suggesting that her control of alveolar pressure was adequate for speech purposes. Her breath group lengths were either normal or abnormal, depending on the task performed. She was able to sustain a vowel for 20 seconds, although only when she used a pressed voice quality. Reading aloud and delivering a brief mock classroom lecture were associated with relatively long breath groups containing as many as 20 syllables. However, such utterances were also produced with a relatively pressed voice quality. After producing five to ten of such breath groups consecutively, JB would stop speaking to "catch her breath." She reported that the speaking difficulty she was having during reading and her mock lecture was typical of what she was experiencing in the classroom.

When JB was asked to "count to 50, putting a comfortable number of words on each breath," she produced only about 10 syllables per breath group, about half as many as she did during her mock lecture. These breath groups were generally preceded by large inspirations and were characterized by a period of speech followed by a nonspeech expiration. This collection of speech breathing signs, although varied in presentation, indicated that JB was using abnormally large lung volume excursions. Her inspirations were slightly longer than normal, primarily because her inspiratory volumes were larger than normal.

JB's perceptions about her breathing discomfort related to physical exertion ("hard work to breathe") and air hunger ("short of breath"). These percepts were more pronounced when she was reading or delivering a mock lecture than when she was performing the comfortable counting task described above.

Physical examination of the breathing apparatus revealed thinness of the body and chacexia (i.e., a wasting in association with her chronic disease). When queried about her physical condition, she reported that she had been gradually losing weight and bulk for about 2 years.

Instrumental examination was performed to gain further insight into JB's speech breathing. Her oxygen saturation was monitored throughout the evaluation and was found to remain above 95% at all times. This was anticipated, given that recent arterial blood draws had shown her blood gases to be normal. Her chest wall behavior and ventilation were monitored with respiratory magnetometers during a subset of her speech breathing activities. Results showed that her starting lung volumes and lung volume excursions were abnormally large, but that all other aspects of her speech breathing performance were normal. Her ventilation (calculated from her lung volume excursions and breathing rate) was higher-than-normal and varied with the speaking activity. More specifically, her ventilation was lower when she read aloud or delivered a mock lecture than when she counted comfortably. She reported that it was "easier to breathe" and that she felt she was "getting more air" during the counting activity.

Given what you know about the client to this juncture, which of the following might you want to do next?

 (a) refer her for a physiological stress test
 (b) observe her in a usual teaching environment
 (c) refer her to a respiratory therapist
 (d) determine what maximizes her speaking-related dyspnea

Arrangements were made to observe JB during one of her class lectures. Observations were generally consistent with her performance during a mock lecture. Her teaching style was essentially a non-stop didactic monologue, high in speaking activity and low in student participation.

After consultation with the client's physician, a management plan was designed with the primary purpose of relieving her speaking-related dyspnea during classroom teaching. This plan incorporated the following three elements: (a) suggested lifestyle changes; (b) strategies for conserving energy; and (c) modifications of speech breathing behavior.

Three recommendations were offered for lifestyle changes. The first was to stop smoking. JB had attempted to quit on several occasions, but was continuing to smoke. She indicated that she wanted to quit, had tried several times, and thought her inability to do so was a "personality weakness." She had decreased her smoking shortly after the death of her husband, but "stresses" had led her to resume smoking. "I don't know why I can't do it. I'm supposed to understand this stuff. I'm a psychology instructor and should be able to beat it." She had significant doubts about being able to conquer her habit alone. Thus, she was referred to a smoking cessation counselor and joined a support group to deal with this aspect of her management.

Understanding a problem and doing something about it are, of course, two quite different things. Matters of addiction, such as to alcohol, drugs, or, in JB's case, tobacco, are often matters of life and death. Knowing that smoking had led to her husband's death and to her breathing discomfort would seem to be enough to make her quit smoking. But it is often not logic that prevails with such problems. There are undoubtedly people reading this who have seen someone who has had his larynx removed because of cancer, but who is still smoking postsurgically through his tracheostomy. The power of such addiction far outweighs the counseling skills and expertise of the speech-language pathologist, and requires the expertise of other professionals who specialize in addiction.

The second lifestyle recommendation targeted JB's physical health. Specifically, she was encouraged to ask her physician if she could participate in a pulmonary rehabilitation program. Her physician supported this idea and wrote a prescription that placed her under the care of a team that included a pulmonologist, a physical therapist with expertise in chronic obstructive pulmonary disease, and a nutritional counselor. It was anticipated that by optimizing her physical health, her breathing comfort might improve as well. This, in fact, turned out to be true. After several weeks in the program, the magnitude of her breathing discomfort had reduced moderately.

The final lifestyle recommendation was to have JB consider requesting a transfer from her existing job site to the main campus of her university. The branch campus where she worked was approximately 7,000 feet above sea level in a heavily forested mountain area. The main campus, by contrast, was approximately 2,400 feet above sea level in a sparsely vegetated desert valley. Living at a lower elevation would ease the physiological stress on her breathing apparatus and probably reduce her speaking-related breathing discomfort. This recommendation surprised JB. She considered it at length and decided not to follow it, mainly because her mother's "world" was in a local nursing home. She did not want to move unless it was absolutely necessary.

The second set of management considerations targeted energy conservation. Several strategies were suggested. One was to adjust her teaching schedule to reduce heavy workloads during any one day. At the time of evaluation, she was teaching all three of her courses and doing most of her student advising on Monday, Wednesday, and Friday. She was encouraged to move one course and most of her student advising to Tuesday and Thursday so that her workload would be more evenly distributed across her workweek and would, therefore, be more manageable. Unfortunately, course scheduling could not be changed because the semester was already in progress, so this had to wait until the following semester. She could, however, change her student advising hours to off-teaching days and did so.

Another energy conservation strategy was to have her eliminate unnecessary voice use. There were certain activities she could easily conduct by electronic mail, rather than in person. For example, certain aspects of routine advising and some departmental committee tasks did not require face-to-face conversations. She chose this strategy and found that not only did it reduce her voice use, but it also resulted in more efficient time management.

Several adjustments were made to help JB conserve energy in the classroom. First, she explained to her students the difficulties she was having with her disease. This lessened the stress on both her and the students and they came to understand why she needed to stop and rest momentarily during lectures.

To relieve her from having to use high driving pressures to "project" her voice during lectures, she began to use a microphone-loudspeaker system. This was especially helpful in large classes.

The work of breathing (defined physically as the product of volume and pressure) is usually greater for running speech activities in which loudness is higher. As the work of breathing increases, the perceived effort to generate speech often increases as well. Keeping the loudness of speech the same, but amplifying it for listeners, is one solution. Roy, Weinrich, Gray, Tanner, Toledo, Dove, Corbin-Lewis, and Stemple (2002) have recommended the use of amplification for classroom teachers to prevent behaviors that are abusive to the voice production apparatus and deleterious to the voice. Amplification also has the advantage of offering an assist to classroom teachers with speaking-related dyspnea.

JB had a habit of walking back and forth in front of the class when she lectured. This in itself sapped some of her energy. It was decided that she would benefit from lecturing in a seated position. She preferred a high stool for this purpose, so that she could see the entire class and maintain a position of authority. Interestingly, she knew that her speech breathing was more uncomfortable when she was doing physical activities, but she had not made the connection that "walking and talking" each had their own demands on her energy. By sitting while lecturing, she was able to allocate more of her energy resources to speaking.

JB was fond of using the chalkboard during her lectures. This was especially tiring for her, but she liked "going to the board" to illustrate a concept or spell out a technical word. To eliminate this need, two adjustments were made. One was to place an overhead projector to the side of the stool. With this arrangement, she could write when she wanted to without having to stand up. She came to like this approach because it not only conserved energy, but also enabled her to write without turning her back on the students (something she had not much thought about before).

The second adjustment took longer to effect, but turned out to be her favorite. She had never taught using visual materials in a computer presentation format. She was not very computer savvy and found the idea to be intimidating. The surplus equipment section of her campus had a laptop Apple computer available that could be used in conjunction with a ceiling-mounted computer projection system already in her classroom. Two of her students helped her prepare some computer-generated visuals and in a short time she was "hooked" on the technology. Using the computer for basic structure and the overhead projector for more spontaneous elaboration, she completely altered her "walking back and forth and going to and from the chalkboard" mode of teaching.

The final suggestion for energy conservation in the classroom involved a modification of JB's general teaching style. For most of her teaching career, she had used a didactic teaching style in which she was essentially the sole speaker throughout the class period. Alternative teaching techniques were introduced that offered her a respite from speaking (and also gave the students opportunities to do more active learning). She was instructed in how to engage students in activities such as group discussions and writing exercises. In one of her courses she began using case examples of individuals with psychological disorders and had students get into small groups to problem-solve the diagnoses. Activities such as these allowed her to stop talking for short periods and concentrate solely on breathing.

The final aspect of management was direct modification of JB's speech breathing behavior during lecturing. Two strategies were implemented, one within-breath-group strategy and one between-breath-group strategy. The within-breath-group strategy had her reduce the number of syllables produced per breath and terminate breath groups with nonspeech expirations. The purpose of this strategy was to shorten expiration time so that she could maintain the high ventilation level she demanded. Although she was concerned that her speech would sound "choppy," she found that with practice she was able to sound quite normal. Nevertheless, this proved a difficult strategy for her and was only modestly successful.

The between-breath-group strategy was much easier for her. This strategy required that she take on a more "relaxed" and "casual" speaking demeanor, allowing for pauses between some breath groups. This meant that, rather than rush from one topic to the next, as was her usual style, JB learned to wait several seconds (enough time to take a nonspeech breath or two) before moving on to another topic. The pause served as a transition signal for the students as well as a speaking break for JB. Another effective way to allow pauses to occur naturally was for her to ask the class a question. She could enjoy several nonspeech breaths while waiting for the student(s) to respond. This strategy also turned out to invigorate the classroom environment by providing yet another means for students to participate actively in the learning process.

The overall management program was quite successful for JB. She ended up incorporating, to at least some degree, nearly all of the strategies suggested to her (save changing job locations). She was able to get through her teaching days without being exhausted. As a side benefit, her teaching ratings improved substantially. Students reported that they enjoyed that the material was presented in a variety of ways and that they were active participants in the classroom. Although JB did not choose to transfer to the main campus of the university, she did confide that she had thought long and hard about the suggestion and believed it was something important to consider if her chronic obstructive pulmonary disease worsened significantly. She also allowed that it might be something to think about as she moved closer to retirement.

JUST THE RIGHT PACE

GT was about to enter college on a wrestling scholarship when he was injured in a diving accident. The accident left him with a C2-level spinal cord injury and paralysis of the rib cage wall, diaphragm, and abdominal wall. Immediately following his injury, he underwent a tracheotomy and was placed on a positive pressure ventilator. He was seen later by a speech-language pathologist who evaluated his swallowing and speech. Swallowing was found to be normal, but speech was found to be characterized by short breath groups, long pauses, variable loudness, and poor voice quality. These problems were managed relatively successfully by making appropriate adjustments to his ventilator. Behavioral strategies were suggested, but GT refused to try them.

It is not uncommon for individuals who have suffered life-changing injuries to refuse certain forms of treatment as they recover. Many different feelings and emotions are at work and it often takes time and patience to get a client ready to help himself or accept help from others. Individuals who have incurred spinal cord injury find their lives instantly changed and they often experience anger and depression. Sometimes the management course the speech-language pathologist would like to follow must be modified or put on hold until the client has worked through certain emotions and is ready to take on new challenges.

During the first year following his injury, GT was extremely angry and depressed. He seldom spoke and was generally uncooperative with rehabilitation efforts. His friends gradually stopped visiting him so that his only regular visitors were his parents and an older cousin. There was a period when he expressed a desire to be removed from his ventilator, but this passed after discussions with his minister. He eventually moved home with his parents and his mother quit her job so she could care for him full-time. She was a competent and attentive caregiver, but she was overbearing and extremely protective. This worsened GT's anger until the situation became intolerable for all concerned. As a result, GT and his parents enrolled in a counseling program that lasted nearly a year. The program was effective and their lives underwent significant positive change. GT grew active in his church. He even gave a short sermon to a youth group at the invitation of his minister. It became his dream to attend a seminary and become a minister himself.

Shortly after the counseling program ended, GT read an article in the press about phrenic nerve pacers. The article, titled "Bionic Breathing," stressed that pacers "let patients breathe almost like they did before they were paralyzed" and that "they free patients of the need to be tied to a ventilator." GT was intrigued and asked his pulmonologist if pacers would work for him. The pulmonologist thought that GT might be a candidate for phrenic nerve pacers, but informed him that he would need to undergo tests before any decision could be made. The pulmonologist discussed the options with GT and his parents. There was the surgery, the cost, the logistics of transferring from a positive pressure ventilator to this different form of ventilation (a process that might take as long as 6 months), and the possibility that his speech might not be as good with the pacers as it currently was with his positive pressure ventilator. GT and his parents expressed a willingness to accept the risk, expense, and inconvenience associated with the procedure because of the potential benefits. The option of being freed from the ventilator was most compelling to GT, especially because he wanted to follow the path of becoming a minister.

Which of the following is a critical factor as to whether or not a client is a candidate for phrenic nerve pacers?

> *(a) ability to tolerate body position shifts*
> *(b) intact phrenic nerves*
> *(c) no tracheostomy*
> *(d) paralyzed abdominal wall*

Electrodiagnostic testing was conducted and confirmed that GT was a good candidate for phrenic nerve pacers. Both phrenic nerves were found to be intact and adequate volume displacement was attained with electrical stimulation. GT got his wish and within a week of his 20th birthday he was implanted with phrenic nerve pacers, bilaterally.

The pacers were set to generate a 10-Hz pulse train lasting 1.2 seconds at a rate of 10 times per minute. Initially, GT used the pacers for just a few hours a day. His pacer use was gradually increased over 4 months until he was able to tolerate continual pacing throughout the day and night. His tracheostomy was retained because he was unable to cough and required periodic suctioning of the pulmonary airways. Also, by retaining the tracheostomy, he could be switched back to positive pressure ventilation if needed. His tracheostomy was fitted with a one-way valve during the day so that he could speak.

Most speech-language pathologists have little exposure to clients who use phrenic nerve pacers and there is little research available on speech breathing with phrenic nerve pacers. However, there are two articles that address this form of speech breathing. One article compares speech breathing with phrenic nerve pacers to speech breathing with invasive positive pressure ventilation in a single subject (Hoit & Shea, 1996). The other article documents the effects of abdominal wall binding on speech breathing in two subjects with phrenic nerve pacers (Hoit, Banzett, & Brown, 2002).

As soon as GT was using his pacers full-time, he was seen for a speech evaluation. During the case history interview, GT stated that he liked the pacers, but that they had taken "some getting used to." He thought his speech seemed more normal in certain ways, especially because he was able to speak on expiration like he did before his accident. However, he thought his speech was not as good as when he used to speak with his "speech settings" on his positive pressure ventilator. He was eager to do whatever it would take to improve his pacer-driven speech.

An auditory-perceptual examination revealed several abnormal features. GT was able to sustain vowel productions for only 2.5 seconds and he produced an average of 6 syllables per breath group when performing running speech activities. His pauses between breath groups were at least 3 seconds long, 1.2 seconds of which was devoted to inspiration. For all speech tasks, his overall loudness was low and faded substantially near the end of breath groups. His voice quality was normal and his upper airway articulation was normal.

A physical examination documented a paralyzed breathing apparatus, intact neck muscle function, and normal laryngeal and upper airway structure and function. GT's tidal volume was measured to be 0.5 L when driven by his phrenic nerve pacers. He was able to supplement his tidal volume by exerting inspiratory

A Breathtaking Experience

On November 4, 1818, Matthew Clydesdale was hanged for murder. His corpse was taken to Glasgow University where Dr. Andrew Ure and an associate performed a variety of "galvinisation" experiments on it. A series of attempts was made to re-animate Clydesdale by passing electricity through his remains. The published account of these experiments (Ure, 1819) makes it clear that Clydesdale was figuratively and literally charged for his crime. In one of the experiments, an attempt was made to restore breathing by passing electricity through rods connected to the left phrenic nerve and the diaphragm. It is reported that breathing took place and that the "chest heaved and fell" each time current was applied. Ure's electrifying account (pun intended) and the macabre gasps of Clydesdale's corpse are crude precursors to the delicate and refined way that phrenic nerve pacing is done today.

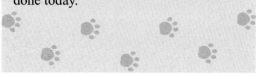

force with his neck muscles. With a maximum effort, he could add 0.3 L to his tidal volume. Thus, with pacers and neck muscles combined, he could breathe with a tidal volume of 0.8 L. The relaxation pressure at tidal end-inspiration was 5 cmH$_2$O when effected by the pacers. It was 8 cmH$_2$O at tidal end-inspiration when effected by the pacers plus maximum neck muscle activation.

At this juncture, what else would you consider to further increase the client's tidal volume in hopes that it would lead to speech improvement?

    (a) supplemental oxygen
    (b) abdominal wall trussing
    (c) rib cage wall binding
    (d) fully erect body positioning

It was noted that GT's abdominal wall was displaced outward because of its paralyzed state and that his rib cage wall tended to move paradoxically inward when his phrenic nerve pacers activated. A decision was made to truss his abdominal wall inward in an attempt to further increase GT's tidal volume. It was assumed that inward displacement of the abdominal wall would lengthen the muscle fibers of his diaphragm and that such lengthening would result in a greater inspiratory force for the same input provided by his pacers. It was also assumed that paradoxical movement of the rib cage wall would be reduced by improving the coupling between the diaphragm and the rib cage wall. A quick test of these assumptions was conducted by pushing against the anterior surface of his abdominal wall while GT performed maximum tidal inspiration and various speech activities. He was able to inspire deeper during manual compression of the abdominal wall than without such compression. Also, it was immediately apparent that his speech was louder and his breath groups were longer during manual compression. The pulmonologist authorized a trial period in which the effects of an abdominal wall truss were tested.

Measurements with the truss in position were favorable. His pacer-driven tidal volume increased to 0.65 L and his relaxation pressure increased to 6.5 cmH_2O. When he assisted the pacers with his neck muscles, his tidal volume was 0.95 L and his relaxation pressure reached 9.5 cmH_2O. GT sustained a vowel for 3.5 seconds and he produced an average of 9 syllables per breath during running speech activities. His speech was louder at the beginning of breath groups with the truss than without it. He reported that "speaking was easier" and that the truss was "comfortable," and he requested to be allowed to continue wearing it. The pulmonologist agreed and authorized the use of the truss during the day when GT was seated upright in his wheelchair.

The following week GT reported that he had been wearing the truss daily and that his mother had commented that his voice was noticeably "stronger." Arterial blood gas measures indicated that his partial pressure of carbon dioxide had decreased slightly, but remained in the low-normal range (substantially higher than it had been when he was using positive pressure ventilation). GT indicated that he was pleased with the improvement, but he was still not satisfied with his speech.

The next phase of management included the introduction of two behavioral strategies designed to further increase his tidal volume. The first of these sought to capitalize on his neck muscle capability. Although GT could activate his neck muscles voluntarily, he did not activate them during speech breathing. Thus, to bring neck muscle activation under more conscious control, myoelectric feedback was used. A pair of surface electrodes was placed in vertical orientation along one side of his neck (it had already been determined that he activated his neck muscles symmetrically) and a ground electrode was fixed to his shoulder. The resultant signal was routed to an amplifier and loudspeaker. GT was encouraged to activate his neck muscles using various levels of effort and listen to the effects on the sound generated. He was then instructed to count to 100 while concentrating on activating his neck muscles during each inspiration. Both he and the clinician noticed immediately that his speech was louder and his breath groups longer when he assisted inspiration with his neck muscles. Once he demonstrated consistent neck muscle activation for counting, he moved on to reciting some of his favorite scripture and was eventually able to generate at least a small myoelectric signal during nearly all of his inspirations. This management approach was continued over several sessions, until he was activating his neck muscles consistently for speech inspirations. Measurement indicated that he generally supplemented the pacer-driven tidal volume by 0.1 to 0.2 L during speech breathing. GT's speech was slightly louder and his breath groups were 2 to 3 syllables longer on average.

Once GT had mastered the neck muscle activation strategy, another behavioral strategy was introduced to further increase his tidal volume for speech production. This strategy was glossopharyngeal breathing. To attempt glossopharyngeal breathing, it was essential that he have a well-sealed tracheostomy. A button was used to achieve occlusion. GT used the button during the day and had it removed at night while sleeping. At first, he was hesitant to attempt glossopharyngeal breathing because he thought it "looked weird." However, after he viewed an instructional videotape about glossopharyngeal breathing, he became convinced of its value for speech, as well as for coughing and for general safety purposes. Management began with GT learning to generate glossopharyngeal volume strokes immediately after the termination of inspiration, starting with one stroke and increasing to multiple consecutive strokes. No attention was given to speech until he was moderately facile at glossopharyngeal breathing and in coordinating it with his pacer-driven breathing. He was eventually able to generate more than a dozen consecutive glossopharyngeal breaths and to achieve a maximum tidal inspiration of 1.7 L. Although such large inspiratory efforts would seldom be required for speech, they were useful for generating the high pressures and flows needed for coughing and airway clearance.

Glossopharyngeal breathing is not especially easy to learn. It takes time to learn it, but it can pay off handsomely for clients who persist and acquire the skill. It is most easily learned in a single-breath context during usual breathing and then later incorporated into running speech activities. Some clients will acquire it spontaneously through their own experimentation without formal instruction. In fact, it is not uncommon to find clients who come to the clinic with the skill in hand. Occasionally, such clients are so skilled at using glossopharyngeal breathing and disguising it in the flow of speech that the lay observer may not even detect it.

The next step was to incorporate glossopharyngeal breathing into GT's speech breathing cycle. To start, he was instructed to add glossopharyngeal breaths to his pacer-driven inspirations during automatic speech activities (e.g., counting, alphabet recitation). He was encouraged to increase the number of syllables he could produce per breath, while minimizing pause duration as much as possible. That is, he needed to strike a balance between how much additional volume he would generate for the subsequent breath group and how much time he would spend in silence to do it. Later, he also learned to insert glossopharyngeal breaths at natural break points (e.g., between words or phrases) during expiration. This allowed him to prolong the breath group without prolonging the pause between breath groups. It also allowed him to maintain a higher average pressure, and, therefore, a greater average loudness.

One final behavioral strategy involving the use of buccal speech was offered to GT before management was terminated. It had been noted that he occasionally "mouthed" the final one or two syllables of a breath group. This most often occurred when he was giving a sermon (he was now asked routinely to give a short sermon directed to the young people in his church). He had a preferred cadence when reciting certain passages and sometimes his obligatory pause came at an awkward point in the text. By using buccal speech, instead of mouthing, to produce the final one or two syllables, he was able to maintain his preferred cadence without sacrificing intelligibility. The use of buccal speech turned out to be a seldom used, but critical, strategy for GT.

GT became impressively adept at incorporating neck muscle activation and glossopharyngeal breathing into his speech breathing cycle, with occasional buccal speech supplementation. In fact, he became so skilled that his speech often passed for normal, with breath groups averaging 20 syllables in length. The only residual speech breathing problem was that his inspiratory pauses were abnormally long. This was because his pacer-driven inspirations lasted 1.2 seconds and could not be made shorter.

GT pursued his dream of becoming a minister. He entered a community college near his home to get started with classes he hoped would lay the groundwork for his eventual application to a theological seminary. His outlook had changed dramatically from what it was just 2 years earlier when he was struggling with anger and despair.

THE EYES HAVE IT

BR was a 61-year-old male with a diagnosis of amyotrophic lateral sclerosis. His neurologist had requested a consult to address what the client had reported as "breathing difficulty when talking." The client had noticed unsteadiness in his gait when playing golf 2 years earlier and within 3 months of that observation he had developed signs and symptoms that prompted a neurologist to offer a tentative diagnosis of spinal muscular atrophy. Within 6 months of the initial diagnosis, bulbar signs began to manifest and the diagnosis was changed to amyotrophic lateral sclerosis. At the time of consultation, the client presented with mixed flaccid-spastic signs throughout the speech production apparatus. His breathing apparatus signs were moderate in severity, whereas his laryngeal and upper airway signs were mild in severity. He had recently begun to use an electric wheelchair and was on disability retirement from his job as a postal worker.

Measurements of lung volumes and lung capacities revealed that BR's vital capacity was 56% of its predicted value. Reduction was on both the inspiratory and expiratory sides of breathing function, with the inspiratory capacity and the expiratory reserve volume being 66 and 40% of their predicted values, respectively. Maximum inspiratory pressure at the resting tidal end-expiratory level was -41 cmH_2O, whereas maximum expiratory pressure at that same level was 23 cmH_2O.

Physical examination of the breathing apparatus revealed moderately impaired diaphragm function. Inspiratory and expiratory rib cage wall function and abdominal wall function also showed moderate impairment. Breathing discomfort during running speech activities was rated as moderate for reading and extemporaneous speaking, and mild-to-moderate for conversational speaking. Discomfort was characterized as "hard work to breathe" and the client reported that he felt fatigued after prolonged engagement in running speech activities. Change in body position influenced the severity of BR's dyspnea, with more downright body positions (e.g., supine) causing him to experience increased breathing discomfort and greater speaking difficulty. BR showed signs of compensatory "neck breathing," especially during inspirations that were larger than resting tidal depth. His neck muscles were moderately hypertrophied and stood out plainly at the surface. Swallowing was judged to be within normal limits, although somewhat slow and weak.

Measurements made with respiratory magnetometers revealed that breath group excursions were slightly restricted and that they involved smaller-than-normal rib cage wall starting volumes and larger-than-normal abdominal wall starting volumes. Relative volume displacements of the rib cage wall and abdominal wall were normal in the upright body position, but abnormal in the supine body position. In supine, coordination between the rib cage wall and the abdominal wall was periodically erratic and characterized by instances of paradoxing.

Why would the client perform in a normal manner when in an upright body position but in an abnormal manner when in a supine body position? Hixon (1982) has suggested that such difference in behavior is related to orthopnea, the sensation of dyspnea when in the supine body position. Orthopnea is often a symptom in clients with significant neuromotor involvement of the breathing apparatus in which the ability of the breathing muscles to perform work is compromised. In the case of motor neuron disease, Hixon has offered three possible reasons for abnormal speech breathing behavior in the supine body position: (a) a need to feel control over perceived breathing embarrassment; (b) the relative novelty of generating speech in such a position with a degenerating neuromotor system; and (c) inadequate or abnormal afferent or sensory information to enable normal neuromotor control.

Auditory-perceptual examination of running speech breathing revealed that BR spoke in slightly short breath groups, with a moderately strained-strangled voice quality, and at a moderately slower-than-normal utterance rate. His articulation was judged to be moderately imprecise, although his intelligibility was not impaired. Hypernasality was occasionally present in his running speech, but only for brief moments and was never more than moderate in severity.

BR was aware of the problems with his speech and voice, but he was mainly concerned with his breathing discomfort during speaking and how quickly he fatigued when involved in conversations with his wife and children. He asked several questions about the reasons for his speech breathing difficulties and what he could expect the future to be for his speech and breathing. He was counseled as to the probable course and potential management options.

Amyotrophic lateral sclerosis is a devastating disease. Its time course is varied and its signs and symptoms may present in different patterns, but the outcome is fatal unless another disease results in death. Advanced stages of the disease wreak havoc on speech production processes and ultimately there is no speech. This eventuality must be planned for and a course of management that considers impending degeneration is best thought out early in the disease, if possible. There are different personal and cultural preferences among clients as to how heroic their medical and communication managements should be during advanced and final stages of the disease. And there are often professional differences of opinion on this matter. The opinion expressed here is that communication is quintessential to human life and that every attempt should be made to meet each client's communication needs, no matter what the effort or cost.

The referring neurologist was advised of the findings of the clinical examination. A suggestion was made that BR's speaking be limited to upright body positions. Four additional suggestions were made to help minimize his speaking-related dyspnea: (a) speak in shorter breath groups; (b) speak only within the tidal volume range; (c) speak only at a conversational loudness level; and (d) speak only in relatively quiet surroundings. A short period of management was conducted to address these suggestions, and the severity of BR's speaking-related dyspnea decreased as a result. Re-referral was recommended for further evaluation 6 months thereafter, or sooner if speech or swallowing signs worsened significantly.

The neurologist made a follow-up referral 10 months later with the statement "speech is getting worse and more aggressive options are needed." Re-evaluation revealed that BR's breathing apparatus signs had become moderate-to-severe, whereas his laryngeal and upper airway signs had become moderate in severity. The most significant change was increased weakness and reduced range of movement of the tongue. Intelligibility was moderately impaired during conversational speaking.

At re-evaluation, BR's vital capacity, inspiratory capacity, and expiratory reserve volume were 36, 47, and 20% of their predicted values, respectively. His maximum inspiratory pressure and maximum expiratory pressure at the resting tidal end-expiratory level were -27 and 15 cmH$_2$O, respectively. All measures were consistent with a significant decline in breathing function since the initial evaluation.

Physical examination indicated that diaphragm function was moderately impaired, and inspiratory and expiratory rib cage wall function and abdominal wall function were moderately to severely impaired. Breathing discomfort for conversational speech was moderate-to-severe and fatigue during conversational speech was a major complaint. Occasional inspiratory struggle was reported by BR and was accompanied by inward paradoxing of the intercostal spaces and pronounced bulging of the neck muscles. Swallowing and choking problems were reported and it was recommended to the neurologist that a comprehensive swallowing evaluation be done.

Auditory-perceptual examination of running speech indicated that the client's breath groups were abnormally short, that his voice quality was moderately breathy and rough, and that his articulatory rate was abnormally slow. Hypernasality was occasionally present, as it had been during the initial evaluation, and it continued to be moderate in severity. Several behavioral adjustments were tried in an attempt to seek some improvement in speech. Only two of these were ameliorating. One was manually compressing his abdomen and one was having him take a deep breath before initiating a breath group. The first was not something he could do on his own and the second was not something he could do without some struggle and a great expenditure of energy.

FADING

Impairment of breathing function is a major prognostic indicator in amyotrophic lateral sclerosis. There are standard measures for documenting such breathing impairment, although other simple measures are sometimes suggested for use along with these. One is the "sniff nasal-pressure test," a test in which the client is asked to perform maximum sniffs (with the mouth closed) from the resting level of the breathing apparatus (Fitting, Paillex, Hirt, Aebischer, & Schluep, 1999). For this test, nasal pressure is recorded through a catheter positioned in a nasal plug fitted into one anterior naris (nostril). The other end of the catheter is coupled to an air pressure transducer and the resultant signal is displayed. The test is easy to perform, inexpensive, and well-suited for documenting the status of disease progression over time.

What now? What do you do next? You are confronted with a client who is undergoing major neuromotor decline and whose disease is likely to end his life within the not-to-distant future. He may soon be in need of a tracheostomy and a mechanical ventilator. At the same time, his laryngeal and upper airway control will eventually be such that he will not be able to generate speech. Given this scenario, which of the following is the course of action you would recommend to the neurologist concerning the client's communication management?

> *(a) discontinue management because loss of speech is inevitable*
> *(b) institute management that involves an alternative mode of communication*
> *(c) encourage the use of noninvasive positive pressure ventilation*
> *(d) encourage the use of a speech amplifier*

It was proposed that alternative modes of communication should be discussed with the client and that these should be tested on him and their function explained in advance of their need. At the same time, it was recommended that the client be provided access to noninvasive positive pressure ventilation to support speech breathing. Two purposes were served by this latter recommendation. First, the client was able to maximize the use of his residual speech production skills, allowing him oral communication with his family and friends for as long as would be possible. Second, the client was introduced to the world of mechanical ventilation and allowed to adjust to it more gradually than would be the case were he abruptly confronted with a life-or-death decision once he could no longer breathe on his own.

The neurologist embraced these recommendations and a pulmonologist was consulted and enlisted to oversee this specialized attention to breathing function. Together the pulmonologist and speech-language pathologist implemented a protocol for noninvasive positive pressure ventilation. Simultaneously, the speech-language pathologist began to introduce the client to alternative modes of communication.

Noninvasive positive pressure ventilation was used to supplement BR's inspiratory capability. Inspirations were delivered through a pipe mouthpiece that the client could access by turning his head slightly and sealing his lips around it. The ventilator was set to deliver a moderately large inspiration (approximately 1.5 L). BR could either inspire the entire 1.5 L or inspire less by coming off the mouthpiece early. Although he had signs of velopharyngeal incompetence, such incompetence did not preclude the delivery of a sizeable volume of air to his pulmonary apparatus. As his disease progressed and velopharyngeal incompetence increased, BR wore a noseclip while using the ventilator.

Which of the following would be possible expected benefits of using non-invasive positive pressure ventilation in this client?

    (a) increased speech loudness
    (b) shortened inspiratory duration
    (c) relief of dyspnea during tidal breathing and speaking
    (d) increased breath group length

BR learned to use noninvasive positive pressure ventilation with ease and under two circumstances initially. One was to take occasional deep breaths when he felt the need for them and one was to take deep breaths during conversation. The first helped to relieve his dyspnea during tidal breathing and the second helped to relieve his dyspnea during speaking as well as to increase the loudness of his utterances and the length of his breath groups. Increased loudness was attributable to larger starting lung volumes and their attendant higher relaxation pressures, and longer breath groups were attributable to larger volume excursions made possible by larger starting lung volumes.

In the meantime, a sleep study revealed that BR's nocturnal ventilation was depressed and he began using noninvasive positive pressure ventilation at night (delivered through a facemask). BR was able to take advantage of supplemental inspiration for speaking for about 9 months. At that juncture, his upper airway signs had worsened to the point that he had difficulty sealing his lips around the pipe mouthpiece. Also, his intelligibility was so impaired by laryngeal and upper airway dysfunction that direct management of speech production was judged not to be profitable. As well, BR's general breathing function had declined to a point where his pulmonologist decided that he was in need of management through invasive positive pressure ventilation. A tracheotomy was performed and BR was placed on permanent invasive positive pressure ventilation with an inflated tracheostomy-tube cuff. In addition, because his swallowing function had become so impaired, a percutaneous endoscopic gastronomy was performed so that BR could be tube fed.

Which of the following is often spared in even profoundly impaired individuals with amyotrophic lateral sclerosis?

    (a) control of lip muscles
    (b) control of eyebrow muscles
    (c) control of eye muscles
    (d) control of toe muscles

At this point in management, BR's prognosis was poor and his speech was non-functional. Control of his eye muscles remained intact and he had been using his eyes to practice operating a speech output device for several weeks prior to his transfer to invasive positive pressure ventilation. This meant that when transfer occurred, he was immediately able to maintain expressive communication.

The device chosen for BR was a commercial unit controlled by eye gaze. The device included a video camera that was trained on one of his eyes and tracked the position of the pupil. This device was programmed to sense when his pupil momentarily fixed on a given visual target. An array of targets was positioned over different portions of a display screen and included alphabet letters, words, and icons representing pre-programmed short sentences. By holding his gaze on a target for a specified duration (which could be adjusted as he increased his efficiency) and then proceeding to other targets in specified sequences, he could generate any number of messages. These messages, created by BR's eye movements, were then transformed by a computer into a synthesized speech output that was played over a small loudspeaker. BR used this form of eye-controlled communication with considerable facility for the remaining year of his life. It served as his main verbal communication link with his wife and children.

STEADY AS SHE GOES

EK was a 67-year-old female who came to the clinic with a medical diagnosis of idiopathic voice tremor. She had been diagnosed 3 years previously by her family physician. EK and her husband had recently sold their farm in a midwestern community, retired, and moved to a southwestern retirement community. Her voice problem had taken on increased significance because her new living situation involved greater socialization. She self-referred and wanted to know if there was some way to make her "voice stop shaking."

Visualization of her larynx and upper airway revealed no signs of tremor. However, her speech and voice exhibited rhythmical and repetitive fluctuations in loudness at a rate of approximately 3 Hz. During sustained vowel utterances, her voice changed in loudness in a beating pattern that was more suggestive of myoclonus than tremor. Each increase in loudness was found to occur in conjunction with a small inward displacement of her abdominal wall.

Given the information provided to this point, which of the following would be your initial course of action?

(a) behavioral management
(b) counseling
(c) referral to a neurologist
(d) referral to a laryngologist

Referral was made to a neurologist who specialized in movement disorders. The returned diagnosis was "idiopathic respiratory myoclonus." The neurologist suspected that the condition might have been caused by an anoxic event attendant to a heart attack several years previously. The neurologist's report indicated that the myoclonic jerks were present bilaterally and that they were confined to muscles of the torso. No medical treatment was prescribed. It was requested that "palliative voice treatment" be provided.

When EK was next seen in the clinic, a comprehensive speech evaluation was conducted. Although her speech and voice were unsteady, the unsteadiness did not significantly affect her intelligibility. Unsteadiness did, however, call attention to her voice. Her speech was somewhat halting in nature and contained many filled pauses. She spoke relatively slowly, which resulted in slightly prolonged voiced segments. Her voice quality was moderately breathy and her demeanor was best described as "soft spoken."

Physical examination of the breathing apparatus was unremarkable, except for recurring involuntary movements of her chest wall. The use of respiratory magnetometers revealed that each myoclonic jerk of her breathing apparatus was associated with an inward movement of her abdominal wall and an outward movement of her rib cage wall. Outward movement of her rib cage wall appeared to be a passive mechanical event (i.e., akin to the pattern observed during a small isovolume maneuver performed with the larynx closed). The magnitude of displacement of the abdominal wall (and correspondingly of the rib cage wall) was found to differ with changes in body position and with changes in the position of the abdominal wall. More upright body positions were associated with more severe signs than were more downright body positions, whereas more outward positioning of the abdominal wall resulted in more prominent signs compared to more inward positioning of the wall.

The effects noted for body position and abdominal wall position presumably had the same bases. More outward positioning of the abdominal wall (caused by gravity in the upright body position) resulted in an increase in the lengths of its muscle fibers. And more outward positioning of the abdominal wall voluntarily (caused by contraction of the diaphragm) also resulted in an increase in the lengths of the muscle fibers of the abdominal wall. One might predict that a similar effect would occur at larger lung volumes, given that larger abdominal wall volumes might be a concomitant. There is, however, the possibility of an inconsistent effect with lung volume change, because increases in lung volume do not nec-

essarily have to be accompanied by increases in abdominal wall volume. Why does all this matter? It matters if you want to try to do something directly about changing the magnitude of the effect of the myoclonic jerks on alveolar pressure. You would probably be better off working on changing abdominal wall position directly, rather than changing it indirectly by adjusting lung volume.

Management of EK focused on behavioral adjustments that were designed to decrease the unsteadiness of her voice. The first of these had to do with changing the background positioning of her abdominal wall during running speech activities. Feedback was provided to EK in the form of an oscillographic display of rib cage wall volume (increasing upward on a vertical axis) against abdominal wall volume (increasing rightward on a horizontal axis). Her usual chest wall shape during running speech production was first shown to her. Then, a vertically oriented ellipse was drawn on the display with a grease pencil to create a target zone that was positioned to the left of EK's usual expiratory limbs. Her task was to talk at a chest wall shape that fell inside the ellipse. To accomplish this, it was necessary for her to position her abdominal wall inward from its usual position at all lung volumes.

The first management session was devoted almost exclusively to helping EK master this adjustment. The task proved to be relatively straightforward for her while watching the graphic display and within about 30 minutes of practice she could make the adjustment consistently. She was gradually weaned from the display during the remainder of the first management session until her own sensations about abdominal wall position could be used alone to guide her performance. By the end of the session, she could speak at will with her abdominal wall pulled inward and had a good general sense of the position of the wall at all times. Auditory-perceptual testing indicated that inward positioning of the abdominal wall had a positive effect on reducing the prominence of EK's voice unsteadiness. Specifically, when listeners in the room were not looking at her, they invariably judged the magnitude of her voice unsteadiness to be less prominent when her abdominal wall was positioned inward than when it was not. EK noted that it was easiest to use this strategy while seated with her arms resting across her lower abdominal wall so that she could feel where it was positioned. EK was instructed to practice using her new strategy during her daily speaking activities.

What options are there for adjusting the voice to make its unsteadiness less obvious? The answer may be different for unsteadiness resulting from dysfunction of the laryngeal apparatus versus dysfunction of the breathing apparatus. In the case under discussion, which involves only breathing dysfunction, the answer may be found in research (Farinella, Hixon, Hoit, & Story, 2004) which indicates that the best way to minimize breathing-based unsteadiness is to have the speaker increase loudness, decrease breathiness, and increase pitch. Also, unsteadiness is less prominent when speaking in sentences than when sustaining a vowel.

During the second and third management sessions, attention was directed to changing EK's loudness and voice quality. An attempt was made to increase loudness and decrease breathiness. The variables of increased loudness and decreased breathiness were chosen because they are associated with increases in muscular opposing pressure provided by the larynx. Higher opposing pressure translates into sound pressure level swings of lesser magnitude. And higher overall sound pressure level renders small alveolar pressure swings (such as those associated with myoclonic jerks) less obvious perceptually. Indeed, this was the result.

Management of loudness and voice quality initially focused on sustained vowel utterances. This allowed EK to develop a feel for the magnitude of the adjustments required to reduce the prominence of her involuntary loudness swings. Loudness proved to be a more influential adjustment than did voice quality, although both were somewhat ameliorative and they tended to vary together. Loudness adjustment also turned out to be easier for EK to perform consistently in a wide range of contexts because it seemed "more natural" to her. Thus, much of the latter part of her third management session was devoted exclusively to the practice of increasing loudness. When asked to increase loudness, EK tended to increase starting lung volume. This ran contrary to her strategy to keep her abdominal wall positioned inward, because increased lung volume tended to be accompanied by an outward positioning of her abdominal wall. To counteract this tendency, EK was encouraged to use only modest increases in lung volume and more prominent increases in the delivery of chest wall muscular pressure. The instruction during this training was to take moderate-sized breaths and "squeeze harder."

While abdominal wall positioning and loudness adjustments were being practiced, additional management strategies were introduced. These strategies were designed to reduce the salience of EK's tremor by minimizing the presence of prolonged voicing in her speech. EK's myoclonic jerks were most noticeable during productions of filled pauses (most often "uh") and during periods of slow speech when vowel segments were lengthened. These periods of slightly sustained voice production tended to expose her myoclonic jerks so that they could be easily heard in her speech. One management strategy was to try to eliminate the filled pauses. However, this was easier said than done. The filled pauses reflected a relatively unconscious strategy to hold the conversational floor and to buy time for linguistic formulation. To help EK reduce the number and length of her filled pauses, she was encouraged to plan her utterances in advance so as to minimize the need to pause for formulation. When EK was able to plan ahead in this way, one of the secondary benefits was that her articulation rate increased slightly. This increase in rate was accompanied by a slight decrease in the duration of voiced segments, which, in turn, helped to make EK's myoclonic jerks less noticeable. It was also suggested that EK attempt to use silent pauses instead of filled pauses when linguistic formulation was required. These strategies were moderately successful.

Another strategy focused on shortening voiced utterances at the ends of breath groups. It had been observed that EK often prolonged the final syllable of a breath group, and when she did, the myoclonus was especially prominent perceptually. To address this, EK was encouraged to "clip" her final syllables. This was first done through the use of reading activities in which the prosodic features were relatively well-defined and alterations could be easily demonstrated. Self-monitoring of syllable clipping was enhanced when the client "chunked" her speech production into smaller units by shortening her breath groups.

Two final sessions were devoted to determining the most effective combination of options for decreasing her voice signs. Perceptual judgments indicated that the four most powerful adjustments in combination were inward positioning of the abdominal wall, loudness increase, reduction in the number and length of filled pauses, and syllable shortening at the ends of breath groups. A follow-up inquiry 3 months after her last management session found EK to be generally satisfied. Especially important to her was the fact that several new friends at her retirement community had commented about how much better her voice sounded.

BITTERSWEET

LJ was a 15-year-old male student in the ninth grade when he was first referred to the clinic. He had been an outstanding student and a gregarious youngster who had been active in the Boy Scouts of America, Youth Soccer, and Little League Baseball. He had excelled at baseball and had been a pitcher of considerable skill, but had begun to show deterioration in speed and coordination near the end of his last eligible season of play (when he was 12 years old). Subtle problems with his hand movements and some slight slurring of his speech prompted his parents to take him to a family physician who referred him for a neurological evaluation. Detailed testing revealed what the neurologist labeled as "decomposition of compound movements, slightly lower-than-normal tone, mild dysmetria during tapping, and speech disorder." Brain imaging revealed a cerebellar tumor and surgical removal was the action of choice. Removal of the tumor was successful, but the size of the tumor and the affected regions were more extensive than had been estimated from brain imaging. Signs and symptoms were worse postoperatively and continued to worsen during a period of other medical therapies.

At the time of his initial speech evaluation, LJ presented with significant limb impairment and was in a wheelchair. His posture was slumped and he tended to drop forward toward his knees. He was able to stand if helped to his feet, but could not ambulate safely. His medical records indicated that he was being treated pharmacologically for depression. He had nystagmus and difficulty with trunk and neck control. His speech was characterized by struggle to initiate utterance, short breath groups, low loudness, and breathy voice quality. At times he was hypernasal and his articulation was imprecise. The intelligibility of his speech and the comprehensibility of his communication efforts were significantly compromised, but were functional with family members (especially his younger brother).

Evaluation of the speech production apparatus revealed neuromotor involvement of the breathing apparatus, larynx, and velopharynx, in particular. Oral airway signs were apparent, but were judged to be less significant contributors to LJ's speech impairment than were the other three subsystem signs. Weighting of the findings suggested that dysfunction of the breathing apparatus and the velopharyngeal apparatus were the main obstacles to improving LJ's speech.

The weighting of clinical data across subsystems is a bit of a science and a bit of an art. Our experience from referrals made to us is that insufficient weight is often given to the velopharynx when multiple subsystems of the speech production apparatus are impaired. For example, articulatory problems routinely tend to be attributed to dysfunction of oral airway structures (i.e., jaw, tongue, lips), even when the control of those structures may be only minimally impaired. Frequently, it is the velopharynx that is the more important contributor to articulatory problems. The reason is that its dysfunction may preclude the normal build-up of oral pressure and the normal manipulation of the air stream, factors critical to the production of stop-plosive, fricative, and affricate consonants and, therefore, speech intelligibility. We believe that a strong case can be made that the velopharynx is the most important of all of the speech production valves when it comes to speech intelligibility.

Physical examination of the breathing apparatus revealed severe paresis of the abdominal wall. The wall was distended outward and showed low tone throughout. The client could not voluntarily reposition the wall consistently and for practical purposes it was nonfunctional. Inspiratory and expiratory muscles of the rib cage wall showed moderate-to-severe weakness with signs that hinted at higher-than-normal compliance of the rib interspaces. The diaphragm was relatively strong, but sniffing was slower than would be expected were the structure functioning normally. The vital capacity was reduced to 60% of its predicted value, with the expiratory reserve volume proportionately more reduced than the inspiratory capacity. The maximum inspiratory pressure was -36 cmH$_2$O and the maximum expiratory pressure was 28 cmH$_2$O. Measurements with respiratory magnetometers indicated that running speech was produced within the midrange of the vital capacity, but with the rib cage wall at a much smaller volume and the abdominal wall at a much larger volume than would be expected for normal function in an upright seated body position. Breath groups were abnormally short (with fewer-than-normal syllables, usually 4 to 6 per breath group) and inspiratory durations between running speech breath groups were longer than normal (typically 0.8 second, as opposed to the 0.5 second that would be expected in normal function). Using manual compression of the abdominal wall as a management probe, it was found that LJ could inspire more deeply, produce about 50% more syllables per breath group, and inspire more quickly.

Velopharyngeal function was analyzed using pressure-flow methods for calculating velopharyngeal orifice area (Warren & Dubois, 1964). Closure was never attained during oralized speech sounds and area calculations during stop-plosive consonants revealed a velopharyngeal orifice area that ranged between 20 and 30 mm^2, depending on the phonetic context. Visualization of the velum during sustained vowel productions revealed only small elevations of the structure and the gag reflex seemed somewhat reduced. Nasal pathway resistance was consistently lower than 3 cmH$_2$O/LPS when measured at inspiratory and expiratory flows typical of resting tidal breathing. Using digital occlusion of the anterior nares as a management probe, it was found that LJ's hypernasality subsided, that he produced more syllables per breath group, and that his articulatory precision and speech intelligibility were somewhat improved. With his anterior nares occluded, LJ's peak oral pressure during /p/ productions averaged 4 cmH$_2$O. Thus, alveolar pressure was just barely adequate for conversational speech production.

A two-pronged management strategy was initiated with LJ. One part of this strategy dealt with the management of his speech breathing and the other part focused on the management of his velopharyngeal function.

Given the information provided thus far, which of the following would you choose as a starting point for the management of the client's speech breathing?

(a) switching to a nasal inspiration strategy
(b) adjusting body posture and body position
(c) adjusting chest wall shape
(d) adjusting speech loudness

Speech breathing management began by addressing LJ's body posture and body position. His slumped presentation was adjusted by positioning his buttocks farther toward the back of his wheelchair and securing his shoulders with straps to help him maintain an upright position. Next, through consultation with his physician and the prescription of a pulmonologist, he was fitted with an abdominal wall truss that was worn during weekdays at school. His mother, who happened to be a nurse, was trained in its application by the pulmonologist. Weekend use was optional, except it could not exceed weekday limits. Positioning of the truss resulted in an inward positioning of the abdominal wall and a lifting of the rib cage wall. At the same time, such positioning forced the diaphragm headward, which improved its contractile effectiveness and coupling to the rib cage wall. Use of the truss resulted in the immediate gains predicted from the management probe. Depth of inspiration, breath group length, and number of syllables per breath group all increased.

Velopharyngeal management was instituted through referral to a prosthodontist who had experience in the fabrication of velar-lift prostheses. Although the initial fitting appeared to be satisfactory (based on pressure-flow testing), the client had some difficulty with gagging when the device was in place and resisted its use. A program of gag reduction was instituted and within several weeks the prosthesis was well-tolerated, except when eating. Minor adjustments had to be made to the prosthesis during management, which included the prosthodontist's sculpting of the lateral borders of the lift to better accommodate nasal breathing. Fitting of the lift prosthesis resulted in an immediate reduction of hypernasality and a moderate improvement in LJ's speech intelligibility.

Having achieved positive results from mechanical adjustments of the breathing apparatus and velopharynx, behavioral components were then added to the client's management program. The first of these sought to increase the magnitude of LJ's driving pressure for speech production by having him attempt to generate oral pressure with a leak tube in place. This component involved the use of the feedback of oral pressure in a time-amplitude display (on a storage oscilloscope) in which progressively higher targets were marked for LJ to reach as he moved through the program. This component lasted 8 weeks and consisted of four half-hour training sessions per week. As a supplement, LJ was shown how to use a water-bubble manometer so he could practice at home between clinical sessions (much to the reported delight of his younger brother who practiced with him). By the end of his 8 weeks of training, he had increased his ability to generate pressure from 4 to 12 cmH_2O in the midrange of the vital capacity and could maintain such pressure over a 5-second period. Given LJ's laryngeal involvement, it did not prove fruitful to attempt to increase his loudness. However, his regained pressure-generating skill had a significant influence on the precision of his articulation and his speech intelligibility. Through behavioral work on his articulation he was able to make additional gains until his speech intelligibility under quiet environmental conditions showed only mild-to-moderate impairment. His comprehensibility to members of his family was now excellent, although he persisted with some modest difficulties with his schoolmates.

Having achieved this success, which of the following might you want to do next?

    (a) *discharge the client from management*
    (b) *refer the client for possible vocal fold medialization*
    (c) *expand the client's management into other areas*
    (d) *teach the client glossopharyngeal breathing*

By this stage of management, LJ was presumed to have benefited near maximally from mechanical and behavioral interventions. It was planned that two additional adjustments would be attempted to try to alleviate two of his remaining signs: (a) his continuing low-level loudness, presumably related to his laryngeal dysfunction; and (b) his tendency to demonstrate tremor in his breathing apparatus near the ends of breath groups, apparently related to the near-termination of a goal-directed activity (a frequent problem in clients with cerebellar disorders). A program was designed that would attempt to increase his starting lung volume modestly for breath groups in the hope of increasing his speech loudness and in the hope of ending his breath groups near his resting tidal end-expiratory level. It was reasoned that the use of a heightened relaxation pressure would increase loudness, and that termination of utterances at lung volumes that did not require substantial muscle activation might reduce his tremor. He loved to sing and asked that some singing be worked into the program to make it more fun for him. An agreement was struck with smiles all around.

Work began on this final clinical thrust with some success, less for the loudness goal than for the tremor reduction goal. At this juncture, an influenza-like illness stopped treatment for several weeks. His mother then reported that he seemed not to be recovering as expected and a return visit to the neurologist had raised the suspicion of recurrence of the tumor. He was placed on additional medications. A telephone call to LJ confirmed that his speech and voice signs had deteriorated since his last visit. His mother reported later that he had again gone into depression and was being treated by a psychiatrist. A conversation with the neurologist confirmed the worst.

Almost a year to the day that LJ was first seen in the clinic, and 4 months after his last visit, his management ceased. On a beautiful morning, his mother called to say that he had passed away in his sleep without signs of struggle. Her message was one of thankfulness for what had been done to help him communicate during the previous year, especially with his younger brother and companion. His life was far too short. His heroes were Garth Brooks, Roger Clemens, Lute Olson, and TJ (his younger brother).

BOOVATION

A referee made a bad call that cost our basketball team a victory. When he was introduced at a later game, he was soundly booed. There were 14,500 fans booing (excluding our President). Each fan booed about five times, with each boo lasting about 4 seconds (standard for our crowd). All booing was done with the vowel /u/ (this is our custom). And the average flow during each boo was about 150 cc/sec (at least in our section). We estimated on the napkin that came with our nachos that about 43,500,000 cc of bad breath were poured on the poor referee. That's about 14,496 gallons, or almost exactly one gallon per person in attendance. We know this exercise was trivial, but presenting it here helped to take our minds off the adjacent bittersweet scenario and the young athlete featured in it. We knew him well enough to know that he would have loved this sidetrack.

IT'S ALL IN THE TIMING

MD was a 42-year-old female living in a long-term care facility. She had been diagnosed with limb-girdle muscular dystrophy in her early 20's, following a period of progressive weakness in her legs. At age 40, after several months of breathing difficulty, MD was counseled to accept ventilatory support. She subsequently underwent tracheotomy and began invasive positive pressure ventilation. At the time of the evaluation, she was quadriplegic and required full ventilatory support 24 hours per day.

MD had several family members and friends who visited her regularly and she participated in a variety of activities at the facility. A recent psychological evaluation indicated that she was "generally well-adjusted." She had requested a referral for a speech evaluation because, as she stated, "My speech is . . . (*4-second pause*) . . . driving me crazy." She had seen a speech-language pathologist soon after she began using a ventilator, but only swallowing function was evaluated at that time (and found to be adequate).

The case history revealed that MD had been speaking routinely only during the past year. During the first year following her tracheotomy, her pulmonologist had insisted that she keep her tracheostomy-tube cuff inflated. Only occasionally, when a nurse or respiratory therapist deflated the cuff, was she able to say a few words. Otherwise, most of her speech had consisted of mouthing words and only a few people could carry on a conversation with her. She was frustrated by her poor communication and found herself becoming depressed and withdrawn because of what she called her "silent prison." However, another pulmonologist eventually took over her care and ordered cuff deflation so that she could speak (the cuff continued to be inflated at night for sleeping). MD immediately began to participate in several in-house activities (Bingo, mouth painting, prayer group). She also ventured out of the facility on field trips to a local museum and to a poetry reading. She reported that being able to speak had completely changed her life. Whereas during her first year of ventilation she had "come to the point . . . (*4-second pause*) . . . of wondering . . . (*5-second pause*) . . . if life was really . . . (*4-second pause*) . . . worth living," she currently reported feeling "much happier" and like she had "regained some . . . (*5-second pause*) . . . enthusiasm . . . (*5-second pause*) . . . for life."

MD's main speech complaint was that she had a "big timing problem." This problem was especially troublesome when using the telephone. Her hope was that "some sort of . . . (*5-second pause*) . . . speech therapy . . . (*5-second pause*) . . . might help" her to learn to time her speech better. She reported that, unless she answered the telephone at just the right point in her breathing cycle, she could not speak, sometimes for several seconds. The same problem occurred when she was making a telephone call. Unless the other person picked up the telephone at just the right moment, she could not respond immediately to the "Hello." In either case, the other party often hung up. This was not a problem with family and friends who were accustomed to her long silences, but it happened frequently when she talked to strangers. She was eager to solve this problem because she wanted to do telephone work for a volunteer organization she had joined which raised money for homeless mothers and children. When asked if people usually understood her speech, she answered that they usually did, "In fact . . . (*5-second pause*) . . . they understand me . . . (*4-second pause*) . . . so well . . . (*5-second pause*) . . . that they often . . . (*4-second pause*) . . . finish my sentences . . . (*4-second pause*) . . . for me." She reported that she had been a high school English teacher until her physical condition had forced her to stop working, and that she prided herself on her "articulate speech."

MD was evaluated in her room. She was using a portable ventilator that was secured to the back of her wheelchair. There was also a larger stationary ventilator in the room that she used while in bed. The initial evaluation focused on her portable unit because she did most of her talking with this ventilator. A brief evaluation with the bedside ventilator was done at a later date.

Analysis of the portable ventilator revealed that only a few adjustments were possible. These included tidal volume, breathing rate, and inspiratory:expiratory (I:E) ratio. The ventilator had been set to deliver a tidal volume of 1 L at a rate of 10 breaths per minute with an I:E ratio of 1:4. MD used a cuffed, unfenestrated tracheostomy tube. The cuff was deflated during the evaluation.

Auditory-perceptual observations revealed that MD's running speech was characterized by short breath groups and intervening pauses that were inordinately long. Actual measurements demonstrated that her breath groups were usually between 3 and 7 syllables in length and her intervening pauses were usually at least 4 seconds long. She often truncated her breath groups so as to break at phrase, clause, and sentence boundaries. She demonstrated occasional bursts of louder-than-usual speech and her voice quality varied substantially, often ranging from breathy to pressed. During sustained vowel productions, she could continue for only about 2 seconds. And during her attempts to "count as far as you can on one breath," her maximum performance was seven (with the final syllable being mouthed).

Which of the following measurements of physiological status would you make during the evaluation of a client of this type (and later, during management) to ensure her safety?

(a) *heart rate*
(b) *blood pressure*
(c) *oxygen saturation*
(d) *end-tidal partial pressure of carbon dioxide*

Baseline measures of physiological status were obtained to ensure the client's safety. Measures of heart rate, blood pressure, and oxygen saturation (SpO_2) were within the normal range while MD sat quietly or performed various speaking activities. Her end-tidal partial pressure of carbon dioxide (PCO_2) was abnormally low (27 mmHg) while at rest, and slightly higher (31 mmHg) immediately after speaking.

The tracheal pressure waveform during the ventilator cycle was found to be typical of that associated with volume-controlled invasive positive pressure ventilation. Pressure rose rapidly during inspiration, reached a maximum of approximately 30 cmH$_2$O, fell rapidly to 0 cmH$_2$O, and remained there until the next inspiration. MD terminated phonation at 8 cmH$_2$O or higher during running speech activities, well above her presumed voicing threshold. She tended to have bursts of loudness and a pressed voice quality at the end of inspiration (when pressure peaked).

Evaluation of MD's maximum inspiratory pressure generating capability was effected by having her close her larynx at the resting tidal end-expiratory level and pull "as hard as possible to try to take in some air." Her tracheal pressure did not change during this task, indicating that she had no inspiratory muscle potential.

Given the information provided thus far, which of the following would you choose as a management approach for this client?

    (a) one-way valve
    (b) laryngeal massage
    (c) talking tracheostomy tube
    (d) ventilator adjustments

Because MD's speech difficulties were primarily related to abnormalities in pressure, a management plan was developed that focused on modifying pressure for speech production purposes. Toward this end, a protocol for potential ventilator adjustments was developed by the speech-language pathologist with the endorsement of MD's respiratory therapist and the approval of her pulmonologist. Ventilator adjustments were selected over a one-way valve because such adjustments were deemed safer for the client. The pulmologist wrote the prescription for the protocol and commented that he was concerned about MD's chronic hyperventilation (as indicated by her abnormally low end-tidal PCO$_2$ values and her previously measured arterial PCO$_2$ values, which were also abnormally low). He suggested that if it were possible to reduce her ventilation in the process of adjusting her ventilator for speech improvement, that this would be an added benefit.

Given this client's breathing and speech problems, which of the following do you think would be the most reasonable ventilator variables to adjust?

    (a) positive end-expiratory pressure
    (b) inspiratory time
    (c) tidal volume
    (d) breathing rate

The primary goal of management was to address MD's "timing problem" by increasing utterance duration and decreasing pause duration. It was reasoned that the ventilator adjustments that would effect these changes could also reduce her loudness fluctuations, improve her voice quality, and reduce her ventilation. Switching the ventilator from control mode to assist-control mode was not an option because MD could not generate inspiratory (negative) pressure and, therefore, could not trigger the ventilator to deliver extra breaths. Three ventilator adjustments were selected to address her speech and ventilation problems. Positive end-expiratory pressure (PEEP) was used to address MD's timing problem. Lengthened inspiratory time (T_I) was used to address her timing problem, reduce loudness variability, and improve voice quality. Finally, reduced tidal volume was chosen to reduce loudness variability, improve voice quality, and decrease ventilation (as per the pulmonologist's request).

If all this sounds complex to you, you are probably not alone. It is only recently that research has been done to try to understand how different ventilator adjustments, alone or in combination, affect speech and voice. The results of this research are really quite encouraging and show that by simply adjusting a ventilator in certain ways, it is possible to instantly improve speech and voice in many clients. Work by the following authors led the way in this regard and a read on their articles should make the adjacent text much less daunting if you are having problems: Hoit and Banzett (1997); Hoit, Banzett, Lohmeier, Hixon, and Brown (2003); Prigent, Samuel, Louis, Abinun, Zerah-Lancner, Lejaille, Raphael, & Lofaso (2003).

The first step involved the addition of PEEP. Because the client's portable ventilator did not have an internal PEEP adjustment, an external PEEP valve was attached to the expiratory line of the ventilator circuit and adjusted to 5 cmH$_2$O. After several minutes, heart rate, blood pressure, SpO$_2$, and end-tidal PCO$_2$ were rechecked and were found to be essentially the same as with her usual ventilator settings. The client reported that her breathing "felt better than usual." The effects of PEEP on speech were tested by having the client sustain a vowel and read a short paragraph aloud. She was able to sustain a vowel for 3 seconds (half again as long as the duration without PEEP). During reading, utterance duration increased by approximately one-third and pause duration shortened to about 3 seconds. All increases in utterance duration occurred during the expiratory phase of the breathing cycle.

The second step involved increasing T_I by adjusting the ventilator's I:E ratio from 1:4 to 1:3. Again, physiological status and client comfort were checked and found to be essentially unchanged. Immediately after the adjustment, MD reported that her breathing "felt a little strange," but then reported feeling comfortable after a few minutes. With T_I adjusted to its new value, MD's utterance duration increased to 3.5 seconds (and pause duration decreased to 2.5 seconds). During reading, she produced from 6 to 11 syllables per breath, with all additional syllables produced during the inspiratory phase of breathing cycles. Loudness bursts were significantly reduced and voice quality was improved. These changes appeared closely linked to a more gradual rise in pressure during inspiration and a somewhat lower peak pressure than under the previous ventilator adjustment conditions.

The final step for the first management session involved a reduction in tidal volume from 1 to 0.8 L. At first, MD expressed slight discomfort – "I'm not sure I'm getting enough air." However, after several breaths, she reported feeling comfortable again. Measurements determined that her physiological status had not changed, except that end-tidal PCO_2 had increased slightly (from 27 to 30 mmHg during quiet breathing) due to the decrease in ventilation. The client's speech was tested and it was found that the timing characteristics were generally the same as with the previous combination of ventilator adjustments, but her loudness variation was reduced (e.g., loudness bursts were gone) and her voice quality was substantially better. All present, including MD, agreed that her speech sounded best with this last set of adjustments (PEEP = 5 cmH$_2$O, I:E = 1:3, tidal volume = 0.8 L).

The pulmonologist was impressed by the results of the ventilator adjustments and with MD's reduced tidal volume in particular. The speech-language pathologist recommended that MD's portable (daytime) ventilator be changed to the new settings for a week. The pulmonologist concurred and wrote orders for the change. He also wrote orders for an arterial blood draw for that day and for 1 week thereafter, so that the effect of the ventilator adjustments on the client's arterial PCO_2 could be determined.

The client was seen for a second management session a week later. She stated that she was extremely happy with her new ventilator settings. She said that she was able to speak more fluently, that the telephone was much easier to use, and that her breathing felt comfortable. Results from the blood draws indicated that her arterial PCO_2 had increased by 4 mmHg (i.e., it was closer to normal). Thus, the goal of this second session was to further refine her speech production skills.

Although her speech was substantially improved, it was believed that the pauses between her utterances were still quite distracting and could be made shorter. An additional adjustment was proposed to the pulmonologist and immediately approved. This adjustment was to increase PEEP to 7.5 cmH$_2$O. The client accepted this change and liked it. When asked to count as continuously as possible, MD was able to produce up to 20 syllables per breath and her pauses were only slightly noticeable (0.5 second). However, when asked to read aloud or speak extemporaneously, she produced fewer syllables per breath and exhibited longer pauses. The speech-language pathologist noted that this was because the client almost always stopped speaking at linguistic junctures and seldom used her full potential speaking time (i.e., when pressure was above the voicing threshold). When queried about this, MD explained that she tried to make her pauses coincide with the "commas and periods" (an appropriate response for a former English teacher).

What behavioral strategy might help the client increase her utterance duration and decrease her pause duration during conversation?

    (a) adopt a continuous-speaking strategy
    (b) increase articulation rate
    (c) decrease speaking rate
    (d) use nonverbal cueing

The speech-language pathologist commended MD for these efforts, but asked her to consider a completely different strategy, at least for carrying on conversations. This strategy was to speak for as long as she could on each breath without concern for where the pauses occurred. It was explained to her that such a strategy had two advantages. One advantage was that more could be said in a given amount of time. The other advantage was that the listener was less apt to interrupt her, especially if a pause occurred at an unexpected point in the sentence (because it would be obvious that the thought was not finished).

MD agreed to try this new strategy. Thus, much of the remainder of the session was spent with the speech-language pathologist and MD engaged in conversation, with MD attempting to use as much of her potential speaking time as she could, even if this meant that her speech occasionally faded out at the end of the breath. This gave the speech-language pathologist opportunities to demonstrate how this strategy was effective in keeping the conversation going and in quelling the listener's temptation to interrupt MD when she spoke. MD became quite effective at implementing this strategy and could appreciate its benefits for conversational interactions. Nevertheless, she was distressed by the idea of using this speech breathing strategy when reading aloud. Her English literature background drove her to respect the grammatical flow of the written word. As well it should! Thus, it was decided that she would adopt the continuous-speaking strategy for conversation and that she would use her elegant and well-crafted oral reading skills as she always had. Fortunately, her new ventilator adjustments allowed her to be adequately fluent so that she could read aloud almost as well as she could before a ventilator dictated her speech breathing cycle.

What, if anything, should be done to the client's bedside ventilator?

    (a) nothing
    (b) it should no longer be used

(c) it should be adjusted to match her portable ventilator settings - permanently

(d) it should be adjusted to match her portable ventilator settings - for speech purposes

---

The third and final management session was held a week later. MD reported that her speech was the best it had been in a year. She had begun her volunteer work and had found that telephone conversations were relatively easy for her. In fact, she reported that "some people don't even seem to know there's anything wrong with me." Her only complaint was that there were times when she wanted to work from her bed, but that she was unable to do so while using her bedside ventilator. Thus, the speech-language pathologist and respiratory therapist determined analogous adjustments for her bedside ventilator and then consulted MD's pulmonologist. It was decided that MD could use what would be designated as her "speech settings" when she was performing her telephone work, but otherwise her bedside ventilator would be returned to her "sleep settings" (with her tracheostomy-tube cuff inflated). The "speech settings" were made to the bedside ventilator and MD conducted several telephone conversations using the ventilator while the speech-language pathologist observed. Physiological status measurements, client report of comfort, and speech performance were all determined to be comparable to when she was using her analogous settings on her portable ventilator. MD was satisfied with her breathing and speech on both ventilators and the speech-language pathologist was satisfied that she had done all she could for MD. Management was, therefore, terminated. When leaving the client's room, MD called out to her, "I'll contact you again when I'm ready for some singing lessons!" (note: no pauses).

REVIEW

Eight clinical scenarios are offered to enhance learning and challenge the reader's knowledge of evaluation and management principles and methods.

The first clinical scenario is about a young male classical singer who adopted a mechanically disadvantageous style of breathing and was managed using exteroceptive feedback and behavioral methods.

The second scenario has to do with a young female smokejumper with a C6 spinal cord injury who was managed using an abdominal wall binder, inspiratory muscle training, and several forms of behavioral training (including work with her service dog).

The third clinical scenario concerns an elderly female college instructor with chronic obstructive pulmonary disease who was managed for speaking-related dyspnea through the use of lifestyle changes, strategies for conserving energy, and modifications to her speech breathing behavior.

The fourth scenario involves a young male college wrestler with a C2 spinal cord injury who was managed through the use of extended counseling, bilateral phrenic nerve pacers, abdominal wall support, myoelectric feedback, glossopharyngeal breathing, and buccal speech.

The fifth scenario describes an elderly male with amyotrophic lateral sclerosis who was managed over a protracted period in a sequence that included elective noninvasive positive pressure ventilation, invasive positive pressure ventilation, and an alternative communication system.

The sixth clinical scenario involves an elderly female with idiopathic respiratory myoclonus and an unsteady voice who was managed through adjustment of the position of her abdominal wall, adjustments of voice variables, and adjustments of the duration of her voiced utterances.

The seventh clinical scenario describes a young male high school student with sequelae from removal of a cerebellar tumor who was managed through the use of a velar-lift prosthesis, body posturing, body positioning, and behavioral adjustments of breathing control.

The eighth scenario involves a middle-aged female with limb-girdle muscular dystrophy who was managed through adjustments to her invasive positive pressure ventilator and behavioral adjustments involving her use of potential speaking time.

REFERENCES

Fitting, J., Paillex, R., Hirt, L., Aebischer, P., & Schluep, M. (1999). Sniff nasal pressure: A sensitive respiratory test to assess progression of amyotrophic lateral sclerosis. *Annals of Neurology, 46*, 887-893.

Farinella, K., Hixon, T., Hoit, J., & Story, B. (March, 2004). Perception of voice tremor induced by forced oscillation of the respiratory system. Paper presented at the Conference on Motor Speech, Albuquerque, NM.

Hixon, T. (1982). Speech breathing kinematics and mechanism inferences therefrom. In S. Grillner, B. Lindblom, J. Lubker, & A. Persson (Eds.), *Speech motor control* (pp. 75-93). Oxford, England: Pergamon Press.

Hixon, T., & Hoffman, C. (1979). Chest wall shape in singing. In V. Lawrence (Ed.), *Proceedings of the Seventh Symposium on Care of the Professional Voice* (pp. 9-10). New York, NY: The Voice Foundation.

Hixon, T., & Putnam, A. (1983). Voice abnormalities in relation to respiratory kinematics. *Seminars in Speech and Language, 5*, 217-231.

Hixon, T., Putnam, A., & Sharp, J. (1983). Speech production with flaccid paralysis of the rib cage, diaghragm, and abdomen. *Journal of Speech and Hearing Disorders, 48*, 315-327.

Hoit, J., & Banzett, R. (1997). Simple adjustments can improve ventilator-supported speech. *American Journal of Speech-Language Pathology, 6*, 87-96.

Hoit, J., Banzett, R., & Brown, R. (2002). Binding the abdomen can improve speech in men with phrenic nerve pacers. *American Journal of Speech-Language Pathology, 11,* 71-76.

Hoit, J., Banzett, R., Lohmeier, H., Hixon, T., & Brown, R. (2003). Clinical ventilator adjustments that improve speech. *Chest, 124,* 1512-1521.

Hoit, J., & Shea, S. (1996). Speech production and speech with a phrenic nerve pacer. *American Journal of Speech-Language Pathology, 5,* 53-60.

Prigent, H., Samuel, C., Louis, B., Abinun, M., Zerah-Lancner, F., Lejaille, M., Raphael, J., & Lofaso, F. (2003). Comparative effects of two ventilatory modes on speech in tracheostomized patients with neuromuscular disease. *American Journal of Respiratory Critical Care Medicine, 167,* 114-119.

Roy, N., Weinrich, B., Gray, S., Tanner, K., Toledo, S., Dove, H., Corbin-Lewis, K., & Stemple, J. (2002). Voice amplification versus vocal hygiene instruction for teachers with voice disorders: A treatment outcomes study. *Journal of Speech, Language, and Hearing Research, 45,* 625-638.

Sataloff, R., Heur, R., & O'Connor, M. (1984). Rehabilitation of a quadriplegic professional singer. *Archives of Otolaryngology, 110,* 682-685.

Ure, A. (1819). An account of some experiments made on the body of a criminal immediately after execution, with physiological and practical observations. *Journal of Science and the Arts, 6,* 283-294.

Warren, D., & DuBois, A. (1964). A pressure-flow technique for measuring velopharyngeal orifice area during continuous speech. *Cleft Palate Journal, 1,* 52-71.

Watson, P., & Hixon, T. (1985). Respiratory kinematics in classical (opera) singers. *Journal of Speech and Hearing Research, 28,* 104-122.

Watson, P., & Hixon, T. (1996). Respiratory behavior during the learning of a novel aria by a highly trained classical singer. In P. Davis & N. Fletcher (Eds.), *Vocal fold physiology: Controlling complexity and chaos* (pp. 325-343). San Diego: Singular Publishing Group, Inc.

Watson, P., & Hixon, T. (2001). Effects of abdominal trussing on breathing and speech in men with cervical spinal cord injury. *Journal of Speech, Language, and Hearing Research, 44,* 751-762.

Watson, P., Hixon, T., Stathopoulos, E., & Sullivan, D. (1990). Respiratory kinematics in female classical singers. *Journal of Voice, 4,* 120-128.

Author Index

Subject Index

About the Authors

Thomas J. Hixon received his Ph.D. degree in speech pathology and audiology from the University of Iowa and did postdoctoral work in respiratory mechanics at Harvard University. He served on the faculty of the University of Wisconsin for 11 years in the Departments of Communicative Disorders and Rehabilitation Medicine. He has since served on the faculty of the University of Arizona for 29 years in the Department of Speech and Hearing Sciences, where he formerly was Head. Hixon is currently Associate Vice President for Research, Dean of the Graduate College, Director of Graduate Interdisciplinary Programs, Research Integrity Officer, Director of the Institute for Neurogenic Communication Disorders, and Professor of Speech, Language, and Hearing Sciences at the University of Arizona. He is a Fellow of the American Speech-Language-Hearing Association, holds its Certificate of Clinical Competence in Speech-Language Pathology, and has received the Honors of the Association. He has been an editorial consultant to more than a dozen journals, is a former Editor of the *Journal of Speech and Hearing Research*, and is currently Editor for Speech of the *Journal of Speech, Language, and Hearing Research*.

Jeannette D. Hoit received her Ph.D. degree in speech and hearing sciences from the University of Arizona and did postdoctoral work in respiratory biology at Harvard University and in speech acoustics at the Massachusetts Institute of Technology. She is currently Professor of Speech, Language, and Hearing Sciences, Research Scientist of the Institute for Neurogenic Communication Disorders, Member of the Committee on Neuroscience, and Coordinator of the Graduate Training Program in Survival Skills and Ethics at the University of Arizona. Dr. Hoit is a former President of the American Association of Phonetic Sciences and holds a Certificate of Clinical Competence in Speech-Language Pathology from the American Speech Language-Hearing Association. She has been an editorial consultant to nearly a dozen journals and is currently Editor of the *American Journal of Speech-Language Pathology*. Dr. Hoit has been awarded Fellowship of the American Speech-Language-Hearing Association.

Hixon and Hoit have professional interests that center on normal and abnormal speech production. Much of their research has been supported by grants from the National Institutes of Health. They have published extensively (individually, together, and with others) about many aspects of speech breathing and its disorders. The authors are married to each other and spend much of their leisure time exploring the Colorado Plateau with their two golden retrievers (Quincy Belle and Charlie Brown) and their beagle (Coogee Mundo). They live together in Tucson, Arizona and in Pagosa Springs, Colorado.